Applications of Optical Coherence Tomography in Ophthalmology

Applications of Optical Coherence Tomography in Ophthalmology

Editor: Harold Anderson

MURPHY & MOORE
www.murphy-moorepublishing.com

www.murphy-moorepublishing.com

MURPHY & MOORE

Cataloging-in-Publication Data

Applications of optical coherence tomography in ophthalmology / edited by Harold Anderson.
p. cm.
Includes bibliographical references and index.
ISBN 978-1-63987-053-0
1. Optical coherence tomography. 2. Ophthalmology. 3. Eye--Diseases. 4. Optical tomography.
5. Coherence (Optics). I. Anderson, Harold.
RE79.I42 A67 2022
616.075 45--dc23

Murphy & Moore Publishing,
1 Rockefeller Plaza,
New York City, NY 10020, USA

ISBN 978-1-63987-053-0 (Hardback)

Contents

Preface

This book has been a concerted effort by a group of academicians, researchers and scientists, who have contributed their research works for the realization of the book. This book has materialized in the wake of emerging advancements and innovations in this field. Therefore, the need of the hour was to compile all the required researches and disseminate the knowledge to a broad spectrum of people comprising of students, researchers and specialists of the field.

Optical coherence tomography is an imaging test which is non-invasive in nature, and makes use of light waves in order to take cross-section pictures of the retina. The different layers of the retina are visible through this technique. There are numerous eye conditions which can be diagnosed through optical coherence tomography. A few of them are glaucoma, diabetic retinopathy, macular edema and macular hole. The disorders of the optic nerve are also examined using this technique. The conditions which interfere with the passage of light through the eye cannot be diagnosed through optical coherence tomography, since it depends on light waves. This book brings forth some of the most innovative concepts and elucidates the unexplored aspects of optical coherence tomography. It strives to provide a fair idea about its clinical applications and to help develop a better understanding of the latest advances within this field. This book is a vital tool for all researching or studying ophthalmology as it gives incredible insights into emerging trends and concepts.

At the end of the preface, I would like to thank the authors for their brilliant chapters and the publisher for guiding us all-through the making of the book till its final stage. Also, I would like to thank my family for providing the support and encouragement throughout my academic career and research projects.

Editor

1

OCT in Lamellar Corneal Transplantation

Mehmet Cüneyt Özmen and
Hüseyin Baran Özdemir

Abstract

Anterior segment optical coherence tomography (AS-OCT) is a valuable tool in corneal transplantation surgery. In deep anterior lamellar keratoplasty (DALK), AS-OCT gives valuable information on preoperative decision process. AS-OCT image of the recipient cornea helps the surgeon to decide whether to proceed with a big bubble DALK or a manual dissection. Preoperative AS-OCT imaging of recipient stroma can also predict Descemet membrane perforation during big bubble induction. Intraoperative AS-OCT assures reaching the proper depth in order, and postoperatively, a surgeon can objectively assess the Descemet membrane and donor association and define complications such as a double anterior chamber. Before deciding for a Descemet membrane endothelial keratoplasty (DMEK), preoperative stromal scars can be identified with an AS-OCT and might affect the decision of the surgical procedure (DMEK or penetrating keratoplasty). After DMEK, graft detachment can be visualized by AS-OCT and treated accordingly.

Keywords: anterior segment optical coherence tomography, AS-OCT, lamellar keratoplasty, deep anterior lamellar keratoplasty, DALK, Descemet stripping automated endothelial keratoplasty, DSAEK, Descemet membrane endothelial keratoplasty, DMEK

1. Introduction

Since lamellar keratoplasty has developed for replacing only a diseased corneal layer, new advantages and challenges showed up [1–4]. Changing only the pathologic tissue brings closed globe surgery, which is safer than conventional penetrating keratoplasty [5]. It also helps to fasten rehabilitation after surgery. The anterior layer of corneal pathologies may be treated by deep anterior lamellar keratoplasty (DALK), and endothelial dysfunctions can be managed by posterior lamellar procedures such as Descemet stripping automated endothelial keratoplasty (DSAEK) and Descemet membrane endothelial keratoplasty (DMEK) [6–8]. Each technique requires specific experience and tricks and has their own difficulties and complications. Beside these challenges, all these procedures provide safer surgery, faster rehabilitation, better functional, and anatomical outcomes [1].

Anterior segment optical coherence tomography (AS-OCT) is a non-contact imaging system that obtains high-resolution images of cornea and anterior chamber [9, 10]. It allows visualizing the shape and depth of corneal lesions such as scarring, measuring central corneal thickness, and lesion size [11, 12]. It can be used before, during, and after lamellar keratoplasty to evaluate the cornea [13]. In this chapter, we discuss the role of AS-OCT on the basis of different corneal lamellar procedures such as DALK, DSAEK, and DMEK.

2. OCT in deep anterior lamellar keratoplasty

DALK has been introduced as an alternative to penetrating keratoplasty (PK) for the diseases that affect anterior layers of cornea [14, 15]. Preserving the endothelium in DALK obtains reduced graft rejections [16, 17]. Many techniques have been described to separate corneal stroma and Descemet's membrane (DM). Peeling stroma up to near DM is called manual dissection [18, 19]. This procedure can be used as the first choice in some situations such as deep scarring, or the second choice intraoperatively when it cannot be progressed with other techniques [20–22]. Other option is the separation of stroma and DM with injection of air, fluid, or viscoelastic into deep stroma [14, 23–25].

Anterior lamellar keratoplasty was described first by Gasset in keratoconus patients which was named as conectomy and included transplantation of DM stripped full thickness graft [26]. Archila et al. introduced deep lamellar keratoplasty, using intrastromal air to separate stroma from DM [27]. After that, different techniques have been described, and today, the most frequently used procedure is "Big Bubble" that Anwar and Teichmann reported [14]. The technique includes 27-gauge needle with air-filled syringe inserted into deep stroma for 3–4 mm centrally and air injection to separate DM from stroma. It has been shown that outcomes of DALK were similar to PK with lower rejection or failure rates. However, Big Bubble can be obtained in only 56–82% of eyes [28–30].

For the improvement of these surgical techniques, new and unique complications beside advantages have emerged. The main purpose during separation of stroma from DM is to obtain a non-damaged DM [31]. But perforation or tears in DM occur in 4–20% of cases which is the most important complication during surgery [28–30, 32]. The risk of perforation is higher if proper big bubble formation is not achieved [33]. Unsuccessful big bubble formation is more frequently seen in patients with keratoconus and deep corneal scar involving DM [34–36]. Microperforations can be managed with air injection to the anterior chamber and careful manual dissection, but most of the macroperforations need to be converted to PK [14, 37]. The other complication is pseudoanterior chamber [38]. It can occur as double or triple anterior chamber [39, 40]. It usually develops after perforation in DM [41]. Remnant viscoelastic material may also cause double anterior chamber [42]. Pseudoanterior chamber may resolve spontaneously when it is shallow but larger chambers should need surgical intervention [43].

The role of AS-OCT in DALK begins at a preoperative assessment. Patient selection and the right indication for surgery can be decided with many variables including AS-OCT findings. AS-OCT images provide central corneal thickness, anterior chamber biometry, angle and iris measurements, and lens thickness [13]. These findings help planning trephination depth during surgery, intraocular lens power assessment if needed combined with phacoemulsification and intraocular lens implantation, detecting narrow angle before surgery [11]. AS-OCT can also visualize corneal pathologies such as scarring in central or periphery, corneal degenerations or dystrophies and cysts. The importance of the imaging is to inform the surgeon about the location, size, and depth of the corneal lesion.

Big bubble procedure in DALK requires well-adjusted trephination depth and centrally inserted air cannula without damaging DM. This technique needs experience and has a steep learning curve. One of the difficulties is reaching the intended depth of the cornea with cannula and advancement to the central stroma. To overcome this challenge, preoperative central and peripheral corneal thickness measurement with AS-OCT is sensible. Busin et al. reported a modified big bubble technique, which needs AS-OCT [44]. They evaluated the thickness of trephination size with AS-OCT and aimed to reach a depth within 50 μm from the internal corneal surface. Air cannula was advanced only 1 mm into the cornea and air injected. They reported a successful pneumatic dissection in 85% of patients with this procedure. AS-OCT was very useful to show the depth of trephination site, and perforation during trephination occurred in only 2.3% (two patients) of patients. Moreover, AS-OCT has superiority over topography with Scheimpflug camera while planning the depth of trephination for DALK. Riss et al. measured corneal thickness with Scheimpflug camera, planned the depth of trephination to 90% of the thinnest pachymetric value, and faced perforation during trephination in 30.1% of patients [45]. Intraoperative AS-OCT seems to increase the choice of DALK rather than PK with easing lack of experience and surgical difficulties.

It is known that corneal stromal scar has effect on the success rate of DALK. Big bubble can be achieved in 56–82% of keratoconus patients without a corneal stromal scar. The success rate varies from keratoconus grade, central corneal thickness, and trephination size in these patients [28, 29, 46]. Corneal stromal scar is a very important risk factor in keratoconus patients and other corneal diseases influencing DALK success rate. Ozmen et al. reported that big bubble formation was achieved in 63.2% of patients and DALK was completed in 91% of patients [47]. The most important factor affecting DALK and big bubble success was the ratio of corneal scar depth and central corneal thickness (scar depth/central corneal thickness) which was calculated with AS-OCT, a cut-off point was given as >53% for scar depth/central corneal thickness, which has an acceptable sensitivity (100%) and specificity (67%). AS-OCT has been evaluated as crucial for measuring this risk factor and planning the right operation for patients. Corneal scar in keratoconus patients may be caused by hydrops. DALK has a relative contraindication for patients with stromal scar [38]. But considering rejection rates after PK, DALK can be an option when carried with great attention in patients with stromal scar. To avoid macroperforation during DALK, preoperative assessment and planning should be proper (**Figure 1**). Nanavaty et al. reported that all of their patients had successful DALK and none required PK even though microperforation occurred in 60% of patients, with the help of AS-OCT at preoperative evaluation [48].

Recent improvements in surgical devices allow us to use AS-OCT at intraoperative evaluation. Several studies point out that visual acuity after DALK is better when stromal dissection is carried to the DM or when there is minimal residual stroma [20, 49–51]. AS-OCT provides intraoperative assessment of the cornea with high resolution. AS-OCT can be used to measure the depth of air cannula while using big bubble technique and may increase the rate of a successful big bubble formation. Scorcia et al. reported the first study in 2013 using intraoperative AS-OCT to visualize air cannula depth and big bubble formation [52]. It was emphasized that if the cannula reached the optimal depth, big bubble could be obtained more probably, but bubble achievement reduced when air was injected superficially. Successful big bubble in 90% of patients was obtained when the cannula reached within 100 μm from the DM. De Benito-Llopis et al. reported similar results and indicated that AS-OCT is also useful when big bubble could not be achieved and manual dissection was performed [53]. AS-OCT images can be used to evaluate a residual stromal bed during the manual dissection of corneal stroma.

Real-time intraoperative AS-OCT device provides imaging of all surgical steps continuously. Steven et al. reported a case series with using intraoperative AS-OCT. They succeeded monitoring big bubble formation in two of six patients [54]. They performed a micro-bubble incision technique in a patient that they could not obtain big bubble and documented with AS-OCT. Half of the patients was complicated with DM rupture. They indicated that the accurate measurement of trephination depth and cannula advancement into the deep central stroma is possible with real-time intraoperative AS-OCT. Sharma et al. published a case report of a patient who has undergone DALK. The procedure was complicated with DM detachment [55]. They used continuous intraoperative AS-OCT while intracameral sulfur

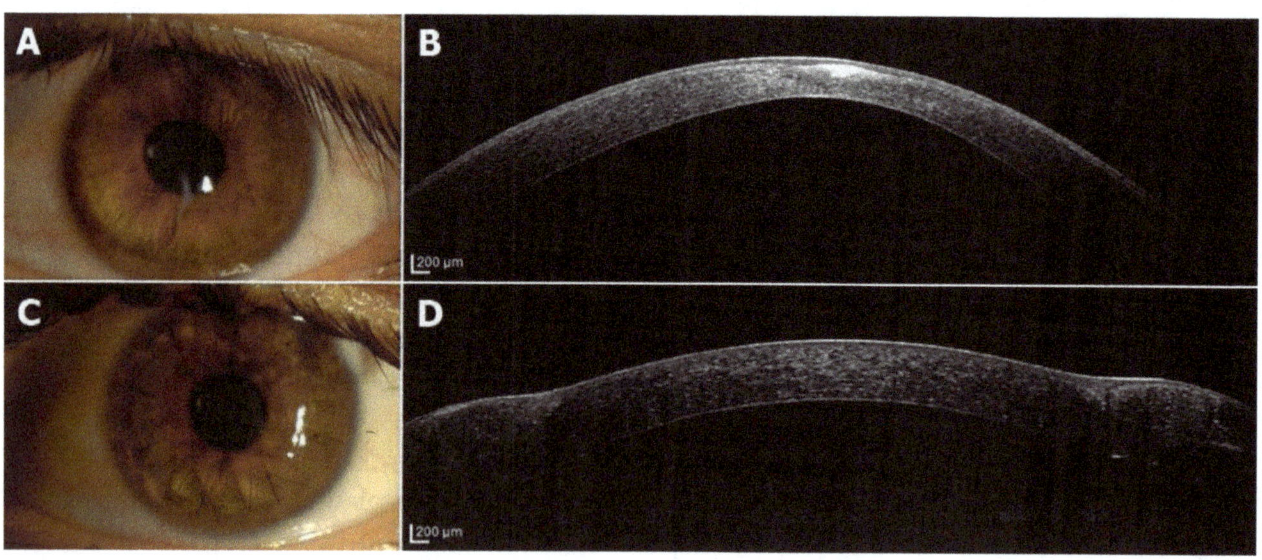

Figure 1. A patient with keratoconus who has an apical scar. (A) Anterior segment photography showing corneal scar. (B) AS-OCT showing corneal scar, which does not involve deep stromal layers and Descemet's membrane. With these findings, DALK was performed. (C) Anterior segment photography after surgery. (D) AS-OCT image of the patient after surgery.

hexafluoride injection and visualized re-attachment of DM with real-time images. Chaniyara et al. reported a complicated DALK case with repair of graft dehiscence with descemetopexy under the guidance of continuous intraoperative AS-OCT [56]. The use of real-time intraoperative AS-OCT seems to increase.

Intraoperative AS-OCT may obtain the depth and central advancement of the cannula while performing surgery. Image distortion caused by metallic objects is the major disadvantage of intraoperative AS-OCT [53]. The depth of the cannula could be assessed with only the image of the tunnel that is created by the cannula. With the manufacturing of plastic needles instead of metallic ones, one may overcome this drawback. Another disadvantage of intraoperative AS-OCT is caused by the devices which are mounted on the operation microscope separately. These devices have a handicap that they need to interrupt the surgery to take AS-OCT images. This disadvantage causes a delay in surgery. New devices that could obtain real-time images that are integrated into the operating microscope are being developed.

Pseudoanterior chamber due to DM detachment is frequently associated with microperforations during surgery, and management includes observation, intracameral gas injection, or reoperation (**Figure 2**). Slit-lamp biomicroscopy is enough to detect clinically significant detachment, but minimal double anterior chamber may not be seen by examination. The decision of treatment type and follow-up requires documentation of the patient. AS-OCT is very helpful to detect DM detachment and follow-up of the patient [57]. It allows to measure the size of pseudoanterior chamber initially and after the treatment [58]. AS-OCT can also visualize Dua's layer in case of triple anterior chamber occurrence [40].

AS-OCT can evaluate other postoperative complications of DALK. Bahadir et al. reported a candida interface keratitis after DALK, showing the keratitis site at AS-OCT [59]. Mukhopadhyay et al. reported a rhinosporidiosis keratitis case and they performed a repeat DALK procedure successfully after determining the site of the infiltrate in corneal stroma with AS-OCT [60]. Muller et al. published a case report with granular corneal dystrophy type-1 and reported that although they achieved pneumatic dissection to predescemetic layer during DALK, AS-OCT showed granular opacities between DM and graft [61]. It is thought that granular deposition occurs at predescemetic layer in granular corneal dystrophy type-1 and PK could be a better alternative than DALK. Costa et al. reported an iris cyst seen after DALK which was documented with AS-OCT and anterior segment photography [62].

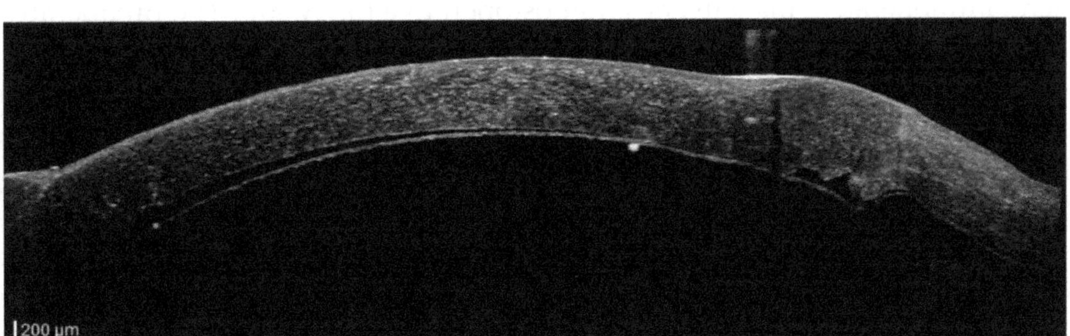

Figure 2. AS-OCT of a patient who had DALK surgery showing pseudoanterior chamber.

3. OCT in posterior lamellar keratoplasty

Posterior lamellar keratoplasty has emerged as an alternative to PK to treat corneal endothelial pathology [63, 64]. Evolution of the posterior lamellar keratoplasty procedures began with Melles et al., who reported deep lamellar endothelial keratoplasty (DLEK) that includes sutureless transplantation of posterior lamellae of cornea from a scleral incision [65]. Following DLEK, Descemet's stripping endothelial keratoplasty (DSEK) and DSAEK were developed [3, 66]. Corneal graft is prepared with automated microkeratome in DSAEK and it has been used worldwide [67]. Recently, DMEK is introduced as the latest posterior lamellar keratoplasty technique by Melles et al. [4]. Today, DSAEK and DMEK are the most popular posterior lamellar keratoplasty procedures [68].

DSAEK and DMEK are completely different interventions and both have different maneuvers [69]. DSAEK needs a 4- or a 5-mm limbal or corneo-scleral incision to insert the donor lamella. Descemet stripping of the host cornea is performed over an 8-mm diameter circle with a reverse Sinskey hook. Preparation of donor cornea is performed with automated microkeratome. Donor button consists of a thin stroma and Descemet's endothelial complex. Femtosecond laser has also been used recently for the preparation of the DSAEK graft. After trephination of donor lamella, it is inserted into the anterior chamber. Graft is attached to the host cornea with an air bubble. By contrast, DMEK provides transplantation of the endothelium with DM layer with minimal or absent stroma [70]. DM is stripped from the posterior stroma [71]. There are two methods of stripping: the first described procedure consists of DM stripping after corneal button trephination and the other technique consists of scoring edge of DM and stripping away from the stroma nearly half way to the center for 360° before trephination. Recently, DM dissection can be performed by an automated microkeratome and called as Descemet's membrane automated endothelial keratoplasty (DMAEK) [72, 73].

Several studies and meta-analysis reported that DMEK has superiority over DSAEK, considering visual outcome and patient satisfaction but DSAEK is used more frequently because of the steeper learning curve of DMEK [1, 74–77]. DMEK and DSAEK have a similar complication profile [78–80]. The most common early complications following posterior lamellar keratoplasty are graft dislocation and primary graft failure [81]. Other complications are graft rejection, endothelial cell loss, iatrogenic pupillary block glaucoma, keratitis, and endophthalmitis.

AS-OCT is a useful tool for posterior lamellar keratoplasty. It is valuable for preoperative assessment, intraoperative maneuvers, and postoperative follow-up. The preoperative duration of corneal stromal edema is found to be an important factor for visual outcome in patients who underwent endothelial keratoplasty [82]. It is known that the long duration of corneal stromal edema causes an increase in fibroblastic activity, irreversible fibrotic changes, and corneal scarring [83–85]. PK can be chosen in patients who have bullous keratopathy more than 12 months, instead of endothelial keratoplasty [82, 86]. AS-OCT may detect these stromal changes and obtain objective data for the decision of a planned surgery (**Figure 3**). AS-OCT images may help to decide which patients with stromal edema more than 12 months will benefit from endothelial surgery. AS-OCT can also obtain fine images of corneal epithelium. Long-standing bullous keratopathy may also cause subepithelial haze and fibrosis [87]. Agarwal et al. reported that endothelial keratoplasty with epithelial debridement provides a

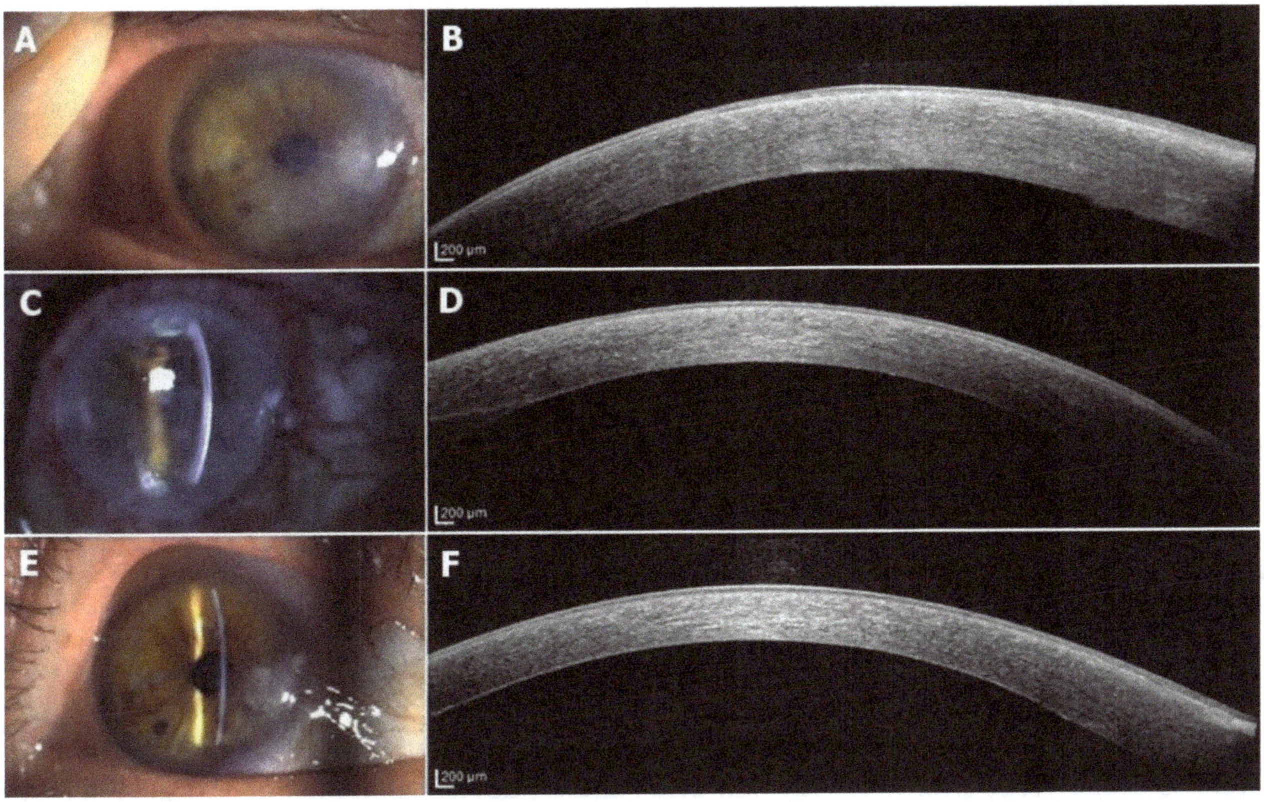

Figure 3. A patient with pseudophakic bullous keratopathy has underwent DMEK. (A) Preoperative anterior segment photography showing corneal edema. (B) Preoperative AS-OCT showing thickened corneal epithelium, subepithelial hyper-reflectance and corneal stromal edema. The central corneal thickness was 771 μm. (C) Early postoperative anterior segment photography shows reduced corneal edema. (D) Early postoperative AS-OCT shows reduced corneal edema and loss of subepithelial hyper-reflectance. The central corneal thickness was 615 μm. (E) Late postoperative anterior segment photography shows a clear cornea. (F) Late postoperative AS-OCT image shows normal corneal reflectance. The central corneal thickness was 555 μm.

better visual outcome in patients with chronic stromal edema [88]. AS-OCT was used to show corneal layers before and after endothelial keratoplasty which indicates that subepithelial haze and opacification of cornea decreased with surgery (**Figure 4**).

DMEK needs special maneuvers to unfold the graft and attach to the host. Attachment of the graft in both DMEK and DSAEK was performed with an air bubble, and there should be no interface fluid. Intraoperative AS-OCT can evaluate the graft orientation and obtain images of interface. Ide et al. reported the successful use of intraoperative AS-OCT in six consecutive patients showing no interface fluid at the end of the DSAEK [89]. Knecht et al. reported that their intraoperative AS-OCT study with six cases underwent DSAEK and indicated that detectable interface space does not mean a failure because the fluid may regress 1 day after surgery [90]. They also reported that detectable interface fluid may disappear with vent incisions by the guidance of intraoperative AS-OCT. In addition to that, PIONEER study published two separate results from DSAEK surgery with intraoperative AS-OCT. The first study indicated that transient interface fluid at the end of the surgery and first postoperative day is more likely to develop textural interface opacity [91]. The second study reported that a larger residual interface fluid volume, area, and thickness at the end of surgery are associated with early-graft detachment [92]. These results emphasize that minimal or no interface fluid should be left at the end of the DSAEK surgery.

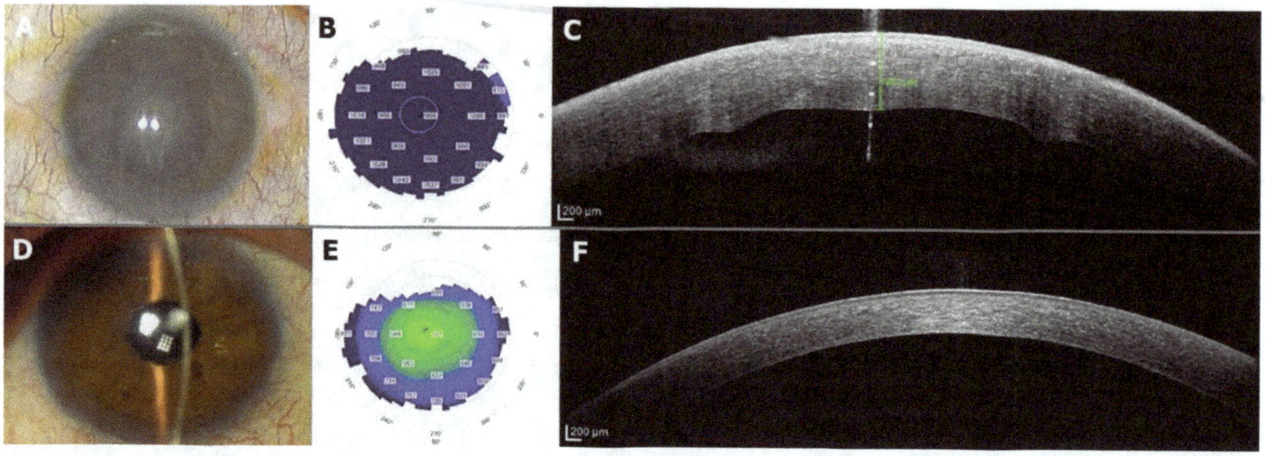

Figure 4. Triple-DMEK was performed successfully to a patient who had Fuchs endothelial dystrophy, severe corneal stromal edema with epithelial bullae, and angle closure glaucoma. (A) Preoperative anterior segment photography showing cataract and severe corneal edema. Visual acuity was hand movements. (B) Preoperative corneal thickness map in corneal topography. (C)preoperative AS-OCT image showing that corneal thickness was 917 μm. (D) Corneal edema was diminished 1 month after surgery and visual acuity was increased to 20/20. (E) Postoperative corneal thickness map showing resolved corneal edema. (F) AS-OCT image showing that corneal layers were returned to normal and the central corneal thickness was 530 μm.

Initial studies were performed with handheld AS-OCT devices, and imaging caused interruption of the surgery. Initial publications were followed by studies with real-time intraoperative AS-OCT which is integrated with the operating microscope [93–96]. Real-time imaging provided more comfortable surgery with simultaneous imaging. Besides evaluating interface fluid during surgery, intraoperative AS-OCT has additional benefits. Intraoperative AS-OCT assists in obtaining images of the nearly opaque corneas caused by stromal edema which could not be assessed well with an operation microscope [95]. This helps the surgeon to manipulate the graft easily in the operation.

DMEK is a relatively new technique than DSAEK, and studies on DMEK with intraoperative AS-OCT are fewer. Steven et al. published a study with 26 patients who underwent DMEK and reported that the usage of intraoperative AS-OCT enhances the graft visibility and surgeon's orientation [97]. Saad et al. reported that intraoperative AS-OCT enables a faster graft positioning with less manipulation in DMEK [96]. DISCOVER study indicated that intraoperative AS-OCT is very useful to confirm graft orientation and to reduce the iatrogenic graft failure [98].

Postoperative follow-up for graft dehiscence and graft failure is crucial in posterior lamellar keratoplasty. The fluid between the cornea and the graft can be seen with a slit-lamp biomicroscopy but Tarnawska and Wylegala reported that half of the interface fluid cannot be seen with examination which was detected by AS-OCT [99]. Early detection of interface fluid and graft detachment provides early intervention. In addition to that, postoperative measurement of graft thickness is an important factor for graft failure in DSAEK patients [100]. Eyes with thick grafts are more prone to graft failure (**Figure 5**). It is important to provide improvement in visual acuity after endothelial keratoplasty but fewer patients achieve excellent quality of vision. Many reasons were suggested including anterior stromal changes, graft-related problems, induced high-order aberrations, and interface-related problems. Turnbull et al. commented that the evolving anterior segment imaging could increase our

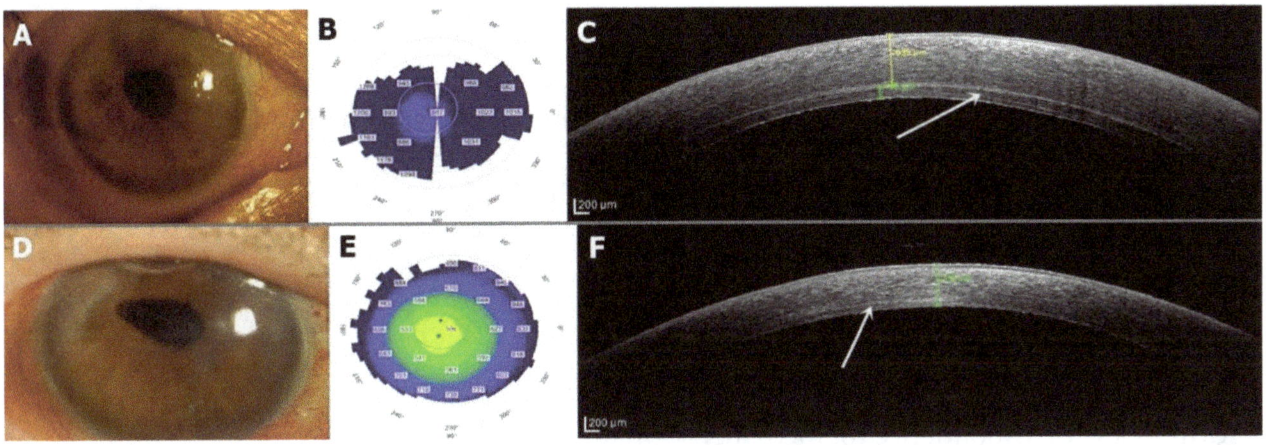

Figure 5. A patient who underwent DSAEK surgery for pseudophakic bullous keratopathy, presented with primary graft failure. DMEK was performed as a second surgery and corneal edema reduced. (A) Anterior segment photography before surgery showing severe edema. (B) Corneal thickness map in corneal topography showing corneal edema. (C) Corneal thickness was 753 μm and DSAEK graft's thickness was 113 μm. Hyperreflective line shown with white arrow shows interphase between posterior corneal stroma and DSAEK graft. (D) Anterior segment photography 1 day after DMEK; there was corneal haze without edema. (E) Corneal thickness map in corneal topography showing thinning in central cornea. (F) AS-OCT image showing that the central corneal thickness was 515 μm. DMEK graft cannot be visualized by AS-OCT. White arrow shows a horizontal hyperreflective posterior corneal stromal scar surface.

understanding of the reason to the solution of these difficulties [85]. Suh et al. reported that the evaluation of epithelial ingrowth in DSAEK patient can be possible with AS-OCT [101]. Kymionis et al. reported a case with residual DM after DSAEK that was shown with AS-OCT [102]. Lopez and Melles et al. published a study that described rebubbling techniques in DMEK, and they showed detached and folded DM with AS-OCT [103]. The assistance of AS-OCT for the assessment and management of complications in DMEK was studied in many publications [104–107].

4. Conclusion

AS-OCT is a valuable tool for assessing lamellar keratoplasty in all steps of the surgery. The use of AS-OCT starts from patient selection to postoperative late complications. Both anterior and posterior lamellar procedures need proper patient selection to obtain desired outcomes. Imaging the graft-host relationship with AS-OCT allows proper assessment of interface and helps surgeon to perform fast and successful surgeries. Some complications such as graft detachment can be visualized with AS-OCT postoperatively, more accurate than a conventional slit-lamp examination. AS-OCT is currently being used widely in corneal surgeries, and its role in lamellar keratoplasty seems to be increasing.

Acknowledgements

The authors thank the technicians of anterior segment imaging, Gazi University Medical School Department of Ophthalmology (Aynur Kartal, Cengiz Aksel, Nilgun Taşçı, Suat Avcı, Şenay Çay, Zafer Yıldırım), for the excellent photographs that have been used in this chapter.

Conflict of interest

None of the authors have any financial interest in any material or method mentioned in this chapter.

Author details

Mehmet Cüneyt Özmen[1]* and Hüseyin Baran Özdemir[2]

*Address all correspondence to: mcozmen@gmail.com

1 Department of Ophthalmology, Faculty of Medicine, Gazi University, Ankara, Turkey

2 Ulucanlar Eye Training and Research Hospital, University of Health Sciences, Ankara, Turkey

References

[1] Kymionis GD, Mikropoulos DG, Portaliou DM, Boboridis KG, Voudouragkaki IC, Dragoumis ND, et al. New perspectives on lamellar keratoplasty. Advances in Therapy. 2014;**31**:494-511. DOI: 10.1007/s12325-014-0121-0

[2] Borderie VM, Sandali O, Bullet J, Gaujoux T, Touzeau O, Laroche L. Long-term results of deep anterior lamellar versus penetrating keratoplasty. Ophthalmology. 2012;**119**:249-255. DOI: 10.1016/j.ophtha.2011.07.057

[3] Gorovoy MS. Descemet-stripping automated endothelial keratoplasty. Cornea. 2006; **25**:886-889. DOI: 10.1097/01.ico.0000214224.90743.01

[4] Melles GR, Ong TS, Ververs B, van der Wees J. Descemet membrane endothelial keratoplasty (DMEK). Cornea. 2006;**25**:987-990. DOI: 10.1097/01.ico.0000248385.16896.34

[5] Maharana PK, Agarwal K, Jhanji V, Vajpayee RB. Deep anterior lamellar keratoplasty for keratoconus: A review. Eye & Contact Lens. 2014;**40**:382-389. DOI: 10.1097/ICL.0000000000000076

[6] Dapena I, Ham L, Lie J, Van-Der-Wees J, Melles GR. Descemet membrane endothelial keratoplasty (DMEK): Two-year results. Archivos de la Sociedad Española de Oftalmología. 2009;**84**:237-243

[7] Shimmura S, Tsubota K. Deep anterior lamellar keratoplasty. Current Opinion in Ophthalmology. 2006;**17**:349-355. DOI: 10.1097/01.icu.0000233953.09595.91

[8] Price MO, Price FW. Descemet's stripping endothelial keratoplasty. Current Opinion in Ophthalmology. 2007;**18**:290-294. DOI: 10.1097/ICU.0b013e3281a4775b

[9] Huang D, Swanson EA, Lin CP, Schuman JS, Stinson WG, Chang W, et al. Optical coherence tomography. Science. 1991;**254**:1178-1181

[10] Izatt JA, Hee MR, Swanson EA, Lin CP, Huang D, Schuman JS, et al. Micrometer-scale resolution imaging of the anterior eye in vivo with optical coherence tomography. Archives of Ophthalmology. 1994;**112**:1584-1589

[11] Ramos JL, Li Y, Huang D. Clinical and research applications of anterior segment optical coherence tomography - a review. Clinical & Experimental Ophthalmology. 2009;**37**: 81-89. DOI: 10.1111/j.1442-9071.2008.01823.x

[12] Maeda N. Optical coherence tomography for corneal diseases. Eye & Contact Lens. 2010; **36**:254-259. DOI: 10.1097/ICL.0b013e3181ef0dbb

[13] Doors M, Berendschot TT, de Brabander J, Webers CA, Nuijts RM. Value of optical coherence tomography for anterior segment surgery. Journal of Cataract and Refractive Surgery. 2010;**36**:1213-1229. DOI: 10.1016/j.jcrs.2010.05.002

[14] Anwar M, Teichmann KD. Deep lamellar keratoplasty: Surgical techniques for anterior lamellar keratoplasty with and without baring of Descemet's membrane. Cornea. 2002;**21**:374-383

[15] Vajpayee RB, Tyagi J, Sharma N, Kumar N, Jhanji V, Titiyal JS. Deep anterior lamellar keratoplasty by big-bubble technique for treatment corneal stromal opacities. American Journal of Ophthalmology. 2007;**143**:954-957. DOI: 10.1016/j.ajo.2007.02.036

[16] Reinhart WJ, Musch DC, Jacobs DS, Lee WB, Kaufman SC, Shtein RM. Deep anterior lamellar keratoplasty as an alternative to penetrating keratoplasty a report by the american academy of ophthalmology. Ophthalmology. 2011;**118**:209-218. DOI: 10.1016/j.ophtha.2010.11.002

[17] Olson EA, Tu EY, Basti S. Stromal rejection following deep anterior lamellar keratoplasty: Implications for postoperative care. Cornea. 2012;**31**:969-973. DOI: 10.1097/ICO.0b013e31823f8a99

[18] Sugita J, Kondo J. Deep lamellar keratoplasty with complete removal of pathological stroma for vision improvement. The British Journal of Ophthalmology. 1997;**81**:184-188

[19] Melles GR, Lander F, Rietveld FJ, Remeijer L, Beekhuis WH, Binder PS. A new surgical technique for deep stromal, anterior lamellar keratoplasty. The British Journal of Ophthalmology. 1999;**83**:327-333

[20] Knutsson KA, Rama P, Paganoni G. Modified big-bubble technique compared to manual dissection deep anterior lamellar keratoplasty in the treatment of keratoconus. Acta Ophthalmologica. 2015;**93**:431-438. DOI: 10.1111/aos.12705

[21] Leccisotti A. Air-assisted manual deep anterior lamellar keratoplasty for treatment of herpetic corneal scars. Cornea. 2009;**28**:728-731. DOI: 10.1097/ICO.0b013e3181930a7e

[22] Chew AC, Mehta JS, Tan DT. Deep lamellar keratoplasty after resolution of hydrops in keratoconus. Cornea. 2011;**30**:454-459. DOI: 10.1097/ICO.0b013e3181f0b1f3

[23] Amayem AF, Anwar M. Fluid lamellar keratoplasty in keratoconus. Ophthalmology. 2000;**107**:76-79 discussion 80

[24] Manche EE, Holland GN, Maloney RK. Deep lamellar keratoplasty using viscoelastic dissection. Archives of Ophthalmology. 1999;**117**:1561-1565

[25] Muftuoglu O, Toro P, Hogan RN, Bowman RW, Cavanagh HD, McCulley JP, et al. Sarnicola air-visco bubble technique in deep anterior lamellar keratoplasty. Cornea. 2013;**32**:527-532. DOI: 10.1097/ICO.0b013e31826cbe99

[26] Gasset AR. Lamellar keratoplasty in the treatment of keratoconus: Conectomy. Ophthalmic Surgery. 1979;**10**:26-33

[27] Archila EA. Deep lamellar keratoplasty dissection of host tissue with intrastromal air injection. Cornea. 1984;**3**:217-218

[28] Feizi S, Javadi MA, Daryabari SH. Factors influencing big-bubble formation during deep anterior lamellar keratoplasty in keratoconus. The British Journal of Ophthalmology. 2016;**100**:622-625. DOI: 10.1136/bjophthalmol-2015-307111

[29] Fogla R, Padmanabhan P. Results of deep lamellar keratoplasty using the big-bubble technique in patients with keratoconus. American Journal of Ophthalmology. 2006; **141**:254-259. DOI: 10.1016/j.ajo.2005.08.064

[30] Fontana L, Parente G, Tassinari G. Clinical outcomes after deep anterior lamellar keratoplasty using the big-bubble technique in patients with keratoconus. American Journal of Ophthalmology. 2007;**143**:117-124. DOI: 10.1016/j.ajo.2006.09.025

[31] El-Danasoury A. Big bubble deep anterior lamellar keratoplasty (BB-DALK). International Ophthalmology Clinics. 2013;**53**:41-53. DOI: 10.1097/IIO.0b013e3182713434

[32] Arslan OS, Unal M, Tuncer I, Yucel I. Deep anterior lamellar keratoplasty using big-bubble technique for treatment of corneal stromal scars. Cornea. 2011;**30**:629-633. DOI: 10.1097/ICO.0b013e3181eeb44a

[33] Jhanji V, Sharma N, Vajpayee RB. Intraoperative perforation of Descemet's membrane during "big bubble" deep anterior lamellar keratoplasty. International Ophthalmology. 2010;**30**:291-295. DOI: 10.1007/s10792-009-9334-7

[34] Michieletto P, Balestrazzi A, Balestrazzi A, Mazzotta C, Occhipinti I, Rossi T. Factors predicting unsuccessful big bubble deep lamellar anterior keratoplasty. Ophthalmologica. 2006; **220**:379-382. DOI: 10.1159/000095864

[35] Huang T, Zhang X, Wang Y, Zhang H, Huand A, Gao N. Outcomes of deep anterior lamellar keratoplasty using the big-bubble technique in various corneal diseases. American Journal of Ophthalmology. 2012;**154**:282-289 e281. DOI: 10.1016/j.ajo.2012.02.025

[36] Shimmura S, Shimazaki J, Omoto M, Teruya A, Ishioka M, Tsubota K. Deep lamellar keratoplasty (DLKP) in keratoconus patients using viscoadaptive viscoelastics. Cornea. 2005;**24**:178-181

[37] Leccisotti A. Descemet's membrane perforation during deep anterior lamellar keratoplasty: Prognosis. Journal of Cataract and Refractive Surgery. 2007;**33**:825-829. DOI: 10.1016/j.jcrs.2007.02.016

[38] Karimian F, Feizi S. Deep anterior lamellar keratoplasty: Indications, surgical techniques and complications. Middle East African Journal of Ophthalmology. 2010;**17**:28-37. DOI: 10.4103/0974-9233.61214

[39] Higaki S, Maeda N, Watanabe H, Kiritoshi A, Inoue Y, Shimomura Y. Double anterior chamber deep lamellar keratoplasty: Case report. Cornea. 1999;**18**:240-242

[40] Selvan H, Patil M, Yadav S, Tandon R. Triple chamber: A clinical rarity after deep anterior lamellar keratoplasty and role of optical coherence tomography in management. International Ophthalmology. 2017. DOI: 10.1007/s10792-017-0755-4

[41] Venkatraman A. Spontaneous resolution of double anterior chamber with perforation of Descemet's membrane in deep anterior lamellar keratoplasty. Oman Journal of Ophthalmology. 2012;**5**:112-114. DOI: 10.4103/0974-620X.99376

[42] Bhojwani RD, Noble B, Chakrabarty AK, Stewart OG. Sequestered viscoelastic after deep lamellar keratoplasty using viscodissection. Cornea. 2003;**22**:371-373

[43] Passani A, Sframeli AT, Loiudice P, Nardi M. Late spontaneous resolution of a double anterior chamber post deep anterior lamellar keratoplasty. Saudi Journal of Ophthalmology. 2017;**31**:58-60. DOI: 10.1016/j.sjopt.2017.01.003

[44] Busin M, Scorcia V, Leon P, Nahum Y. Outcomes of air injection within 2 mm inside a deep trephination for deep anterior lamellar Keratoplasty in eyes with Keratoconus. American Journal of Ophthalmology. 2016;**164**:6-13. DOI: 10.1016/j.ajo.2015.12.033

[45] Riss S, Heindl LM, Bachmann BO, Kruse FE, Cursiefen C. Pentacam-based big bubble deep anterior lamellar keratoplasty in patients with keratoconus. Cornea. 2012;**31**:627-632. DOI: 10.1097/ICO.0b013e31823f8c85

[46] Feizi S, Javadi MA, Jamali H, Mirbabaee F. Deep anterior lamellar keratoplasty in patients with keratoconus: Big-bubble technique. Cornea. 2010;**29**:177-182. DOI: 10.1097/ICO.0b013e3181af25b7

[47] Ozmen MC, Yesilirmak N, Aydin B, Ceylanoglu KS, Atalay HT, Akata F. Prediction of descemet membrane perforation during deep anterior lamellar keratoplasty in patients with keratoconus with stromal scar. Eye & Contact Lens. 2017. DOI: 10.1097/ICL.0000000000000434

[48] Nanavaty MA, Daya SM. Outcomes of deep anterior lamellar keratoplasty in keratoconic eyes with previous hydrops. The British Journal of Ophthalmology. 2012;**96**:1304-1309. DOI: 10.1136/bjophthalmol-2012-302110

[49] Sarnicola V, Toro P, Gentile D, Hannush SB. Descemetic DALK and predescemetic DALK: Outcomes in 236 cases of keratoconus. Cornea. 2010;**29**:53-59. DOI: 10.1097/ICO.0b013e3181a31aea

[50] Feizi S, Javadi MA, Rastegarpour A. Visual acuity and refraction after deep anterior lamellar keratoplasty with and without successful big-bubble formation. Cornea. 2010;**29**:1252-1255. DOI: 10.1097/ICO.0b013e3181d83710

[51] Tan DT, Anshu A, Parthasarathy A, Htoon HM. Visual acuity outcomes after deep anterior lamellar keratoplasty: A case-control study. The British Journal of Ophthalmology. 2010;**94**:1295-1299. DOI: 10.1136/bjo.2009.167528

[52] Scorcia V, Busin M, Lucisano A, Beltz J, Carta A, Scorcia G. Anterior segment optical coherence tomography-guided big-bubble technique. Ophthalmology. 2013;**120**:471-476. DOI: 10.1016/j.ophtha.2012.08.041

[53] De Benito-Llopis L, Mehta JS, Angunawela RI, Ang M, Tan DT. Intraoperative anterior segment optical coherence tomography: A novel assessment tool during deep anterior lamellar keratoplasty. American Journal of Ophthalmology. 2014;**157**:334-341 e333. DOI: 10.1016/j.ajo.2013.10.001

[54] Steven P, Le Blanc C, Lankenau E, Krug M, Oelckers S, Heindl LM, et al. Optimising deep anterior lamellar keratoplasty (DALK) using intraoperative online optical coherence tomography (iOCT). The British Journal of Ophthalmology. 2014;**98**:900-904. DOI: 10.1136/bjophthalmol-2013-304585

[55] Sharma N, Aron N, Kakkar P, Titiyal JS. Continuous intraoperative OCT guided management of post-deep anterior lamellar keratoplasty descemet's membrane detachment. Saudi Journal of Ophthalmology. 2016;**30**:133-136. DOI: 10.1016/j.sjopt.2016.01.001

[56] Chaniyara MH, Bafna R, Urkude J, Sharma N. Rescuing the host Descemet's membrane in full-thickness traumatic wound dehiscence in deep anterior lamellar keratoplasty: Intraoperative optical coherence tomography (iOCT)-guided technique. BML Case Reports. 2017;**2017**. DOI: 10.1136/bcr-2017-221495

[57] Lim LS, Aung HT, Aung T, Tan DT. Corneal imaging with anterior segment optical coherence tomography for lamellar keratoplasty procedures. American Journal of Ophthalmology. 2008;**145**:81-90. DOI: 10.1016/j.ajo.2007.08.019

[58] Wylegala E, Nowinska A. Usefulness of anterior segment optical coherence tomography in Descemet membrane detachment. European Journal of Ophthalmology. 2009; **19**:723-728

[59] Bahadir AE, Bozkurt TK, Kutan SA, Yanyali CA, Acar S. Candida interface keratitis following deep anterior lamellar keratoplasty. International Ophthalmology. 2012;**32**: 383-386. DOI: 10.1007/s10792-012-9545-1

[60] Mukhopadhyay S, Datta H, Sen D. Intracorneal rhinosporidiosis managed with deep anterior lamellar keratoplasty. Middle East African Journal of Ophthalmology. 2014; **21**:361-362. DOI: 10.4103/0974-9233.142282

[61] Muller EG, Gomes JAP, Nose W, Nose RM. Persistence of granular corneal dystrophy type-1 deposits in the predescemetic layer after big-bubble deep anterior lamellar keratoplasty. Arquivos Brasileiros de Oftalmologia. 2018;**81**:66-69. DOI: 10.5935/0004-2749.20180015

[62] Costa JF, Rego M, Rosa A, Costa E, Fonseca P, Cachulo ML, et al. Anterior chamber epithelial cyst after uneventful deep anterior lamellar Keratoplasty. Cornea. 2016;**35**: 1372-1374. DOI: 10.1097/ICO.0000000000000866

[63] Maier P, Reinhard T, Cursiefen C. Descemet stripping endothelial keratoplasty–rapid recovery of visual acuity. Deutsches Ärzteblatt International. 2013;**110**:365-371. DOI: 10.3238/arztebl.2013.0365

[64] Grottone GT, Pereira NC, Gomes JA. Endothelial keratoplasty: Evolution and horizons. Arquivos Brasileiros de Oftalmologia. 2012;**75**:439-446

[65] Melles GR, Lander F, van Dooren BT, Pels E, Beekhuis WH. Preliminary clinical results of posterior lamellar keratoplasty through a sclerocorneal pocket incision. Ophthalmology. 2000;**107**:1850-1856 discussion 1857

[66] Price FW Jr, Price MO. Descemet's stripping with endothelial keratoplasty in 50 eyes: A refractive neutral corneal transplant. Journal of Refractive Surgery. 2005;**21**:339-345

[67] Veldman PB, Terry MA, Straiko MD. Evolving indications for Descemet's stripping automated endothelial keratoplasty. Current Opinion in Ophthalmology. 2014;**25**:306-311. DOI: 10.1097/ICU.0000000000000073

[68] Dapena I, Ham L, Melles GR. Endothelial keratoplasty: DSEK/DSAEK or DMEK--the thinner the better? Current Opinion in Ophthalmology. 2009;**20**:299-307. DOI: 10.1097/ICU.0b013e32832b8d18

[69] Talajic JC, Straiko MD, Terry MA. Descemet's stripping automated endothelial keratoplasty: Then and now. International Ophthalmology Clinics. 2013;**53**:1-20. DOI: 10.1097/IIO.0b013e31827eb6ba

[70] Terry MA, Straiko MD, Veldman PB, Talajic JC, VanZyl C, Sales CS, et al. Standardized DMEK technique: Reducing complications using Prestripped tissue, novel glass injector, and sulfur hexafluoride (SF6) gas. Cornea. 2015;**34**:845-852. DOI: 10.1097/ICO.0000000000000479

[71] Birbal RS, Sikder S, Lie JT, Groeneveld-van Beek EA, Oellerich S, Melles GRJ. Donor tissue preparation for descemet membrane endothelial keratoplasty: An updated review. Cornea. 2018;**37**:128-135. DOI: 10.1097/ICO.0000000000001368

[72] Kymionis GD, Yoo SH, Diakonis VF, Grentzelos MA, Naoumidi I, Pallikaris IG. Automated donor tissue preparation for descemet membrane automated endothelial keratoplasty (DMAEK): An experimental study. Ophthalmic Surgery, Lasers & Imaging. 2011;**42**:158-161. DOI: 10.3928/15428877-20101223-01

[73] Pereira Cda R, Guerra FP, Price FW Jr, Price MO. Descemet's membrane automated endothelial keratoplasty (DMAEK): Visual outcomes and visual quality. The British Journal of Ophthalmology. 2011;**95**:951-954. DOI: 10.1136/bjo.2010.191494

[74] Green M, Wilkins MR. Comparison of early surgical experience and visual outcomes of DSAEK and DMEK. Cornea. 2015;**34**:1341-1344. DOI: 10.1097/ICO.0000000000000590

[75] Hamzaoglu EC, Straiko MD, Mayko ZM, Sales CS, Terry MA. The first 100 eyes of standardized Descemet stripping automated endothelial Keratoplasty versus standardized Descemet membrane endothelial Keratoplasty. Ophthalmology. 2015;**122**:2193-2199. DOI: 10.1016/j.ophtha.2015.07.003

[76] Maier AK, Gundlach E, Gonnermann J, Klamann MK, Bertelmann E, Rieck PW, et al. Retrospective contralateral study comparing Descemet membrane endothelial keratoplasty with Descemet stripping automated endothelial keratoplasty. Eye (London, England). 2015;**29**:327-332. DOI: 10.1038/eye.2014.280

[77] Tourtas T, Laaser K, Bachmann BO, Cursiefen C, Kruse FE. Descemet membrane endothelial keratoplasty versus descemet stripping automated endothelial keratoplasty. American Journal of Ophthalmology. 2012;**153**:1082-1090 e1082. DOI: 10.1016/j.ajo.2011.12.012

[78] Thiel MA, Bochmann F, Schmittinger-Zirm A, Banninger PB, Schmid MK, Kaufmann C. Complications of descemet stripping automated endothelial keratoplasty (DSAEK). Der Ophthalmologe. 2015;**112**:969-973. DOI: 10.1007/s00347-015-0166-8

[79] Gorovoy MS. DMEK complications. Cornea. 2014;**33**:101-104. DOI: 10.1097/ICO.0000000000000023

[80] Straiko MD, Terry MA, Shamie N. Descemet stripping automated endothelial keratoplasty under failed penetrating keratoplasty: A surgical strategy to minimize complications. American Journal of Ophthalmology. 2011;**151**:233-237 e232. DOI: 10.1016/j.ajo.2010.08.017

[81] Pavlovic I, Shajari M, Herrmann E, Schmack I, Lencova A, Kohnen T. Meta-analysis of postoperative outcome parameters comparing Descemet membrane endothelial Keratoplasty versus Descemet stripping automated endothelial Keratoplasty. Cornea. 2017;**36**:1445-1451. DOI: 10.1097/ICO.0000000000001384

[82] Morishige N, Chikama T, Yamada N, Takahashi N, Morita Y, Nishida T, et al. Effect of preoperative duration of stromal edema in bullous keratopathy on early visual acuity after endothelial keratoplasty. Journal of Cataract and Refractive Surgery. 2012;**38**:303-308. DOI: 10.1016/j.jcrs.2011.08.032

[83] Morishige N, Yamada N, Teranishi S, Chikama T, Nishida T, Takahara A. Detection of subepithelial fibrosis associated with corneal stromal edema by second harmonic generation imaging microscopy. Investigative Ophthalmology & Visual Science. 2009;**50**:3145-3150. DOI: 10.1167/iovs.08-3309

[84] Ljubimov AV, Burgeson RE, Butkowski RJ, Couchman JR, Wu RR, Ninomiya Y, et al. Extracellular matrix alterations in human corneas with bullous keratopathy. Investigative Ophthalmology & Visual Science. 1996;**37**:997-1007

[85] Turnbull AM, Tsatsos M, Hossain PN, Anderson DF. Determinants of visual quality after endothelial keratoplasty. Survey of Ophthalmology. 2016;**61**:257-271. DOI: 10.1016/j.survophthal.2015.12.006

[86] Morishige N, Nomi N, Morita Y, Nishida T. Immunohistofluorescence analysis of myofibroblast transdifferentiation in human corneas with bullous keratopathy. Cornea. 2011;**30**:1129-1134. DOI: 10.1097/ICO.0b013e318213798d

[87] Chaurasia S, Price MO, McKee Y, Price FW Jr. Descemet membrane endothelial keratoplasty combined with epithelial debridement and mitomycin-C application for fuchs

dystrophy with preoperative subepithelial fibrosis or anterior basement membrane dystrophy. Cornea. 2014;**33**:335-339. DOI: 10.1097/ICO.0000000000000078

[88] Agarwal A, Narang P, Kumar DA, Agarwal A. Young donor-graft assisted endothelial keratoplasty (PDEK/DMEK) with epithelial debridement for chronic pseudophakic bullous keratopathy. Canadian Journal of Ophthalmology. 2017;**52**:519-526. DOI: 10.1016/j.jcjo.2017.03.004

[89] Ide T, Wang J, Tao A, Leng T, Kymionis GD, O'Brien TP, et al. Intraoperative use of three-dimensional spectral-domain optical coherence tomography. Ophthalmic Surgery, Lasers & Imaging. 2010;**41**:250-254. DOI: 10.3928/15428877-20100303-15

[90] Knecht PB, Kaufmann C, Menke MN, Watson SL, Bosch MM. Use of intraoperative fourier-domain anterior segment optical coherence tomography during descemet stripping endothelial keratoplasty. American Journal of Ophthalmology. 2010;**150**:360-365 e362. DOI: 10.1016/j.ajo.2010.04.017

[91] Juthani VV, Goshe JM, Srivastava SK, Ehlers JP. Association between transient interface fluid on intraoperative OCT and textural interface opacity after DSAEK surgery in the PIONEER study. Cornea. 2014;**33**:887-892. DOI: 10.1097/ICO.0000000000000209

[92] Hallahan KM, Cost B, Goshe JM, Dupps WJ Jr, Srivastava SK, Ehlers JP. Intraoperative interface fluid dynamics and clinical outcomes for intraoperative optical coherence tomography-assisted descemet stripping automated endothelial keratoplasty from the PIONEER study. American Journal of Ophthalmology. 2017;**173**:16-22. DOI: 10.1016/j.ajo.2016.09.028

[93] Kobayashi A, Yokogawa H, Mori N, Sugiyama K. Visualization of precut DSAEK and pre-stripped DMEK donor corneas by intraoperative optical coherence tomography using the RESCAN 700. BMC Ophthalmology. 2016;**16**:135. DOI: 10.1186/s12886-016-0308-z

[94] Siebelmann S, Bachmann B, Lappas A, Dietlein T, Hermann M, Roters S, et al. Intraoperative optical coherence tomography in corneal and glaucoma surgical procedures. Der Ophthalmologe. 2016;**113**:646-650. DOI: 10.1007/s00347-016-0320-y

[95] Pasricha ND, Shieh C, Carrasco-Zevallos OM, Keller B, Izatt JA, Toth CA, et al. Real-time microscope-integrated OCT to improve visualization in DSAEK for advanced bullous keratopathy. Cornea. 2015;**34**:1606-1610. DOI: 10.1097/ICO.0000000000000661

[96] Saad A, Guilbert E, Grise-Dulac A, Sabatier P, Gatinel D. Intraoperative OCT-assisted DMEK: 14 consecutive cases. Cornea. 2015;**34**:802-807. DOI: 10.1097/ICO.0000000000000462

[97] Steven P, Le Blanc C, Velten K, Lankenau E, Krug M, Oelckers S, et al. Optimizing descemet membrane endothelial keratoplasty using intraoperative optical coherence tomography. JAMA Ophthalmology. 2013;**131**:1135-1142. DOI: 10.1001/jamaophthalmol.2013.4672

[98] Cost B, Goshe JM, Srivastava S, Ehlers JP. Intraoperative optical coherence tomography-assisted descemet membrane endothelial keratoplasty in the DISCOVER study. American Journal of Ophthalmology. 2015;**160**:430-437. DOI: 10.1016/j.ajo.2015.05.020

[99] Tarnawska D, Wylegala E. Monitoring cornea and graft morphometric dynamics after descemet stripping and endothelial keratoplasty with anterior segment optical coherence tomography. Cornea. 2010;**29**:272-277. DOI: 10.1097/ICO.0b013e3181b61496

[100] Shih CY, Ritterband DC, Palmiero PM, Seedor JA, Papachristou G, Harizman N, et al. The use of postoperative slit-lamp optical coherence tomography to predict primary failure in descemet stripping automated endothelial keratoplasty. American Journal of Ophthalmology. 2009;**147**:796-800, 800 e791. DOI: 10.1016/j.ajo.2008.12.015

[101] Suh LH, Shousha MA, Ventura RU, Kieval JZ, Perez VL, Wang J, et al. Epithelial ingrowth after Descemet stripping automated endothelial keratoplasty: Description of cases and assessment with anterior segment optical coherence tomography. Cornea. 2011;**30**:528-534. DOI: 10.1097/ICO.0b013e3181fb8149

[102] Kymionis GD, Suh LH, Dubovy SR, Yoo SH. Diagnosis of residual Descemet's membrane after Descemet's stripping endothelial keratoplasty with anterior segment optical coherence tomography. Journal of Cataract and Refractive Surgery. 2007;**33**:1322-1324. DOI: 10.1016/j.jcrs.2007.03.029

[103] Fernandez Lopez E, Baydoun L, Gerber-Hollbach N, Dapena I, Liarakos VS, Ham L, et al. Rebubbling techniques for graft detachment after Descemet membrane endothelial Keratoplasty. Cornea. 2016;**35**:759-764. DOI: 10.1097/ICO.0000000000000829

[104] Werkmeister RM, Sapeta S, Schmidl D, Garhofer G, Schmidinger G, Aranha Dos Santos V, et al. Ultrahigh-resolution OCT imaging of the human cornea. Biomedical Optics Express. 2017;**8**:1221-1239. DOI: 10.1364/BOE.8.001221

[105] Leon P, Parekh M, Nahum Y, Mimouni M, Giannaccare G, Sapigni L, et al. Factors associated with early graft detachment in primary Descemet membrane endothelial Keratoplasty. American Journal of Ophthalmology. 2018;**187**:117-124. DOI: 10.1016/j.ajo.2017.12.014

[106] Satue M, Idoipe M, Sanchez-Perez A, Liarakos VS, Mateo A, Garcia-Martin E, et al. Evaluation of early graft detachment after Descemet membrane endothelial Keratoplasty using new swept-source optical coherence tomography. Cornea. 2016;**35**:1279-1284. DOI: 10.1097/ICO.0000000000000925

[107] Ang M, Dubis AM, Wilkins MR. Descemet membrane endothelial keratoplasty: Intraoperative and postoperative imaging spectral-domain optical coherence tomography. Case Reports in Ophthalmological Medicine. 2015;**2015**:506251. DOI: 10.1155/2015/506251

2

Cross-Polarization OCT for In Vivo Diagnostics and Prediction of Bladder Cancer

Elena Kiseleva, Gladkova Natalia, Streltzova Olga, Kirillin Mikhail, Maslennikova Anna, Dudenkova Varvara, Yunusova Katerina and Sergeeva Ekaterina

Abstract

This chapter contains three parts covering recent efforts to increase the accuracy of optical coherence tomography (OCT) differential diagnostics of bladder pathologies. The first part compares the diagnostic efficacy of traditional OCT and cross-polarization OCT (CP OCT); CP OCT and fluorescence cystoscopy (FC) for detecting flat lesions in the bladder at the early stages of cancer. The second part contains a report on achievements in application of CP OCT for detection of recurrent carcinoma in the scar area that is a hardly distinguishable form of bladder cancer using an optimized CP OCT image analysis. The third part of the chapter reviews the results on CP OCT usage for in vivo diagnosis of the bladder cancer after radiation therapy of cervical cancer.

Keywords: cross-polarization optical coherence tomography (CP OCT), bladder cancer, collagen, laser scanning microscopy (LSM), radiation damage

1. Introduction

Bladder cancer can manifest in a variety of different forms, and chronic inflammation plays the key role in its development [1]. One of the origins of bladder cancer development is the side-effect of radiation therapy. The radiation therapy of the uterus or prostate cancer frequently induces substantial alterations in the bladder wall that may progress to bladder cancer. Such side-effects of the radiation therapy of pelvic organs are of particular interest, as they occur in the patients with predicted long life expectancy, and preservation of the life quality is of comparable importance with recurrence prevention [2]. In this situation, early detection of bladder cancer or pre-cancer manifestations, preferably non-invasive, is the key for timely treatment.

Traditionally, white-light cystoscopy is employed for detection of bladder cancer. Besides the invasiveness and potential risks, white light cystoscopy drawbacks include difficult detection of flat lesions, inaccurate tumor delineation, which leads to complete resection and inability to differentiate between inflammation and malignancy and to determine the tumor grade and stage. In clinical practice, the overcoming of these drawbacks strongly depends on the surgeon's experience [3].

In the last decade, the techniques for diagnosing bladder pathologies were complemented by optical coherence tomography (OCT) being actively introduced into clinical practice [4–6]. OCT is a modern optical non-invasive imaging technique based on the principles of reflectance low-coherence interferometry, which can provide a tissue image to the depths up to several millimeters with spatial resolution down to units of μm. Cross-polarization OCT (CP OCT) is an OCT modality where probing is performed by polarized light; and two conjugated images are being registered in the channels with polarization parallel and orthogonal to initial one (co- and cross-polarization channels, respectively).

Many OCT research groups develop their own approaches for differential diagnostic of early bladder cancer [3, 7, 8]. The combination of OCT diagnostics with image analysis and signal processing (e.g., histograms analysis [9, 10], extraction of optical properties [11], texture analysis [12, 13]) has a high potential for automated differential diagnostics. To bridge the gap between research and clinical use, the potential of CP OCT was systematically investigated for real-time and label-free imaging. Nowadays, the studies are focused on challenging problems such as hardly distinguishable forms of bladder disorders related with cancer. Alterations in normal tissue that occur in the early and late periods after radiation therapy are an actual problem of modern radiation oncology [14] where high potential of the CP OCT was demonstrated.

This chapter contains three parts covering recent efforts to increase the accuracy of OCT differential diagnostics of bladder pathologies. The first part compares the diagnostic efficacy of traditional OCT (equivalent to obtaining co-polarized image only), CP OCT (employing combination of cross-polarized and co-polarized images), and fluorescence cystoscopy (FC) for detecting flat lesions in the bladder at early stages of cancer. In the second part, we report on the recent achievements in application of CP OCT for detection of carcinoma recurrence in scar area using an optimized CP OCT image analysis/quantification platform. The platform is based on detecting alterations in the collagen compartment of interrogated tissue's extra-cellular matrix (ECM). The third part reviews the pilot results of CP OCT employment for in vivo evaluation of the severity of the bladder mucosa damage after radiation therapy of cervical cancer. In addition to morphological analysis with hematoxylin and eosin (H&E) and picrosirius red (PSR) staining, nonlinear laser scanning microscopy (LSM) study was performed to confirm the level of collagen damage and remodeling as a consequence of cancer invasion and radiation therapy.

CP OCT studies of human urinary bladder mucosa during in vivo endoscopic examination described in this chapter were performed with the "OCT 1300-U" system (IAP RAS, Nizhny

Novgorod, Russia). CP OCT device has a forward-looking (en-face) endoscopic probe with outer diameter 2.7 mm that is placed vertically to the mucous surface leaving an imprint on it, so the tissue is taken for histology from the same area and has the same orientation. The CP OCT system is based on superluminiscent diode with central wavelength 1300- and 100-nm bandwidth and has axial resolution ~15 μm and lateral resolution ~25 μm. Using the circular polarized probing light and two signal acquisition channels to detect scattered light that maintained initial polarization and change it to orthogonal one gave an advantage to assess co- ("co-polarized image") and cross-scattering ("cross-polarized image") properties of the tissue up to 1.8 mm in depth. CP OCT image size is 2.5 × 4.0 mm (width × height), image acquisition rate is 0.5 frames per sec. Refer to previous publications [15, 16] for more detailed system descriptions, including the optical phase retardation particulars to enable CP operation.

The fragments of the bladder mucosa from the sites of CP OCT inspection extracted in course of surgery and biopsy were subjects for further histological and LSM examination. Later, CP OCT images were compared to the morphological images. Histologic study included light microscopy with H&E staining and polarized light transmission microscopy with PSR staining for evaluation of structural and spatial organization of collagen fibers; LSM was applied in second harmonic generation (SHG) mode with excitation at the wavelength of 800 nm and spectral detection in the range of 362–415 nm to reveal the distribution of collagen fibers in the bladder mucosa.

The Ethics Committee of Nizhny Novgorod State Medical Academy for scientific research involving human subjects approved the clinical study. All patients voluntarily signed the informed consent for the study.

2. Efficacy of cross-polarization OCT in bladder cancer diagnosis: comparison with traditional OCT, fluorescence cystoscopy, and immunohistochemical study

The early OCT studies of bladder mucosa were performed with traditional time-domain modality equipped with an endoscopic probe. Diagnosis of early bladder cancer was the central topic of OCT studies in urology [4]. After 25 years, the OCT technique significantly improved resulting, in particular in cross-polarization time-domain OCT with common-path optical layout and two signal acquisition channels and in spectral CP OCT modification with the similar characteristics enabling 3D imaging.

2.1. Cross-polarization OCT and traditional OCT at bladder cancer

In course of introduction of CP OCT into clinical practice, the capabilities of this new technique for early bladder cancer detection were assessed in a comparative study with the traditional OCT. To assess the efficacy, the special test was developed. It consisted of two independent stages: assessing diagnostic capabilities of OCT (using a set of co-polarized images) for detecting neoplasia and assessing diagnostic capabilities of CP OCT (using a set of the same clinical cases, but with two images: in co- and in cross-polarization) for the same task. Statistical evaluation of the diagnostic efficacies of OCT and CP OCT was also performed independently. A total of 116 patients with localized flat suspicious lesions in the bladder were enrolled, 360 CP OCT images were acquired and analyzed. Statistical parameters and general results of the blind recognition tests of CP OCT and OCT images of flat suspicious lesions in the bladder are listed in Ref. [17].

Briefly, it was shown that CP OCT demonstrated higher sensitivity of 93.7% (vs. 81.2%, $p < 0.0001$), specificity 84% (vs. 70.0%, $p < 0.001$), and diagnostic accuracy 85.3% (vs. 71.5%, <0.001) in detecting early malignant changes in flat suspicious zones compared to the traditional OCT technique. The interobserver agreement index *kappa* increased from 0.68 to 0.82 when images in cross-polarization were added. The earlier analysis of more than 500 traditional OCT [4] and CP OCT images of benign and malignant states of the bladder [18] enabled us to formulate visual criteria for assessing CP OCT images in co- and in cross-polarization (**Table 1**).

Higher diagnostic efficacy of CP OCT in detecting early bladder cancer is associated with the ability to detect changes in epithelium and connective tissues. In previous works (see Refs. [17, 19]), it was demonstrated that OCT signal in cross-polarization (**Figure 1a**, upper image) is formed primarily due to cross-scattering from unaltered, well-organized type I collagen. This statement is based on the comparison of the signal level in cross-polarization with the brightness of PSR-stained collagen fiber luminescence in polarized light (**Figure 1j**).

It is known that collagen stained with PSR and examined with polarized light microscopy reveals its birefringent properties, visualized as bright pixels against the background of dark surrounding tissue elements (reference). Collagen type I has red and red-yellow color (thick fibers with thickness ~2–5 μm and higher) and collagen type III—green and green-white color (thin fibers with thickness ~1 μm). Red-orange color of thick-collagen fibers is also associated with densely packed collagen fibers indicative of their maturity [20].

CP OCT image characteristics		**Benign processes in the bladder**	**Malignant processes in the bladder**
In co-polarization:	OCT features	Sharp, high contrast between epithelium and connective tissue in more than 75% of the lateral range of image. The epithelial layer has lower signal level than the connective tissue layer	No or weak contrast between horizontal layers
	OCT type images	Benign	Cancer
In cross-polarization:	OCT features	Uniform signal that may have the structure of horizontal layers	No or weak signal, in some images in the form of isolated spots
	OCT type images	Benign	Cancer

Table 1. Visual criteria for assessing CP OCT images in co- and in cross-polarizations.

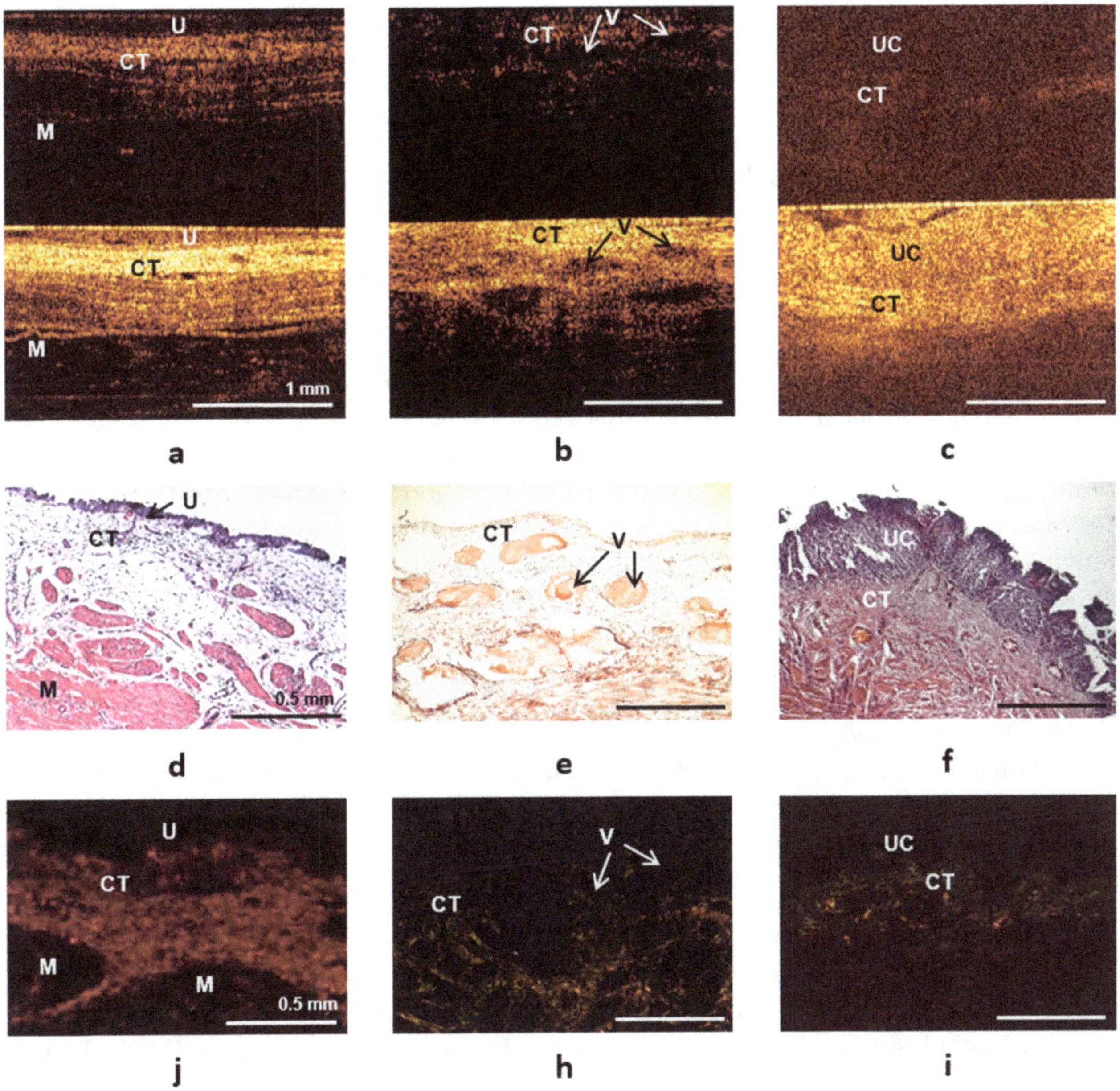

Figure 1. Bladder mucosa in normal state and in pathology. Normal (a, d, j), chronic exudative cystitis (b, e, h) and urothelial carcinoma Ia (c, f, i). CP OCT images (upper panel = cross-polarization, lower panel = co-polarization) (a, b, c), the corresponding histological slides stained with hematoxylin and eosin was used to confirm the diagnosis (d, e, f), stained with picrosirius red and examined with polarized light—to reveal the presence and type of collagen (j, h, i). U—urothelium, CT—connective tissue, M—muscle, V—vessel, UC—urothelial carcinoma.

The loss of collagen polarization properties due to its disorganization at neoplasia (**Figure 1f** and **i**) and massive inflammatory cellular infiltration significantly reduces OCT signal level in cross-polarization (**Figure 1c**, upper image). At the same time, CP OCT images at chronic cystitis in cross-polarization have regions with high-level signal (**Figure 1b**). It is caused by diffuse excessive synthesis and accumulation of collagen fibers (its assembly/bunching in the background of reduced degradation), especially around vessels (sclerosis of vessel wall; **Figure 1e** and **h**).

Based on the qualitative considerations above, it appears that morphological and polarization changes of collagen fibers properties in various pathological states are complex and interrelated.

2.2. Cross-polarization OCT, fluorescence cystoscopy, and immunohistochemical study at bladder cancer

Fluorescence cystoscopy (FC) is one of the techniques to search for regions suspicious for cancer on the inner bladder surface. However, it has low-positive predictive value [21, 22]. Immunohistochemical (IHC) markers for bladder cancer Ta-T2a have potential to improve the diagnostics and help in understanding of carcinogenesis at molecular level [23]. Unfortunately, this technique can be employed only ex vivo. Recent studies of years [19] were aimed to assess the diagnostic accuracy of the combined use of FC and CP OCT with quantitative estimation of OCT signal in cross-polarization for diagnosis of superficial bladder cancer in flat suspicious lesions and analyze epithelial and carcinoma cells proliferation activity by using IHC markers. A total of 26 patients with bladder cancer were enrolled in the study. Total amount of regions of interest was 92; 41 sites with urothelial carcinoma (28 cases of cancer in bladder tissue/13 cases of recurrent cancer in scar tissue) and 51 sites with inflammation (16 mild/35 severe).

The results of the study show that the combined use of FC and CP OCT with quantitative estimation of the OCT signal yields the diagnostic accuracy in detecting bladder cancer in flat suspicious zones of 93.6%, the sensitivity of 96.4%, specificity of 92.1%, positive predictive value of 87%, and negative predictive value of 97.9%, which indicates that the efficacy of this approach is close to that of biopsy.

Since chronic inflammation in the bladder is manifested by the increased proliferative activity of uroteliocytes, IHC study using cell proliferation markers (Ki-67, p53, and p63) allows for more accurate quantification of the urothelium state and the risk of developing urothelial neoplasm. Ki-67, p53, and p63 immunohistochemistry is suggested to be helpful to distinguish dysplastic changes and carcinoma in situ from reactive atypia. These IHC markers were applied for the study of areas where CP OCT images can be classified as cancer type.

The IHC study demonstrated a high level of p53 expression and high proliferation activity (the number of the cells positively stained for Ki-67, p53, and p63 exceeded 50%) in the regions of bladder cancer. Those indices were significantly higher ($p < 0.0001$) comparing to the regions with severe inflammation. In the regions with mild inflammation, the level of Ki-67, p53, and p63 did not differ significantly ($p > 0.05$) from those with severe inflammation [23]. This confirms that the increased urothelium proliferation level in patients with bladder cancer is typical for the entire mucosa and does not depend on the visual manifestations of the inflammatory process [1, 24].

The expression of p63 only in the areas of red fluorescence was significantly higher ($p = 0.038$) than in the areas without fluorescence. The expression of Ki-67 and p53 did not depend on fluorescence.

The study confirms enhanced expression of p53, p63, and Ki-67 in patients with recurrent, highly differentiated superficial (without invasion into the muscular layer) urothelial carcinoma with a low or moderate risk of disease progression [25–28].

Also, a correlation between CP OCT data and IHC markers data was demonstrated. High inverse correlation ($r = -0.732$; $r = -0.647$ and $r = -0.481$, respectively, $p < 0.002$) was demonstrated between the expression of p63, Ki-67, and p53 markers and the CP OCT signal in cross-polarization. The obtained correlations allow suggesting why signal in cross-polarization alters in cases of inflammation and neoplasia. Healthy tissue in co-polarization has a layered structure featuring the epithelium and connective stroma. A neoplastic process characterized by excessive proliferation of urothelial cells losing specificity is accompanied by activation of p53, p63, and Ki-67 expression. On the one hand, active proliferation can change optical properties of epithelial cells; on the other hand, it eventually leads to disorganization of collagen matrix. It was found that the higher the expression of the markers of cellular proliferation and adherence, the more intense loss of cross-scattering properties by connective tissue collagen is registered by CP OCT. However, it is still unclear which process is primary.

3. CP OCT for diagnostics of recurrent bladder cancer

Recurrent forms of bladder cancer are hard to distinguish by routine diagnostic approaches (cystoscopy). In the majority of cases, cancer recurrence at scar is hard to be distinguished from the scar tissue. In this situation, even OCT inspection may fail to provide adequate information due to visual similarity of scar and cancer in a diagnostic OCT image.

To develop an approach to distinguish the recurrence of bladder cancer and the scar, parallel in vivo CP OCT and morphological study of the level of cross scattering and state of collagen was performed for scar tissue (group 1, $n = 30$) and carcinoma in the scar area (group 2, $n = 28$). **Figure 2** shows that sometimes CP OCT images in the scar tissue (a) and in recurrence of carcinoma in scar area (d) look quite similar. In cross-polarization, the OCT signal is heterogeneous: in both cases, there are areas with high, reduced, or absence of signal (**Figure 2a** and **d**, upper images). Analysis of the structural organization of collagen fibers at fiber and tissue levels in the scar tissue (group 1) showed that in condition of chronic inflammation of the bladder mucosa areas of excessive synthesis and accumulation of collagen (see **Figure 2**, red and yellow color on PSR image (b) and intense green color on SGH image (c)) might alternate with not yet formed collagen fibers areas (see **Figure 2**, pale green color or dark areas on PSR image (b) and week or no SHG signal (c)). Analysis of the recurrence of carcinoma on a post-operation scar region (Group 2) revealed that on PSR image areas of carcinoma are dark, and collagen fibers are thin of pale-red color (**Figure 2e**); some of collagen fibers are destroyed. The collagen fibers are loosely stacked and surround cancer cells in SGH image (**Figure 2f**).

OCT image processing and quantification may give an additional valuable information for differentiation these two conditions. A number of previous studies demonstrate that the changes in polarization properties correlate with changes in collagen state [6, 23, 29–31] while

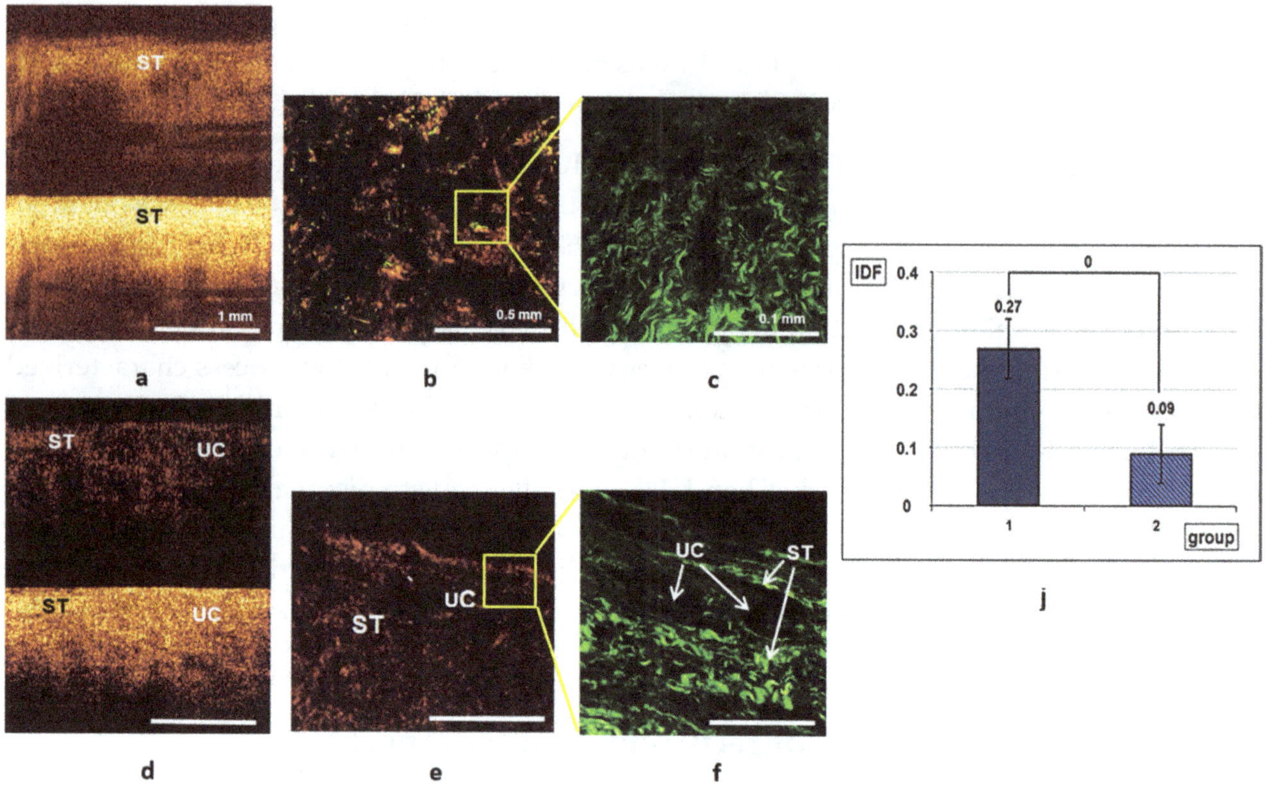

Figure 2. Scar tissue on the bladder mucosa and recurrence of urothelial carcinoma in the scar region. Group 1 (the upper row of images and left column on the diagram), Group 2—recurrence of carcinoma in the scar region (the lower row and left column on the diagram). CP OCT images (upper panel = orthogonal polarization, lower panel = initial polarization) (a, d); corresponding histological slides stained with picrosirius red and examined with polarized light (b, e); SHG images (c, f). ST—scar tissue, UC—urothelial carcinoma.

orientation and the degree of structural organization of collagen at fiber and tissue levels allowed to conclude on the presence of pathology [30]. Quantitative processing of CP OCT images was based on analysis of the cross-scattering properties of the bladder tissue [6]. An integral depolarization factor (IDF) was developed and successfully applied to quantify the collagen state within tissue [31]. IDF is defined as a ratio of the OCT signals in cross-polarization to co-polarization, both averaged over the transverse coordinates.

The results of comparing IDF in the groups of scar tissue (Group 1) and recurrence of urothelial carcinoma in the scar region (Group 2) are presented in **Figure 2j**. A statistically significant difference in IDF values between these two conditions is demonstrated ($p < 0.0001$), which testifies to the possibility of effective cystoscopic recognition of carcinoma in the region of post-operation scar with the IDF/CP OCT platform. It is known that collagen fibers are destroyed under the influence of tumor cell enzymes [32]; this likely decreased the resultant cross-polarization OCT signal. The quantitative assessment of CP OCT images obtained from the suspicious areas of postoperation scars can thus help in distinguishing the appearance of tumor in scar region.

Sensitivity, specificity, and diagnostic accuracy of separating recurrence of carcinoma in region of the bladder scar by quantitative assessment of CP OCT images with IDF are 93, 99, and 97%, respectively.

Intraoperative CP OCT monitoring of completeness of tumor removal was introduced into clinical practice (N.A. Semashko Nizhny Novgorod Regional Hospital) allowing minimizing the number of cancer recurrences at postoperative scar regions.

4. CP OCT for in vivo detection of bladder cancer after radiation therapy

The third paragraph of the chapter reviews the pilot results on CP OCT employment for in vivo detection of the bladder cancer after radiation therapy of cervical cancer.

Bladder cancer that occurs after radiation therapy of malignant neoplasms of the pelvic organs is a special problem in clinical urology. According to European Association of Urology, there is a two- to four-fold increase in the risk of secondary malignant tumors development in the bladder after radiotherapy of tumors of pelvic organs [33]. Recent studies [34, 35] confirmed the increase in the risk of bladder cancer for 1.5–4 times after the course of radiotherapy.

Alterations of normal bladder tissue occurring in the early and late periods after radiotherapy are an unsolved problem in modern radiation oncology [36]. The early side-effects include changes developed in the course of radiotherapy and 100 days after it. Radiation damages that appear after 3 months since radiotherapy procedure are treated as late; sometimes, they may occur in years after irradiation. In addition, in recent years, late effects resulting from long-term persistent severe acute radiation damage called "consequential late effects" are distinguished separately [37]. Specifically, late radiation-induced adverse events are of significant clinical importance [14]. Their severity can vary from clinically insignificant structural abnormalities to severe complications that have a great impact on the quality of patient's life (Cancer Therapy Evaluation Program) [38]. Different classifications including CTCAE, RTOG/EORTC, RILIT, and LENTSOMA were employed to determine the severity of post-radiation damage to normal tissues. Currently, the classification developed by Radiotherapy Oncology Group in collaboration with the European Organization for Research and Treatment of Cancer (RTOG/EORTC, 1995) is the most common classification scale for radiation complications (**Table 2**).

When bladder cancer appears in the irradiated and altered tissues, it becomes extremely difficult to diagnose cancer against edema, hemorrhage, and pronounced changes in the mucosa. Therefore, there is a challenge to differentiate changes induced by ionizing radiation and the changes caused by the tumor growth by standard clinical methods. In this situation, optical diagnostic techniques can play a crucial role in establishing the correct diagnosis.

In our clinical practice during last 2 years, a situation where CP OCT inspection allowed to diagnose bladder cancer in patients previously received radiotherapy for cervical cancer was met twice. Both patients have tumors developed at the background of severe (Grades 3 and 4) late side-effects of radiotherapy (**Table 2**).

Patient T., 65 years old, was hospitalized in urology department for vesico-urinary fistula. In January 2014, she was diagnosed with cervical cancer T3N0M0 (stage III). She received a concurrent chemoradiation therapy (external beam irradiation in a dose of 40 Gy, single dose

Organ tissue	Bladder
Grade 0	None
Grade 1	Slight epithelial atrophy, minor telangiectasia (microscopic hematuria)
Grade 2	Moderate frequency Generalized telangiectasia Intermittent macroscopic hematuria
Grade 3	Severe frequency and dysuria Severe generalized telangiectasia (often with petechiae) Frequent hematuria Reduction in bladder capacity (<150 cc)
Grade 4	Necrosis/contracted bladder (capacity <100 cc) Severe hemorrhagic cystitis
Grade 5	Death directly related to radiation late effects

Table 2. Classification of late radiation bladder damage (RTOG/EORTC, 1995).

2 Gy), brachytherapy in a dose of 25 Gy, single dose 5 Gy). In 18 months after radiation therapy, urine outflow from the vagina and blood in urine appeared. Ultrasound study revealed serozometra and right-side hydronephrosis. Laboratory blood tests showed signs of kidney failure. The right-side nephrostomy under ultrasound control and optical inspection of the bladder was made in November 2015. Cystoscopy revealed an organized blood clot within the bladder cavity. After bladder cavity dilatation, it was found that the bladder bottom was absent resulting in, a fistula defect of 3.5–4.0 cm in diameter. Bullous fabric with disintegration was revealed at the edge of the fistula. Mucosa of the bladder walls was hyperemic and hydropic (**Figure 3a**). Ureteral orifices were not visualized. Therefore, cystoscopy picture was consistent with the picture of Grade 4 radiation bladder damage (fistula, bleeding).

At the same time, bladder mucosa was studied with CP OCT; images of back left and right walls and around the fistula defect were acquired. CP OCT image of the back wall (**Figure 3c**) demonstrates the classic picture of chronic inflammation. Despite contrasted layers in co-polarization and high-level signal from connective tissue fibrosis in cross-polarization, both images feature edema (dark elongated areas, which have vertical shadows) and homogeneous areas originating from inflammatory cell infiltration of the stroma.

CP OCT image of the fistula edge (**Figure 3b**) manifests bullous features: in co-polarization, the image is mostly structureless: only the small area of image in the left has layers of epithelium (the first layer, may be with dysplastic changes), underlying connective tissue (the second layer, brighter) and below the signal abruptly falls (this area is suspicious to cancer); the central and the right side of the image are structureless, indicating neoplasia (**Figure 3b**). In cross-polarization, there is no pronounced signal, which approves the presence of neoplasia, and only small area in left side of the image corresponding to connective tissue demonstrates low-level signal. This flat zone is the suspicious area of the CP OCT image and transurethral biopsy was taken from this site. Morphologically, invasive

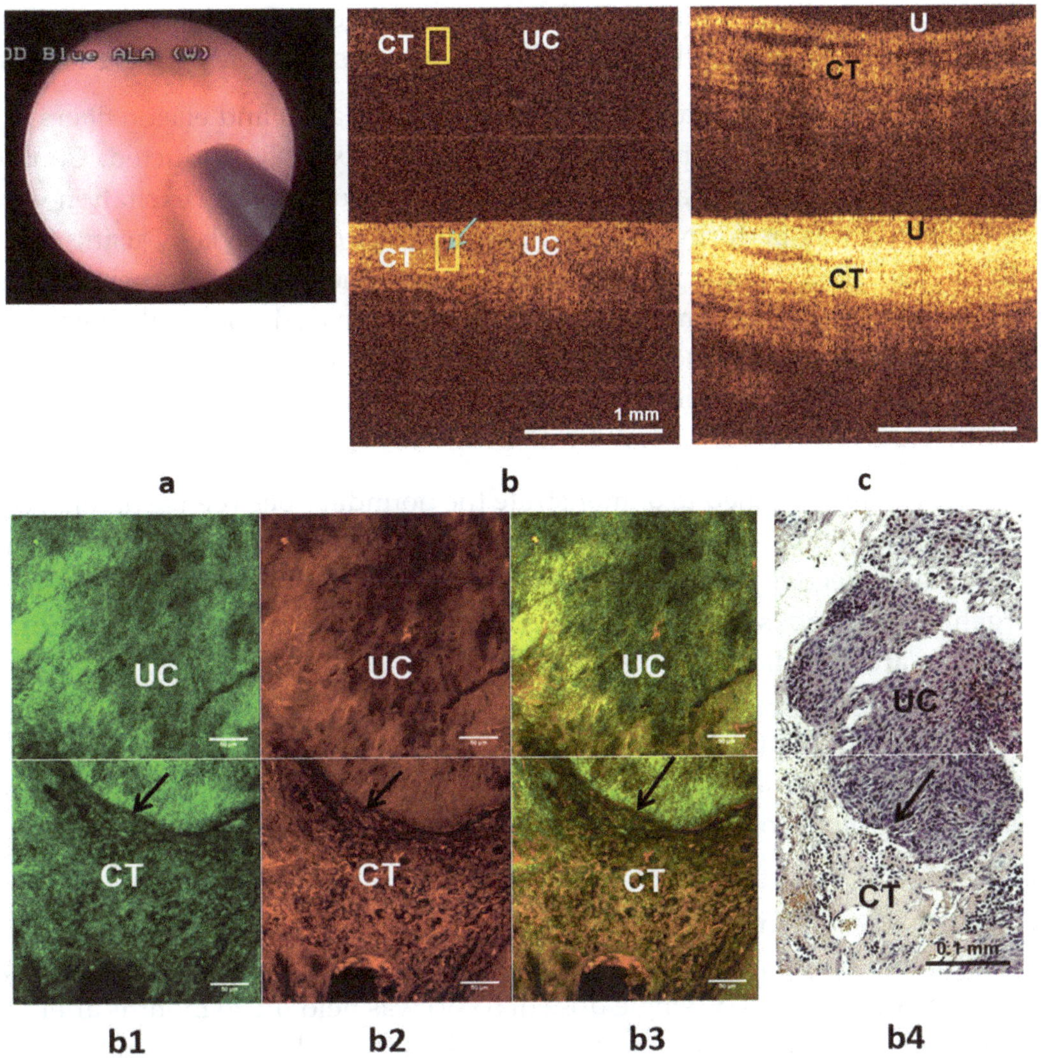

Figure 3. CP OCT guided biopsy of bladder mucosa and LSM study of extracellular matrix in 18 months after the end of radiation therapy. Cystoscopy image of the back wall in a moment of CP OCT study (a), CP OCT images (upper panel = cross-polarization, lower panel = co-polarization): image of tissue suspicious to cancer from border of fistula b), image of benign tissue from the back wall (c), LSM images (SHG (b1), 2PEF (b2) and combined SHG-2PEF (b3)) and histology (H&E) (b4) corresponding to CP OCT image (b). CT—connective tissue; U—urothelium; UC—urothelial carcinoma; arrows indicate border of carcinoma growth; yellow rectangle in (b) indicates area of LSM imaging (b1–b3).

transitional cell carcinoma Grade 2 was diagnosed (**Figure 3b4**). Conglomerates of cancer cells grow into the mucosa and submucosa layers of the bladder wall (area with low signal in co- and dark area in cross-polarization in **Figure 3b**, border of connective tissue is indicated with blue arrow). Carcinoma cells were localized deeper in connective tissue at the one side, whereas at the other side, it starts from the surface. Owing to CP OCT, biopsy was performed and urothelial carcinoma Grade 2 was detected while visually this area looked like inflammation.

We suppose that radiation induced damage of bladder connective tissue induced carcinoma development. In cross-polarization (left side of image), a low level signal from connective tissue is observed, originating from exudative inflammation process. Morphological analysis revealed congestion, swelling, lymphoid cell infiltrates in mucosa, and, important to mention, degenerative changes in collagen that cause decrease in cross-polarization OCT signal.

In order to determine more accurately the condition of collagen and elastic fibers in connective tissue of mucosa layer multiphoton, microscopy study was conducted. Confocal laser scanning microscope (LSM 710, Carl Zeiss, Germany) was used at the excitation wavelength of 800 nm. Detection was performed simultaneously in two channels by using filters in the wavelength ranges of 362–415 nm and 480–554 nm, with the aim to detect signals indicating SHG emission (green color in the images) and 2PEF emission (red color in the images), respectively. This approach allowed visualization of the collagen (seen in SHG) and primary elastin (seen in 2PEF) fibers in the walls of the bladder within the unstained, dewaxed sections with a thickness of 10 μm.

Two LSM images were combined to demonstrate the boundary between urothelial carcinoma and connective tissue (**Figure 3b1–b3**, the boundary is indicated with black arrow). Numerous small holes in the connective tissue corresponded to inflammatory infiltration, collagen is primary disorganized and looks homogeneous without clearly distinguished fibers (**Figure 3b1**), and elastic fibers are also damaged: they produced weak signal and are presented by fragments in a small amount (**Figure 3b2**). LSM study confirms that the connective tissue of the bladder after radiation therapy of pelvic organs has destructive changes that are preserved for the long time after treatment and in conjunction with chronic inflammation such condition can serve as a background for the cancer development.

Patient N., 41 years old, was urgently hospitalized in urology department with the diagnosis of chronic urinary retention. In 2014, she was diagnosed with cervical cancer T2bN0M0 (stage II), concurrent chemoradiation therapy (external beam irradiation in a dose of 40 Gy, brachytherapy in a dose of 25 Gy, single dose of 5 Gy) was held. In 20 months after the end of chemoradiotherapy, the patient became complaining of difficulty in urinating.

An ultrasound revealed pelvic adhesions, as well as the fact of bladder atony. Trocar cystostomy and cystoscopy study was done. Cystoscopically (**Figure 4a**), the mucous membrane of the bladder was shiny, whitish, trabecular, with tissue granulation on the back wall and in the triangle area; the bladder neck is loose, with a rough surface. Visually, three areas on mucosa were suspicious: in the center of the neck, in the neck close to the right wall, and close to the back wall. The CP OCT study of these areas was conducted, and then three biopsies were taken. Histology revealed presence of urothelial carcinoma Grade 3 complexes in two locations: in the center of the neck and in the neck close to the right wall (**Figure 4b4** and **c4**), where suspicious type of CP OCT images was obtained (**Figure 4b** and **c**). Both images have some features are not common for benign states. They contain structureless low signal areas without clear borders in co- and cross-polarizations at the lower part of the mucosa layer (first layer with a high level signal), and there is no epithelium layer usually manifested by middle intensity signal above the mucosa layer. Moreover, OCT signal from connective tissue in cross-polarization is homogeneous, whereas in norm and inflammation state, an image shows more or less distinct horizontally orientated structures.

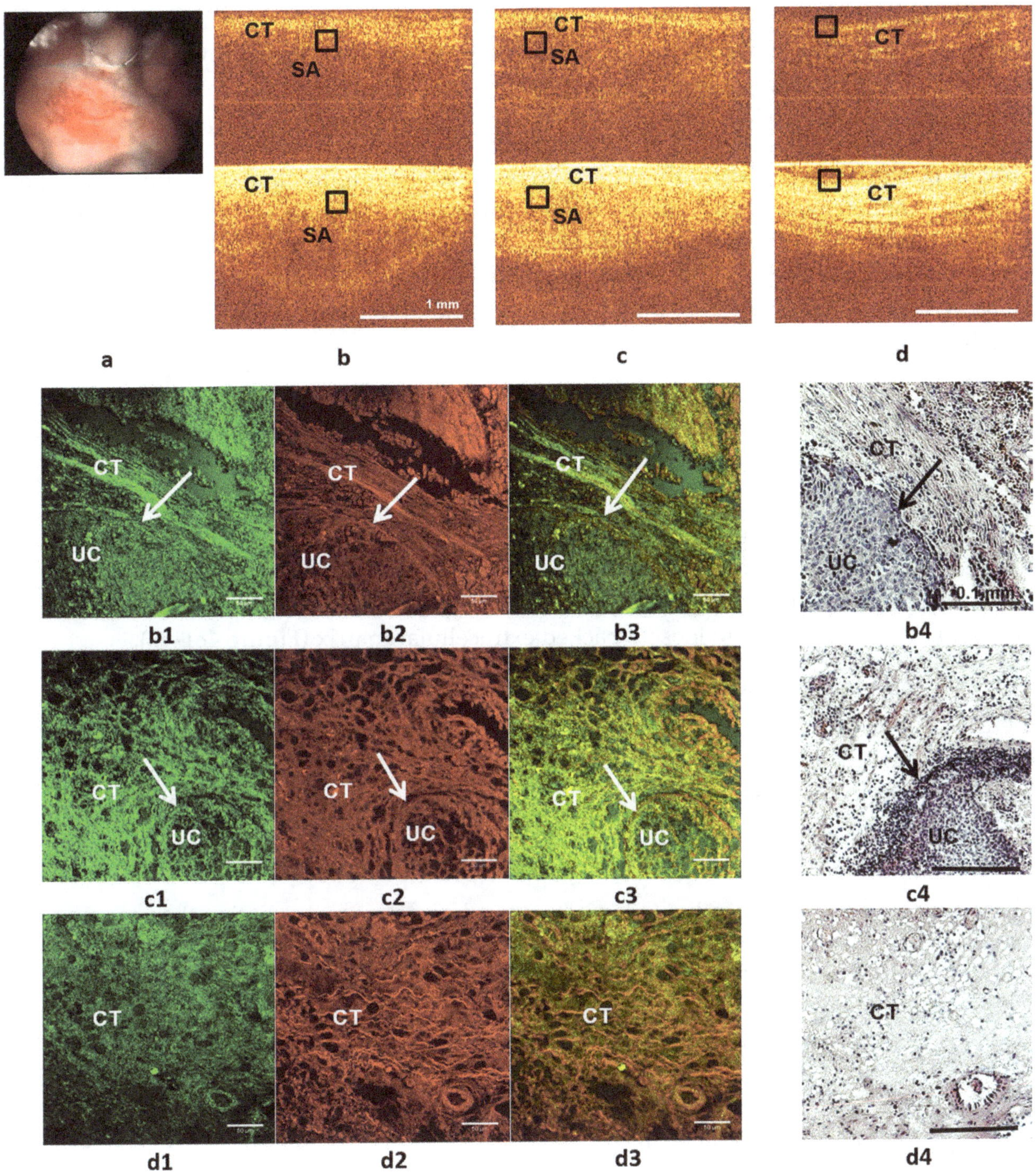

Figure 4. CP OCT of suspicious areas of bladder mucosa and LSM study of extracellular matrix in 20 months after the end of radiation therapy. Cystoscopy image of bladder neck with a loop of resectoscope at the time of biopsy (a), CP OCT images (upper panel = cross-polarization, lower panel = co-polarization): image of suspicious tissue at the bladder neck (b), image of suspicious tissue at the right wall close to the neck (c), image of bening tissue at the back wall (d), LSM images (SHG (b1, c1, d1), 2PEF (b2, c2, d2) and combined SHG-2PEF (b3, c3, d3)) and histology (H&E) (b4, c4, d4) corresponding to CP OCT images (b, c, d). CT—connective tissue; SA—suspicious area; UC—urothelial carcinoma; arrows indicate borders of carcinoma growth; black rectangle in (b, c, d) indicates area of LSM imaging (b1–b3, c1–c3, d1–d3, correspondingly).

CP OCT image of the third visually suspicious area (bladder neck close to the back wall) demonstrates the picture of chronic inflammation (**Figure 4d**) described above. Histology confirms supposed diagnosis: edemas, acute plethora, and round cells infiltration in the mucosa were present (**Figure 4d4**).

LSM images of bladder wall for the patient N. revealed that predominant amount of the fibers produces homogeneous signal similar to the previous case (**Figure 4c1–c3** and **d1–d3**). Only a few individual fibers of collagen and elastin are distinguished. This indicates disorganization processes in extracellular matrix. Loose network and holes in connective tissue in LSM images correspond to morphologically verified inflammation: edema and round a (**Figure 4c4** and **d4**).

Urothelial carcinoma in LSM images looks different: in the bladder neck, collagen in carcinoma is not organized (homogeneous SHG signal, **Figure 4b1**); however, close to the tumor, collagen fibers are straight, densely arranged, and have a prevailing orientation. This may point to aggressive and long-time growth of the carcinoma that starts to produce its own stroma and change the environment around to facilitate the invasion [32, 39]. In the neck close to the right wall, the carcinoma contains no elastic fibers and minimal amount of collagen organized in thin wavy fibers like in surrounding connective tissue, what may indicate infiltrative dissemination of carcinoma cells into loosely packed extracellular matrix **(Figure 4c1–c3**).

The described clinical cases show that extracellular matrix of bladder mucosa after radiation therapy of pelvic organs manifests dystrophic changes that could originate from the side-effects of radiation exposure and subsequent chronic inflammation. Rate of the bladder synchronic cancer in this case is up to 1.5–4 times larger as compared to nonirradiated bladder [34]. We suppose that disorganized collagen and elastic network in mucosa could also promote carcinoma fast growth and facilitate its invasion.

These examples demonstrate that to the patients, who undergone radiation therapy, a special attention and monitoring in the follow-up are required to prevent possible development of radiation induced urothelial carcinoma or detects it as early as possible. In this situation, CP OCT is an excellent minimally invasive tool for bladder mucosa inspection and evaluation of connective tissue state based on data in cross-polarization.

5. Conclusions

This chapter highlighted a novel diagnostic method, CP OCT, with high potential application for bladder pathology diagnosis. CP OCT can be considered an effective complementary in vivo technique to assess flat suspicious lesions in the bladder initially detected by white light or/and fluorescence cystoscopy, whereas the efficacy of these cystoscopy modalities alone or combined with traditional OCT is much lower.

Analysis and quantitative assessment of CP OCT images confirmed the presence of cross-scattering properties of connective tissue stroma in human mucosa that are determined by well-defined spatial and structural organization of collagen matrix. Collagen fibers undergo significant changes as a result of pathological processes which affect their cross-scattering properties that can be detected and quantified in vivo with CP OCT.

An approach to quantitative, robust, and potentially automated assessment of CP OCT images reflecting the state of bladder collagen fibers was developed. It was shown that IDF can be applied to in vivo detection of clinically relevant pathological states in urology. Differentiating between carcinoma recurrence at post-operation scar and tumor-free scar resulted in diagnostic accuracy of 97%. Thus, CP OCT and IDF quantification have promising potential to visualize and quantify the structural and spatial organization of CF in bladder tissues for clinical disease assessment including differential diagnosis applications.

Acknowledgements

This study was financially supported by the Russian Science Foundation, agreement no. 14-15-00538 (EBK, NDG, VVD) and the grants of the Russian Foundation for Basic Research No. 15-32-20250 (MYuK) and No. 16-07-00655 (OSS, AVM, KEYu).

Author details

Elena Kiseleva[1]*, Gladkova Natalia[1], Streltzova Olga[1], Kirillin Mikhail[2], Maslennikova Anna[1], Dudenkova Varvara[1], Yunusova Katerina[1] and Sergeeva Ekaterina[2]

*Address all correspondence to: kiseleva84@gmail.com

1 Nizhny Novgorod State Medical Academy, Institute of Biomedical Technologies, Nizhny Novgorod, Russia

2 Institute of Applied Physics of the Russian Academy of Sciences, Nizhny Novgorod, Russia

References

[1] Gakis G. The role of inflammation in bladder cancer. Adv Exp Med Biol. 2014;**816**:183-196. DOI: 10.1007/978-3-0348-0837-8_8.

[2] Fiorino C., Valdagni R., Rancati T., Sanguineti, G. Dose-volume effects for normal tissues in external radiotherapy: pelvis. Radiother Oncol. 2009;**93**(2):153-167. DOI: 10.1016/j.radonc.2009.08.004.

[3] Liu J.J., Droller M.J., Liao J.C. New optical imaging technologies for bladder cancer: considerations and perspectives. J Urol. 2012;**188**(2):361-368. DOI: 10.1016/j.juro.2012.03.127.

[4] Zagaynova E., Gladkova N., Shakhova N., Gelikonov G., Gelikonov V., Zagaynova E. Endoscopic OCT with forward-looking probe: clinical studies in urology and gastroenterology. J Biophotonics. 2008;**1**(2):114-128. DOI: 10.1002/jbio.200710017.

[5] Lee C.S., Yoon C.Y., Witjes J.A. The past, present and future of cystoscopy: the fusion of cystoscopy and novel imaging technology. BJU Int. 2008;**102**(9 Pt B):1228-1233. DOI: 10.1111/j.1464-410X.2008.

[6] Kiseleva E.B., Kirillin M.Yu., Feldchtein F.I., Vitkin I.A., Sergeeva E.A., Zagaynova E.V., Streltzova O.S., Shakhov B.E., Gubarkova E.V., Gladkova N.D. Differential diagnosis of human bladder mucosa pathologies in vivo with cross-polarization optical coherence tomography. Biomed Opt Express. 2015;**6**(4):1464-1476. DOI: 10.1364/BOE.6.001464.

[7] Ren H., Yuan Z., Waltzer W., Shroyer K., Pan Y. Enhancing detection of bladder carcinoma in situ by 3-dimensional optical coherence tomography. J Urol. 2010;**184**(4):1499-1506. DOI: 10.1016/j.juro.2010.05.087.

[8] Ikeda M., Matsumoto K., Choi D., Nishi M., Fujita T., Ohbayashi K., Shimizu K., Iwamura M. The impact of real-time 3d imaging by ultra-high speed optical coherence tomography in urothelial carcinoma. BMC Urol. 2013;**13**(65). DOI: 10.1186/1471-2490-13-65.

[9] Kirillin M., Panteleeva O., Yunusova E., Donchenko E., Shakhova N. Criteria for pathology recognition in optical coherence tomography of fallopian tubes. J Biomed Opt. 2012;**17**(8):081413-081421. DOI: 10.1117/1.JBO.17.8.081413.

[10] Yang Y., Wang T., Biswal N.C., Wang X., Sanders M., Brewer M., Zhu Q. Optical scattering coefficient estimated by optical coherence tomography correlates with collagen content in ovarian tissue. J Biomed Opt. 2011;**16**(9):090504. DOI: 10.1117/1.3625247.

[11] Ejofodomi O. Measurement of optical scattering coefficient of the individual layers of the human urinary bladder using optical coherence tomography. ISRN Biomed Imaging. 2014;**2014**. 1-4. DOI: 10.1155/2014/591592.

[12] Kirillin M., Panteleeva O., Agrba P., Pasukhin M., Sergeeva E., Plankina E., Dudenkova V., Gubarkova E., Kiseleva E., Gladkova N., Shakhova N., Vitkin A. Towards advanced OCT clinical applications. In: Lilge L.D., Sroka R., editors. Medical Laser Applications and Laser-Tissue Interactions VII; July 15, 2015; Munich, Germany. Proc. SPIE; 2015. p. 9542. DOI: 10.1117/12.2183794.

[13] Lindenmaier A.A., Conroy L., Farhat G., DaCosta R.S., Flueraru C., Vitkin I.A. Texture analysis of optical coherence tomography speckle for characterizing biological tissues in vivo. Opt Lett. 2013;**38**(8):1280-1282. DOI: 10.1364/OL.38.001280.

[14] Dorr W. Pathogenesis and repair of normal tissue damage. Radiother Oncol. May 2011;**99**(Supp 1):S135. DOI: 10.1016/S0167-8140(11)70460-1.

[15] Gelikonov V.M., Gelikonov G.V. New approach to cross-polarized optical coherence tomography based on orthogonal arbitrarily polarized modes. Laser Phys Lett. 2006;**3**(9):445-451. DOI: 10.1002/lapl.200610030.

[16] Gubarkova E.V., Dudenkova V.V., Feldchtein F.I., Timofeeva L.B., Kiseleva E.B., Kuznetsov S.S., Shakhov B.E., Moiseev A.A., Gelikonov G.V., Vitkin A., Gladkova N.D. Multi-modal optical imaging characterization of athero-sclerotic plaques. J Biophotonics. 2016;**9**(10):1009-1020. DOI 10.1002/jbio.201500223.

[17] Gladkova N.D., Streltsova O.S., Zagaynova E.V., Kiseleva E.B., Gelikonov V.M., Gelikonov G.V., Karabut M.M., Yunusova K.E., Evdokimova O.V. Cross polarization optical coherence tomography for early bladder cancer detection: statistical study. J Biophotonics. 2011;**4**(7–8):519-532. DOI: 10.1002/jbio.201000088.

[18] Gladkova N.D., Zagaynova E.V., Streltsova O.S., Kiseleva E.B., Karabut M.M., Snopova L.B., Yunusova E.E., Tararova E., Gelikonov V.M. Advantages of cross-polarization endoscopic optical coherence tomography in diagnosis of bladder neoplasia. In: Kollias N., Choi B., Zeng H., Malek R.S., Wong B.J.F., Gregory K.W., Tearney G.J., Marcu L., Hirschberg H., Madsen S.J., Mandelis A., Mahadevan-Jansen A., Jansen E.D., editors. Photonic Therapeutics and Diagnostics VI; January 23, 2010; San Francisco, California. Proc SPIE; 2010. p. 754813. DOI: 10.1117/12.841810.

[19] Gladkova N., Kiseleva E., Robakidze N., Balalaeva I., Karabut M., Gubarkova E., Feldchtein F. Evaluation of oral mucosa collagen condition with cross-polarization optical coherence tomography. J Biophotonics. 2013;**6**(4):321-329. DOI: 10.1002/jbio.201200059.

[20] Lattouf R., Younes R., Lutomski D., Naaman N., Godeau G., Senni K., Changotade S. Picrosirius red staining: a useful tool to appraise collagen networks in normal and pathological tissues. J Histochem Cytochem. 2014;**62**(10):751-758. DOI: 10.1369/0022155414545787.

[21] Mowatt G., N'Dow J., Vale L., Nabi G., Boachie C., Cook J.A., Fraser C., Griffiths T.R. Photodynamic diagnosis of bladder cancer compared with white light cystoscopy: systematic review and meta-analysis. Int J Technol Assess Health Care. 2011;**27**:3-10. DOI: 1017/s0266462310001364.

[22] Elferink O.P., Witjes J.A. Blue-light cystoscopy in the evaluation of non-muscle-invasive bladder cancer. Ther Adv Urol. 2014;**6**(1):25-33. DOI: 10.1177/1756287213510590.

[23] Gladkova N., Kiseleva E., Streltsova O., Prodanets N., Snopova L., Karabut M., Gubarkova E., Zagaynova E. Combined use of fluorescence cystoscopy and cross-polarization OCT for diagnosis of bladder cancer and correlation with immunohistochemical markers. J Biophotonics. 2013;**6**(9):687-698. DOI: 10.1002/jbio.201200105.

[24] Acar Ö., Özkurt E., Demir G., Saraç H., Alkan C., Esen T., Somel M., Lack N.A. Determining the origin of synchronous multifocal bladder cancer by exome sequencing. BMC Cancer. 2015;**15**(1):871. DOI: 10.1186/s12885-015-1859-8.

[25] Charfi S., Khabir A., Mnif H., Ellouze S., Mhiri M.N., Boudawara-Sellami T. Immunohistochemical expression of HER2 in urothelial bladder carcinoma and its correlation with p53 and p63 expression. J Microscopy Ultrastruct. 2013;**1**(1–2):17-21. DOI: 10.1016/j.jmau.2013.06.001.

[26] Goebell P.J., Groshen S.G., Schmitz-Drager B.J. p53 immunohistochemistry in bladder cancer—a new approach to an old question. Urol Oncol. 2010;**28**(4):377-388. DOI: 10.1016/j.urolonc.2010.03.021.

[27] Shariat S.F., Bolenz C., Godoy G., Fradet Y., Ashfaq R., Karakiewicz P.I., Isbarn H., Jeldres C., Rigaud J., Sagalowsky A.I., Lotan Y. Predictive value of combined immunohistochemical markers in patients with pT1 urothelial carcinoma at radical cystectomy. J Urol. 2009;**182**(1):78-84. DOI: 10.1016/j.juro.2009.02.125.

[28] Yalçin Ö., Sağlican Y., Özdemir S., Özkan N., Mangir N., Eren F. The Relationship of p16, Ki-67, Bcl-2, P53 and CK20 immune expressions with recurrence in superficial bladder tumors. World J Pathol. 2015;**4**:44-51.

[29] Nadkami S.K., Pierce M.C., Park B.H., de Boer J.F., Whittaker P., Bouma B.E., Bressner J.E., Halpern E., Houser S.L., Tearney G.J. Measurement of collagen and smooth muscle cell content in atherosclerotic plaques using polarization-sensitive optical coherence tomography. J Am Coll Cardiol. 2007;**49**(13):1474-1481. DOI: 10.1016/j.jacc.2006.11.040.

[30] Giattina S.D., Courtney B.K., Herz P.R., Harman M., Shortkroff S., Stamper D.L., Liu B., Fujimoto J.G., Brezinski M.E. Assessment of coronary plaque collagen with polarization sensitive optical coherence tomography (PS-OCT). Int J Cardiol. 2006;**107**(3):400-409. DOI: 10.1016/j.ijcard.2005.11.036.

[31] Gubarkova E.V., Kirillin M.Y., Sergeeva E.A., Kiseleva E.B., Snopova L.B., Prodanets N.N., Sharabrin E.G., Shakhov E.B., Nemirova S.V., Gladkova N.D. Cross-polarization optical coherence tomography in evaluation of atherosclerotic plaque structure. Sovrem Tehnol Med. 2013;**5**(4):45-54. DOI: 10.17691/stm2015.7.4.05.

[32] Provenzano P.P., Eliceiri K.W., Campbell J.M., Inman D.R., White J.G., Keely P.J. Collagen reorganization at the tumor-stromal interface facilitates local invasion. BMC Med. 2006;**4**:38. DOI: 10.1186/1741-7015-4-38.

[33] Chrouser K., Leibovich B., Bergstralh E., Zincke H., Blute M. Bladder cancer risk following primary and adjuvant external beam radiation for prostate cancer. J Urol. 2008;**159**(5 Suppl):S7-S11. DOI: 10.1016/j.juro.2008.03.131.

[34] Jacobs B.L., Lee C.T., Montie J.E. Bladder cancer in 2010: how far have we come?. CA Cancer J Clin. 2010;**60**(4):244-272. DOI: 10.3322/caac.20077.

[35] Suriano F, Altobelli E, Sergi F, Buscarini M. Bladder cancer after radiotherapy for prostate cancer. Rev Urol. 2013;**15**(3):108-112.

[36] Dorr W. Radiation effect in normal tissue—principles of damage and protection. Nuklearmedizin. 2010;**49**(1):S53-S58.

[37] Hendry J.H., Jeremic B., Zubizarreta E.H. Normal tissue complications after radiation therapy. Rev Panam Salud Publica. 2006;**20**(2–3):151-160. https://dx.doi.org/10.1590/S1020-49892006000800012.

[38] Cancer Therapy Evaluation Program. Common Terminology Criteria for Adverse Events (CTCAE) v4.0 [Internet]. 2010. [Updated: 2016.08.07]. Available from: https://ctep.cancer.gov/protocoldevelopment/electronic_applications/ctc.htm#ctc_40 [Accessed: 2016.08.10].

[39] Thrasivoulou C., Virich G., Krenacs T., Korom I., Becker D.L. Optical delineation of human malignant melanoma using second harmonic imaging of collagen. Biomed Opt Express. 2011;**2**(5):1282-1295. DOI: 10.1364/BOE.2.001282.

3

Clinical Use of OCT in the Management of Epiretinal Membranes

Nur Acar

Abstract

Epiretinal membranes (ERM) are frequently seen in an aging eye, especially after posterior vitreous detachment, and can cause decreased vision, and/or metamorphopsia. Not all of the ERMs detected in routine ophthalmological examination are indicated to be removed with surgery. Optical coherence tomography (OCT) examination reveals the microanatomy of all the retinal layers and enables the vitreoretinal surgeon to make decision to follow-up or to perform a vitrectomy to peel the ERM. OCT imaging clearly shows all the tractions on the retina and the intraretinal layers; and can have a prognostic value for the surgery. OCT imaging is also very valuable in the differential diagnosis of pseudoholes with macular and lameller holes; much better than the clinical examination. It is a routine part of the detailed retinal examination of an eye with an ERM. This chapter covers OCT findings in ERMs, and examples of cases with ERMs indicated for surgery of follow-up will be shown, explaining the clinical results of the cases.

Keywords: central macular thickness, external limiting membrane idiopathicepiretinal membrane, internal limiting membrane, lamellar macular hole, optical coherence tomography, OCT, pars plana vitrectomy, photoreceptor, posterior vitreous detachment, pseudohole, secondary epiretinal membrane

1. Introduction

Optical coherence tomography (OCT) is a noninvasive imaging technique that has very important advantages in the diagnosis, treatment, and management of a variety of macular disorders [1]. Since its first use in the clinics, there has been continuous advancements in OCT technology, and current spectral-domain (SD) OCT, and swept-source (SS) OCTs demonstrate macular structures on a microscopic level further clarifying the pathophysiology of many diseases and enabling novel therapeutic options. OCT evaluation has become the routine imaging method for any vitreomacular disease in retinal evaluation of the patients in the clinics as well as the essential component in any study design regarding the treatment of retinal diseases. Recently, OCT has also been integrated into our operating rooms by supporting our decision-making during vitrectomy known as intraoperative OCT (iOCT).

Epiretinal membrane (ERM), which has also been named as epimacular membrane, cellophane maculopathy, preretinal macular fibrosis, and surface-wrinkling retinopathy, is a disorder of the vitreomacular interface. It is a fibrocellular membrane lying on the inner surface of the retina, which can cause decreased vision and/or metamorphopsia. Epiretinal membranes are frequently seen in an aging eye, especially after posterior vitreous detachment (PVD), and its prevalence increases with increased age [2]. The mean age of ERM diagnosis is 65 years old, affecting both sexes equally [3]. The prevalence of ERM varies from 2.2 to 28.9% depending on the population being studied [4, 5]. The incidence of developing an ERM in the primary eye is 1.1% per year, whereas its incidence in the fellow eye is 2.7% per year. Bilaterality changes between 19 and 31% of the eyes, and mostly with asymmetric involvement.

2. ERM classification

Epiretinal membranes are classified as idiopathic, and secondary regarding their etiology. Idiopathic ERM is the most common form. Secondary ERMs are associated with posterior uveitis, retinal vascular occlusions, diabetic retinopathy, trauma, retinal tear or detachment, and their repair, argon laser photocoagulation, cataract surgery [6]. Other risk factors include age, PVD, and history of ERM in the fellow eye. Secondary ERMs tend to occur in younger patients [7]. Clinically, ERMs are classified as cellophane macular reflex or preretinal macular fibrosis according to their severity [8]. Cellophane macular reflex is an early form, including a thin transparent membrane overlying the macula usually clinically asymptomatic, whereas preretinal macular fibrosis is the later form with thickened and contracted membrane causing visual impairment in most eyes.

3. ERM-pathogenesis

The diagnosis of PVD, which is defined as separation between the posterior vitreous cortex and the internal limiting membrane (ILM) of the retina, has been described in up to 95% of cases of idiopathic ERM [9]. Residual cortical vitreous secondary to a PVD or anomalous PVD leading to vitreoschisis with only partial separation of the posterior hyaloid remain to be factors allowing proliferation of glial cells. Inflammation is a central component of disorders leading to secondary ERMs, with increased inflammatory mediators promoting fibrocellular growth. Retinal glial cells, hyalocytes, fibroblasts, myofibroblasts are the predominant cell types found in the ERMs. Retinal pigment epithelial cells, macrophages, T-, and, B-cells are identified in secondary ERMs [6]. Extracellular matrix production and remodeling are predominant. The extracellular matrix components that have been described in ERMs include collagen types I, II, III, IV, and VI, fibronectin, and laminin [10–12]. Extracellular fibrils are thin in cellophane macular reflex and are much thicker in preretinal macular fibrosis [10].

4. ERM clinical findings

Epiretinal membrane is relatively common especially after 60 years of age, and both sexes are equally affected. A careful history should be obtained to evaluate for secondary causes of ERMs. The patient more often presents without any symptoms diagnosed on a routine ophthalmological examination especially with very early and thin membranes. He can also present with the symptoms of metamorphopsia, blurred vision, monocular diplopia, and micropsia [13]. Contrast sensitivity is frequently decreased.

In the ophtalmological examination, best corrected visual acuity (BCVA) is noted. Amsler grid test is also performed. On slit lamp examination lens status with any form of cataract is noted. Dilated fundus examination is performed. Careful examination of the macular area for any subtle membrane is important as it can easily be missed on routine examination. The presence of PVD is noted. Detailed examination of the peripheral retina for any missed retinal tear should be performed. The examination of the vitreous for any cells, and of retinal vessels for secondary causes should also be performed. The same examination should also be done for the fellow eye.

Clinically, an ERM can be seen as a loss in the normal convex contour of the fovea, an abnormal reflectivity of the macular area, or as wrinkling on the macular area in fundoscopy. As cellophane macular reflex is a thin membrane without causing any distortions in the retina, it usually does not cause visual impairment, and usually observed as an incidental finding in routine fundus examination. More advanced ERMs classified as preretinal macular fibrosis can be easily seen as they are often opaque and whitish in color, obscuring the underlying retina (**Figure 1**). There may be traction, or tortuosity in the vessels in thick membranes

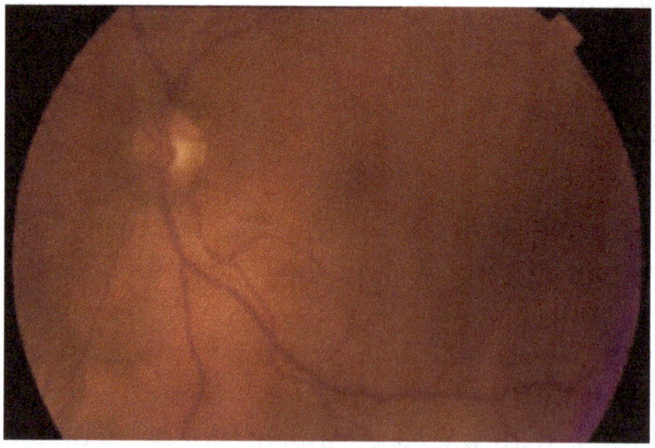

Figure 1. Epiretinal membrane. Color fundus image of the left eye showing grayish tissue over the macula obscuring the details of the underlying retina and causing tortuosity in the retinal vessels. The patient complains of blurred vision and metamorphopsia.

sometimes with intraretinal hemorrhages, or exudates in severe cases. Macular edema can be observed. Preretinal macular fibrosis usually distorts the retina causing visual impairment in nearly 80% of cases [14]. ERMs can give an impression of a macular hole, when there is proliferation on both sides of the fovea, but a gap in the center which looks like a macular hole gives the name as a "pseudohole". The best method to examine it is with a contact macular or a goniolens, though it may be difficult in a busy daily practice. ERMs can also be associated with lamellar macular holes or less commonly with macular holes. The usual course is slow progression over the years with VA decreasing to 0.1.

5. ERM diagnostic tests

5.1. Optical coherence tomography

Despite the fact that ERM can be diagnosed clinically, OCT imaging has become a routine part of the vitreomacular surface examination. OCT has proven to be more sensitive than clinical examination for the diagnosis of numerous disorders of the vitreomacular interface, including ERM [15]. OCT imaging shows the macular area in cross section, and three dimensionally in high resolution, and is extremely helpful in detecting subtle, very thin membranes, associated findings as macular edema, traction on the macula, lamellar macular hole, changes in the contour and the thickness of the macula, or any other macular pathology. 3D OCT imaging can help to evaluate the degree of traction, identify points of attachment and of detachment of the ERM to the retina [16]. OCT not only shows clearly if a lamellar hole is present, but also helps the differential diagnosis of ERMs, macular holes, lamellar macular holes, pseudoholes, and macular edema. OCT evaluation of eyes with ERM has also a prognostic value. It is ideal to follow the patient with the same OCT device and through the same baseline point.

5.1.1. OCT findings

ERMs are observed as highly reflective layer on the retinal surface. ERMs in early stage are seen as thin hyperreflective line with normal foveal contour and retinal architecture (**Figure 2a**, **b**). Idiopathic ERMs mostly are globally adherent to the retina seen as hyperreflective band, but in some cases (20–25%), they are clearly separated from the retina with focal points of attachment (**Figure 3a**, **b**) [17]. Secondary ERMs are more frequently (50%) seen with focal attachments. ERM causes increase in central macular thickness. Usually there is diffuse retinal thickening without any cystic changes in cases with ERM. Especially, the retinal layers above the outer plexiform layers increase in thickness. Increased central macular thickness alone is not usually correlated with VA of the patient. Normal foveal contour is lost. The characteristic foveal depression is not seen (**Figure 4a–c**). Hyperreflectivity between ILM and inner plexiform layers is increased especially in longstanding ERMs, which is a typical finding (**Figure 3b**). This type of fibrosis generally produces traction in retinal layers, causing visual impairment. They may be associated with underlying corrugation of the retinal surface. The surface of the retina where the ERM is more pronounced has a distinctive saw-toothed appearance corresponding to retinal striae from ERM traction [18]. ERMs can also cause irregularities in retinal layers (**Figure 4a**). This feature is seen more frequently

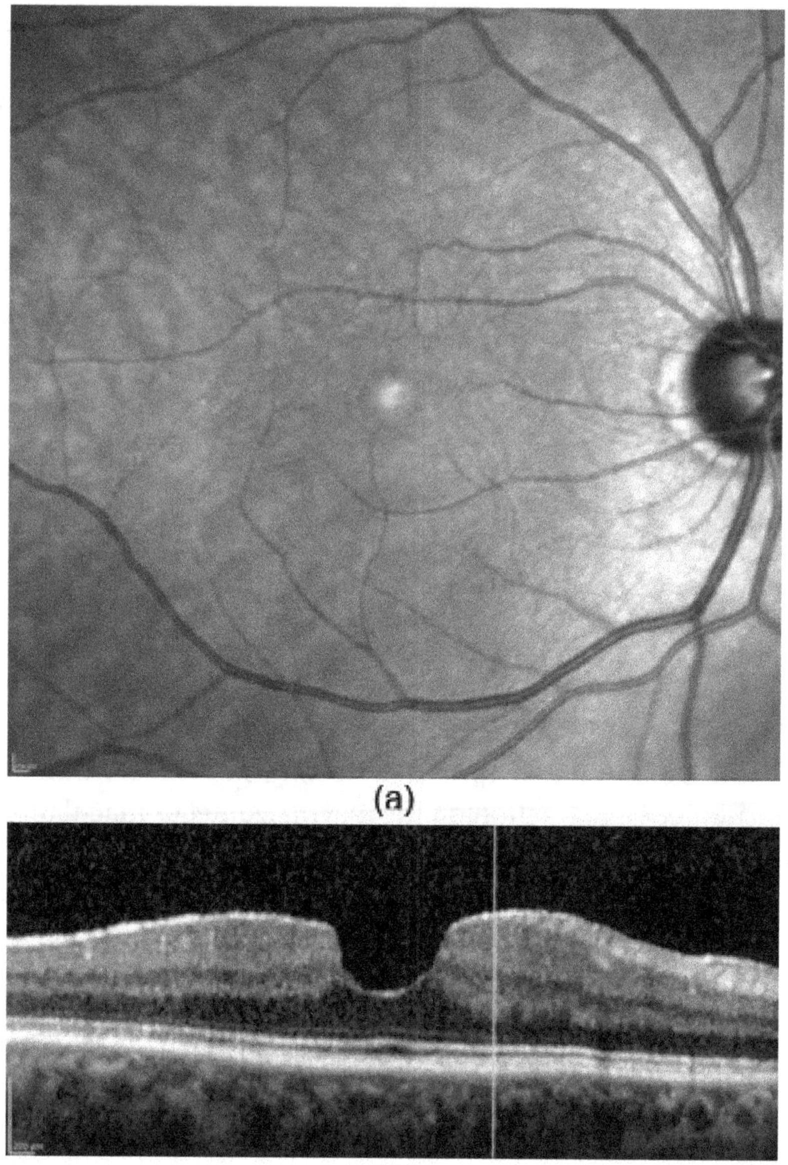

(a)

(b)

Figure 2. (a) Infrared (IR) photography of an asymptomatic patient with visual acuity of 20/20, and a thin ERM observed in routine fundoscopy. IR imaging shows a pseudo hole image at the fovea with slight wrinkling of the retina. The retinal vasculature looks normal. (b) SD-OCT image of the same eye. A thin hyperreflective line is seen on the retina which is globally adherent. There is no increase in foveal thickness, with the foveal pit contour being steeper, and wider than usual indicating an early form of a pseudohole. The retinal layers are normal. The retinal tissue at the base of the fovea is intact unlike a lamellar hole.

with partially attached ERMs. Also, slight elevation of photoreceptor layer above RPE layer has been described as "outer retinal defect", which may be related with traction of retina (**Figure 5a**). Cystoid changes in the retina observed as hyporeflective round spaces are usually accompanying longstanding ERMs as a result of intraretinal traction in idiopathic ERMs. If cystoid retinal thickening is more dominant, vascular reasons of a secondary ERM should be kept in mind. Pseudohole formation is usually accompanied by globally attached membranes (**Figure 6**). There is abnormally steep and wide foveal pit contour. The retinal tissue at the base of the fovea is preserved differentiating it from a lamellar (**Figure 7a**) or a full-thickness macular hole, and ERM is seen as hyperreflective band on the macular surface.

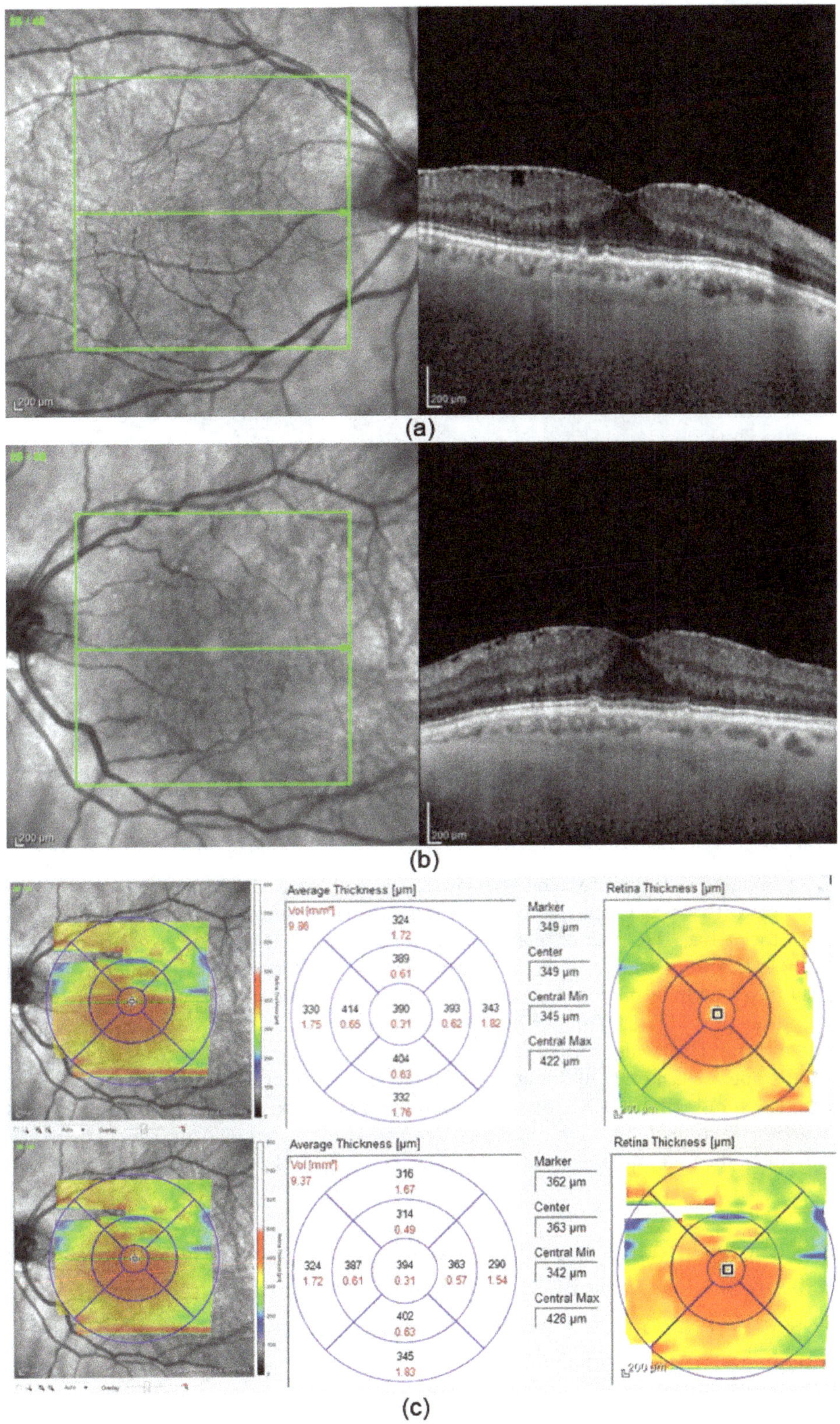

Figure 3. The SD-OCT imaging of both eyes of a patient with a complaint of slight blurring in vision, but no metamorphopsia. The VA in both eyes are 20/32 with early nuclear sclerosis in both eyes. The patient has also drusen bilaterally. (a) RE; ERM is seen as a hyperreflective layer on the macula, and we can clearly see the separated areas of ERM from the retina. There is also associated corrugation of the underlying retinal surface prominent on the temporal side. Slight intraretinal traction can be seen, and the normal foveal depression is decreased. (b) LE; The similar appearance is seen. Hyperreflectivity between ILM and inner plexiform layers is also increased at the nasal side as a typical finding. (c) The central macular thickness map shows that the central foveal thickness is increased to 390 μ in RE, and to 394 μ in LE.

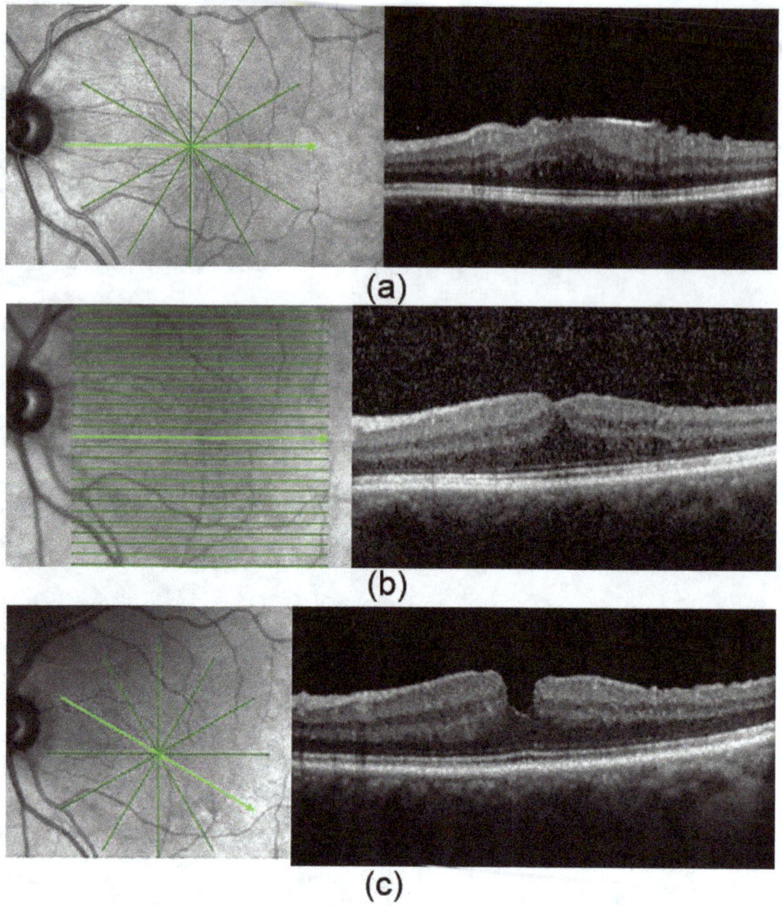

Figure 4. (a) SD-OCT imaging of a symptomatic eye with decreased VA of 0.3, and metamorphopsia shows increased central macular thickness with loss of foveal depression. Especially the inner retinal layers are increased in thickness with associated traction of the retina. The inner segment ellipsoid band and ELM can be seen undisrupted associated with better postoperative VA. The retinal surface is irregular due to ERM, and there is traction on the retinal vasculature at the temporal side of the fovea seen in IR photograph on the left. The 62-year-old male underwent 23 g pars plana vitrectomy with ERM and ILM peeling. (b) SD-OCT image at postoperative month 1 shows decreased central macular thickness with no traction of the retina. The retinal surface is smooth. The VA increased to 0.5. However, during follow-up, the VA decreased to 0.2 at postoperative month 10 due to nuclear cataract formation. Following phacoemulsification and IOL implantation, VA increased to 1.0. (c) SD-OCT image 3 months following lens surgery shows the intraretinal architecture is almost normal with normal retinal thickness and foveal depression is formed. The focal small depressions on the retinal surface of temporal side of the fovea are seen probably associated with ILM peeling. The VA is 1.0 with no symptoms.

There is still no internationally approved OCT-based classification system of ERMs. In one study, classification of idiopathic ERM based on the morphologic characteristics of the fovea has been proposed [19]. In another one, the anatomical structure of the vitreoretinal interface and the macula was studied and divided into two major groups according to the presence of PVD, and subdivided by the presence of contraction, edema, lamellar macular hole, and vitreomacular traction [20]. However, their clinical relevance is unclear.

OCT imaging is also helpful for decision-making in the management of an ERM. If the membrane is thin showing near normal contour in OCT not associated with metamorphopsia or blurred vision clinically the patient is usually followed up with periodically checking for symptoms and with OCT. However, some clinically subtle ERMs are better observed with OCT for accompanying vitreomacular traction. These cases may be offered earlier surgery or

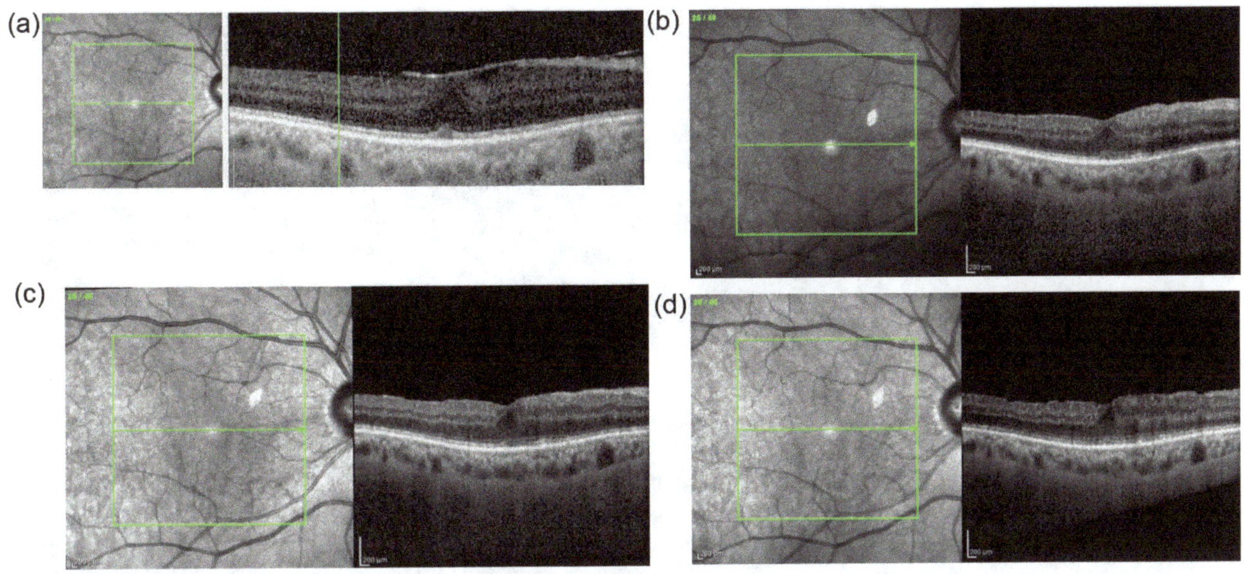

Figure 5. (a) SD-OCT image of a 69-year-old male presenting with decreased vision, and metamorphopsia on the RE. The patient had an ERM with nuclear cataract. ERM is seen as a hyperreflective layer on the macula. The central macular thickness is increased to 398 μ with loss of normal contour of fovea. The ERM is partially attached. Also, there is slight elevation of photoreceptor layer above the RPE layer, which has been described as "outer retinal defect" at the center of the fovea. This feature may be related with traction of retina. The VA was 0.3. (b) The patient underwent combined lens surgery with ERM, and ILM peeling. At postoperative week 2, SD-OCT shows decreased macular thickness, with foveal depression appearing. The photoreceptor layer is still a bit irregular at the fovea. (c) Postoperative month 1, the VA increased to 1.0. Intraretinal architecture is getting better. (d) Postoperative month 3. The photoreceptor and ELM layers look normal and intact.

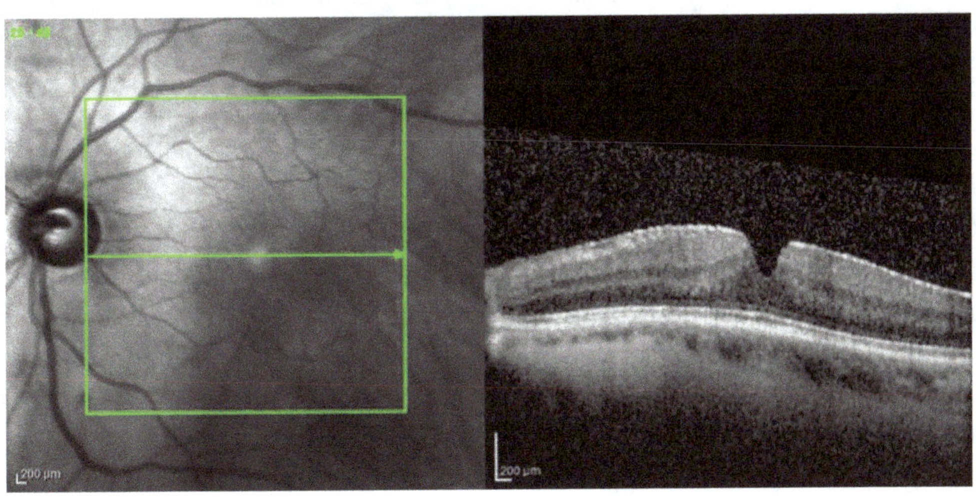

Figure 6. SD-OCT image of a patient shows an ERM as a thin hyperreflective layer on the macula on both sides of the fovea, but there is a gap in the foveal center. Foveal depression is steeper, giving the image of a pseudohole. There is no loss of outer retinal tissue at the base of the fovea.

at least followed up more closely for worsening of symptoms. On the other hand, with OCT imaging, we can assess the vitreoretinal interface in detail and note how diffuse or how tight is the adherence of the ERM and can decide to approach which site to start peeling of the ERM surgically. 3D OCT imaging can also be helpful in identifying any free edges of the ERM that may help in starting membrane peeling during surgery [16, 21]. A new report using en-face

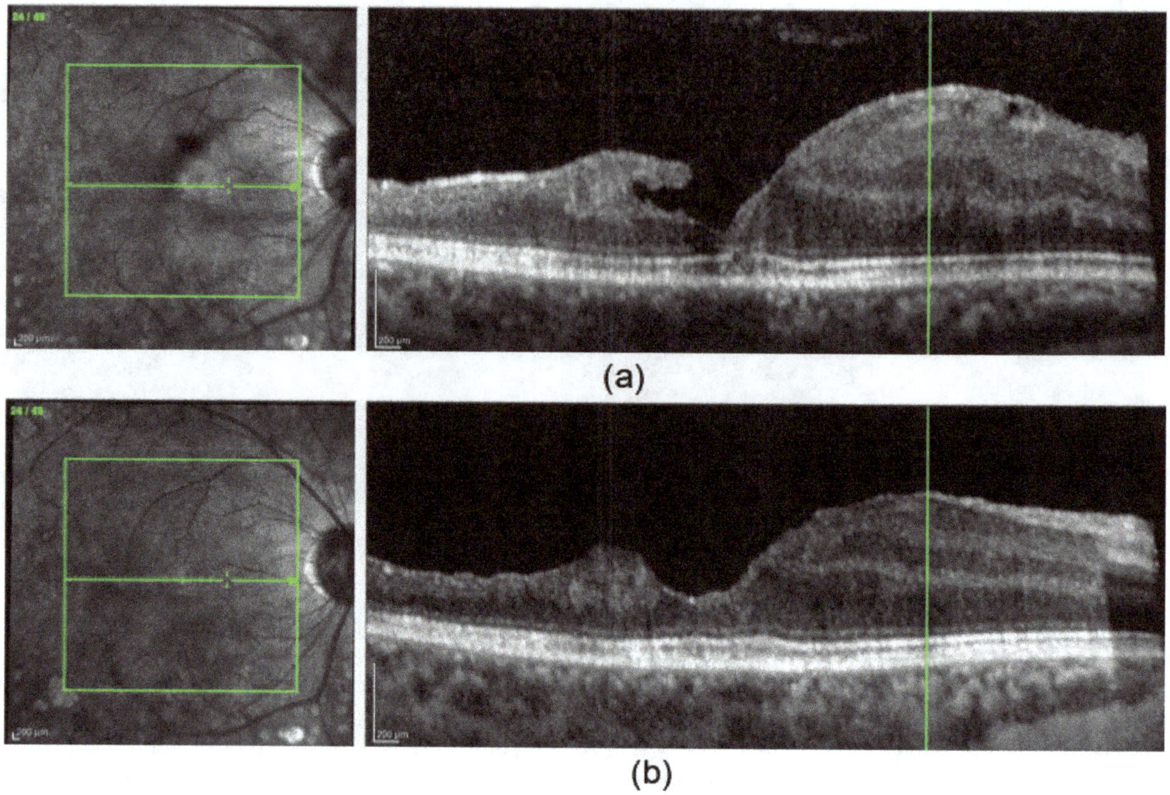

Figure 7. (a) SD-OCT image of a 39-year-old female with an ERM and a lamellar macular hole (LMH) secondary to tractional retinal detachment. There is a hyperreflective layer of ERM on both sides of the fovea, retinal thickness is increased at the nasal side. There is loss of retinal inner layers at the temporal side of the fovea compatible with LMH. The outer layer is also decreased at the center, and disruption of the photoreceptor segment layer is noted. The retinal thickness is decreased due to atrophy at the temporal side of the fovea. The VA decreased to 0.6 during follow-up with symptoms of metamorphopsia. The patient underwent vitrectomy with ERM, and ILM peeling due to TRD, and vitreous hemorrhage from active vessels despite argon laser treatment. (b) At postoperative month 6, SD-OCT image demonstrates that LMH is closed. The retinal layers are better defined at the nasal side. Photoreceptor and ELM layers are continuous with no disruption. The VA increased to 1.0 with totally attached retina.

OCT scans and generating a map, which is called the GapMap, showing the elevated and attached areas between an ERM and the macula stated that this imaging can help surgeons detect elevated areas of ERM preoperatively to avoid excessive retinal contact during surgical manipulation [22]. They commented that in the future, such en-face gliosis reports may be incorporated into computer-assisted surgery systems installed in the operating microscope's oculars, serving as a source of intraoperative guidance for surgeons to facilitate the removal of ERM with reduced trauma [23].

OCT imaging also demonstrates all the layers of the retina, which is also important for the prognosis of the surgical outcome of an ERM removal. These features will be outlined below in "*Surgical Prognosis*" section.

5.1.2. Intraoperative OCT

OCT has become an essential imaging in guiding our clinical decision-making, and it has recently been adapted to use during surgery, known as intraoperative OCT (iOCT). Prospective studies performed have already shown the safety and feasibility of iOCT imaging [24, 25]. The most common posterior segment procedure was vitrectomy with membrane peeling, in 43% of which iOCT informed surgeon decision-making [24]. The following study, performed to evaluate a microscope-integrated iOCT system with a heads-up display, showed that iOCT data conflicted with the surgeon's impression of membrane peel completeness in 19% of cases [25]. The surgeons reported that use of iOCT provided valuable feedback in 71% posterior-segment surgeries [26]. The author's experience is also compatible with the findings of the studies that, iOCT can show residual membranes if any, unconnected areas between ERM and the retina, and confirm if ERM/ILM peel is completed during ERM surgery. Although iOCT is a nice instrument to supplement surgical assessment, it is not available in most ORs, is costly, and is apt to further advancements of the system in the future.

5.2. Optical coherence tomography angiography

Optical coherence tomography angiography (OCTA) is a new technology for imaging the microvasculature of the retina and choroid, using laser light reflectance of the surface of moving red blood cells to demonstrate vessels noninvasively. The vessels through different segmented areas of the eye can be imaged, and differences can be analyzed between scans. The image is segmented into four zones, namely, the superficial retinal plexus, the deep retinal plexus, the outer retina and the choriocapillaris. OCTA can show the changes in the retinal vasculature caused by macular traction of an ERM. OCTA can help to evaluate the depth and extent of foveal capillary distortion. Reduction in VA is found to be associated with this distortion [27]. Differences in foveal avascular area and decrease in parafoveal vascular density both in superficial and deep capillary plexus are also reported in the eyes following ERM surgery, and these changes were associated with worse postoperative VAs [28]. As more studies will be performed with OCTA imaging, more prognostic findings may be available for surgeons to help decision-making for removal of ERM as well as to determine visual prognosis.

5.3. Fundus fluorescein angiography

Fundus fluorescein angiography (FFA) is usually not necessary in routine evaluation of ERMs, but it is helpful in secondary ERMs following retinal vascular occlusions or inflammations to assess not only the macular area but also the peripheral retinal circulation. It can demonstrate leakage, traction on the vessels, ischemia, or secondary neovascularizations.

6. ERM-management

6.1. Indication for surgery

Most thin ERMs are visually asymptomatic and can be followed up for a long time with periodical visits and with amsler card testing by the patient himself. In reported series regarding the natural evolution of an idiopathic ERM, it is reported that in a mean follow-up of 21 months, there was no significant change in mean VA of CRT or central volume of the macula [29]. The author's experience is also similar, especially for the initial severity, thin membranes without major tractional components. In asymptomatic cases, the OCT may reveal thickened macula with loss of central depression, and a CRT of higher than 330 microns with a VA of 20/20. So, only thickened macula due to ERM, which is measured with OCT imaging, does not correlate with the complaints of the patients. The retinal distortions induced by ERM contraction are believed to be the primary reason for visual impairment in idiopathic ERM, which can easily be observed with OCT imaging.

When indicated, the management of idiopathic ERMs is surgical. There are still no strict recommendations regarding the exact timing of the surgery. However, the most important indication is deciding the presence of visual complaints of the patients are related with ERMs, but not cataractous or refractive changes. As the mean age of patients with ERM is usually around their 70s, their lenses have frequently cataractous changes, which should be considered as a cause of blurred vision. On the other hand, the complaint of metamorhopsia is often more intolerable for the patient and is an indication for surgical removal of an ERM even though the visual acuity is high. If the tractional distortions in the retinal layers are not prominent, and the patient has cataract without any metamorphopsia, the patient can be offered a lens surgery first, and the ERM can be followed-up, informing the patient has a higher risk of having postoperative macular edema. On the other hand, if the surgical removal is indicated, a combined surgery of a pars plana vitrectomy and a lens surgery is usually preferred as cataractous changes usually increase fastly following PPV, necessitating a lens surgery soon after.

6.2. Surgery

Epiretinal membrane surgery involves a pars plana vitrectomy procedure with ERM peeling. Internal limiting membrane peeling (ILM) is usually performed to prevent secondary membrane formation. It is already reported that ILM peeling decreased secondary membrane formations significantly [30]. A meta-analysis reported that vitrectomy with ILM peeling resulted in better visual improvement in long-term follow-ups and lower ERM recurrence rates [31]. On the other hand, other meta analyses reports found that although additional ILM peeling could result in a significantly lower ERM recurrence rates, it does not significantly influence postoperative best-corrected VA and central macular thickness [32, 33]. The postoperative VA is not found to be different in two groups with or without ILM peeling in idiopathic ERMS in a prospective trial [34]. The author's experience is also similar. In a prospective interventional case series, the efficacy and safety of combined peeling of ERM and ILM membranes with the single injection of mixture of tryphan blue and brilliant blue G dyes in eyes with idiopathic ERM was evaluated (Video). Seven (three pseudophakic and four phakic) eyes underwent vitrectomy and eight eyes had combined phacoemulsification and vitrectomy. Four phakic patients needed lens surgery with a mean of 10 months postoperatively. At postoperative month 6, the mean CMT decreased significantly from 502 ± 35 to 277 ± 43 μ. The mean VA significantly increased from 20/64 to 20/32 in all eyes with no recurrent ERM observed (**Figure 8**) [35].

ILM peeling maneuver should be performed cautiously to avoid secondary complications as a retinal hole formation, traumatic defects in the macular area, as well as phototoxicity. The surgery itself has the possible complications of a PPV, such as retinal tear and detachment, endophthalmitis, loss of ganglion cells, and others, which must be discussed with the patient.

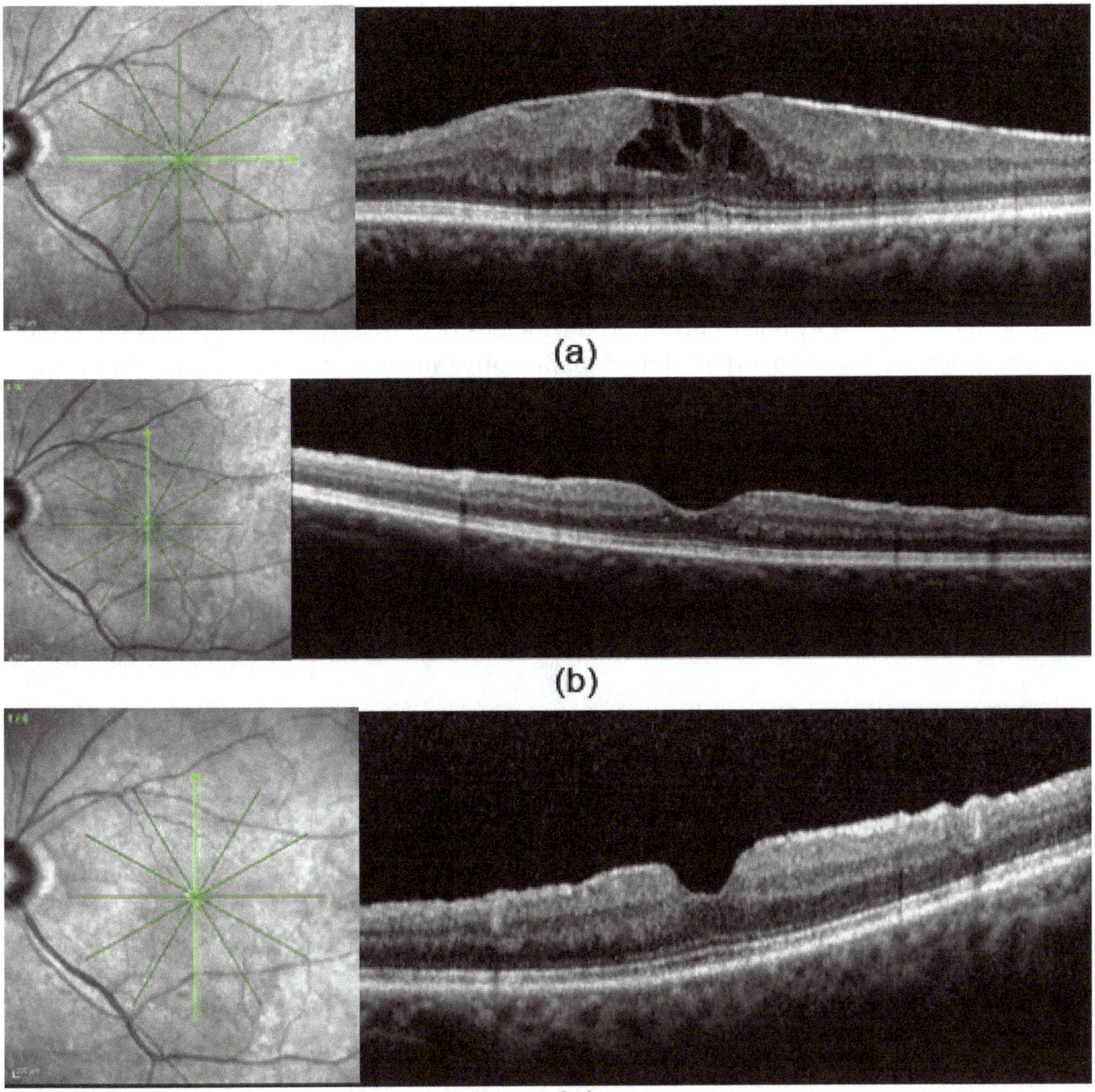

(a)

(b)

(c)

Figure 8. (a) SD-OCT image of a 73-year-old female presented with visual blurring and metamorphopsia with a VA of 0.6 shows a tightly adherent hyperreflective layer of ERM on the macula. The central retinal thickness is increased with traction on the fovea causing intraretinal cystic changes seen as hyporeflective spaces in the inner retina. The outer retinal layers are intact. The symptomatic patient underwent vitrectomy with ERM and ILM peeling. (b) SD-OCT at postoperative month 1 shows normal retinal architecture with normal retinal thickness. There is small depression on the superior side. The patient's metamorphopsia decreased with a VA of 1.0. (c) SD-OCT image at postoperative year 5 is the same with no recurrent ERM observed during 5 years of follow-up.

6.3. Surgical prognosis

Following ERM removal increase in VA of two or more lines in 60–85% of cases 6–12 months postoperatively with around 50% gaining a VA of 20/50 or better [36]. The mean preoperative and postoperative VA has been reported to be 20/110 and 20/55 [37]. This data were a meta-analysis of three studies reporting surgical results following small incision pars plana vitrectomy, in which the recurrence of ERM was around 1% [37]. Those with worse VA preoperatively gain more lines postoperatively. However, the eyes with higher preoperative VA tend to have a higher postoperative VA [38–40]. Poor preoperative VA, and long duration of symptoms are poor prognostic factors [36, 38–39]. Visual acuity improves in 1–6 months postoperatively. However, VA improvement can continue to increase following 1–2 years of surgery. Successful surgical intervention is associated with both decreased central foveal thickness (CFT) and improved VA [30–42]. However, central macular thickness is not necessarily correlated with postoperative VA [4–43]. Although CFT may be useful for evaluating the impact of ERM on baseline VA, it is probably not useful for predicting postoperative VA [6]. The preoperative OCT characteristics are more important. Intact preoperative inner segment ellipsoid (ISe) band is associated with a better postoperative VA than a disrupted preoperative ISe band in both idiopathic and secondary ERMs [38, 41–49]. The longer photoreceptor outer segment (PROS) length is also reported to be a good prognostic factor for the postoperative VA [39, 42]. It has also been shown that the integrity of outer photoreceptor cell layer as well as of ELM is related with better postoperative VA [50]. Postoperative increase in contrast sensitivity is associated with the thickness of outer retinal layer [44]. The preoperative degree of metamorphopsia was also found to be a prognostic factor for the postoperative degree of metamorphopsia, suggesting that surgery for ERM should be performed before development of severe metamorphopsia [39].

7. Conclusion

In conclusion, OCT provides a very detailed information of all the retinal layers, and the vitreomacular interface. Epiretinal membranes are a frequent clinical finding in an aging eye, and sometimes result in decreased vision, and/or metamorphopsia. OCT, as a noninvasive, fast imaging system of the macula being more sensitive than the clinical examination has become the routine evaluation of ERMs. OCT imaging is used to diagnose, differentiate, manage, and follow ERMs. It also gives valuable information regarding the visual prognosis of the operated eye. Intact and continuous preoperative inner segment ellipsoid band, the longer photoreceptor outer segment, and the integrity of ELM are reported to be good prognostic signs. On the other hand, preoperative three-dimensional OCT evaluation of an ERM can also help the surgeons to identify any free edges of the ERM that may help in starting membrane peeling with reduced trauma. Lastly, OCT has recently been integrated into our operating rooms as intraoperative OCT and may support our decision-making during vitrectomy.

Author details

Nur Acar

Address all correspondence to: nuracarr@gmail.com

School of Medicine, Acıbadem Mehmet Ali Aydınlar University, Maslak Hospital, Sarıyer, Istanbul, Turkey

References

[1] Huang D, Swanson EA, Lin CP, et al. Optical coherence tomography. Science. 1991;**254**: 1178-1181

[2] Aung KZ, Makeyeva G, Adams MK, et al. The prevalence and risk factors of epiretinal membranes: The Melbourne Collaborative Cohort Study. Retina. 2013;**33**(5):1026-1034

[3] Fraser-Bell S, Guzowski M, Rochtchina E, et al. Five-year cumulative incidence and progression of epiretinal membranes: The Blue Mountains Eye Study. Ophthalmology. 2003;**110**(1):34-40

[4] You Q, Xu L, Jonas JB. Prevalence and associations of epiretinal membranes in adult Chinese: The Beijing eye study. Eye (London, England). 2008;**22**(7):874-879

[5] Ng CH, Cheung N, Wang JJ, et al. Prevalence and risk factors for epiretinal membranes in a multi-ethnic United States population. Ophthalmology. 2011;**118**(4):694-699

[6] Stevenson W, Prospero Ponce CM, Agarwal DR, Gelman R, Christoforidis JB. Epiretinal membrane: Optical coherence tomography-based diagnosis and classification. Clinical Ophthalmology. 2016;**10**:527-534

[7] Yazici AT, Alagöz N, Celik HU, et al. Idiopathic and secondary epiretinal membranes: Do they differ in terms of morphology? An optical coherence tomography-based study. Retina. 2011;**31**(4):779-784

[8] Klein R, Klein BE, Wang Q, Moss SE. The epidemiology of epiretinal membranes. Transactions of the American Ophthalmological Society. 1994;**92**:403-425

[9] Wiznia RA. Posterior vitreous detachment and idiopathic preretinal macular gliosis. American Journal of Ophthalmology. 1986;**102**(2):196-198

[10] Kritzenberger M, Junglas B, Framme C, et al. Different collagen types define two types of idiopathic epiretinal membranes. Histopathology. 2011;**58**(6):953-965

[11] Okada M, Ogino N, Matsumura M, Honda Y, Nagai Y. Histological and immunohistochemical study of idiopathic epiretinal membrane. Ophthalmic Research. 1995; **27**(2):118-128

[12] George B, Chen S, Chaudhary V, Gonder J, Chakrabarti S. Extracellular matrix proteins in epiretinal membranes and in diabetic retinopathy. Current Eye Research. 2009; **34**(2):134-144

[13] Ghazi-Nouri SM, Tranos PG, Rubin GS, Adams ZC, Charteris DG. Visual function and quality of life following vitrectomy and epiretinal membrane peel surgery. The British Journal of Ophthalmology. 2006;**90**(5):559-562

[14] Ryan SJ. Epiretinal membrane. In: Ryan SJ, Schachat AP, Wilkinson CP, Hinton DR, Sadda SR, Wiedemann P, editors. Retina. 5th ed. Philadelphia, PA: Saunders (Imprint) Elselvier; 2013. pp. 1955-1957

[15] Do DV, Cho M, Nguyen QD, et al. The impact of optical coherence tomography on surgical decision making in epiretinal membrane and vitreomacular traction. Transactions of the American Ophthalmological Society. 2006;**104**:161-166

[16] Koizumi H, Spaide RF, Fisher YL, Freund KB, Klancnik JM, Yannuzzi LA. Three-dimensional evaluation of vitreomacular traction and epiretinal membrane using spectral-domain optical coherence tomography. American Journal of Ophthalmology. 2008;**145**(3):509-517

[17] Wilkins JR, Puliato CA, Hee MR, et al. Characterization of epiretinal membranes using optical coherence tomography. Ophthalmology. 1996;**103**(12):2142-2151

[18] Mori K, Gehlbach PL, Sano A, Deguchi T, Yoneya S. Comparison of epiretinal membranes of differing pathogenesis using optical coherence tomography. Retina. 2004;**24**(1):57-62

[19] Hwang JU, Sohn J, Moon BG, et al. Assessment of macular function for idiopathic epiretinal membranes classified by spectral-domain optical coherence tomography. Investigative Ophthalmology & Visual Science. 2012;**53**(7):3562-3569

[20] Konidaris V, Androudi S, Alexandridis A, Dastiridou A, Brazitikos P. Optical coherence tomography-guided classification of epiretinal membranes. International Ophthalmology. 2015;**35**(4):495-501

[21] Elbendary AM. Three-dimensional characterization of epiretinal membrane using spectral domain optical coherence tomography. Saudi Journal of Ophthalmology. 2010; **24**(2):37-43

[22] Pavlidis M, Georgalas I, Körber N. Determination of a new parameter, elevated membrane, by en face OCT as a prognostic factor for pars plana vitrectomy and safer epiretinal membrane peeling. Journal of Ophthalmology. 2015;**2015**:838646;1-7. DOI: 10.1155/2015/838646

[23] Kreatsoulas J. Enhancing retinal surgery with augmented reality technology. Retina Today. 2011;**6**(3):18

[24] Ehlers JP, Dupps WJ, Kaiser PK, et al. The prospective intraoperative and perioperative ophthalmic imaging with optical coherence tomography (PIONEER) study: 2-year results. American Journal of Ophthalmology. 2014;**158**:999-1007

[25] Ehlers JP, Goshe J, Dupps WJ, et al. Determination of feasibility and utility of microscope-integrated optical coherence tomography during ophthalmic surgery: The DISCOVER study RESCAN results. JAMA Ophthalmology. 2015;**133**:1124-1132

[26] Ehlers JP, Tao YK, Farsiu S, et al. Integration of a spectral domain optical coherence tomography system into a surgical microscope for intraoperative imaging. Investigative Ophthalmology & Visual Science. 2011;**52**:3153-3159

[27] Nelis P, Alten F, Clemens C, Heiduschka P, Eter N. Quantification of changes in foveal capillary architecture caused by idiopathic epiretinal membrane using OCT angiography. Graefe's Archive for Clinical and Experimental Ophthalmology. 2017;**255**(7):1319-1324

[28] Kim YJ, Kim S, Lee JY, Kim JG, Yoon YH. Macular capillary plexuses after epiretinal membrane surgery: An optical coherence tomography angiography study. The British Journal of Ophthalmology. 2017. DOI: 10.1136/bjophthalmol-2017-311188. pii: bjophthalmol-2017-311188

[29] Hejsek L, Stepanov A, Dohnalova A, Rehakova T, Jiraskova N. The natural evolution of idiophatic epimacular membrane. Biomedical Papers of the Medical Faculty of the University Palacky, Olomouc, Czech Republic. 2017;**161**(1):100-106

[30] Sandali O, El Sanharawi M, Basli E, et al. Epiretinal membrane recurrence: Incidence, characteristics, evolution, and preventive and risk factors. Retina. 2013;**33**(10):2032-2038

[31] Chang WC, Lin C, Lee CH, Sung TL, Tung TH, Liu JH. Vitrectomy with or without internal limiting membrane peeling for idiopathic epiretinal membrane: A meta-analysis. PLoS One. 2017;**12**(6):e0179105

[32] Fang XL, Tong Y, Zhou YL, Zhao PQ, Wang ZY. Internal limiting membrane peeling or not: A systematic review and meta-analysis of idiopathic macular pucker surgery. The British Journal of Ophthalmology. 2017;**101**(11):1535-1541

[33] Azuma K, Ueta T, Eguchi S, Aihara M. Effects of internal limiting membrane peeling combined with removal of idiopathic epiretinal membrane: A systematic review of literature and meta-analysis. Retina. 2017;**37**(10):1813-1819

[34] Tranos P, Koukoula S, Charteris DG, Perganda G, Vakalis A, Asteriadis S, Georgalas I, Petrou P. The role of internal limiting membrane peeling in epiretinal membrane surgery: A randomised controlled trial. The British Journal of Ophthalmology. 2017; **101**(6):719-724

[35] Acar N. Combined peeling of epiretinal and internal limiting membranes with the single injection of membraneblue-dual® in eyes with idiopathic ERM. In: Proceedings of 13th Annual Meeting of European Vitreo Retinal Society; Rhodes, Greece; 2013

[36] Wong JG, Sachdev N, Beaumont PE, Chang AA. Visual outcomes following vitrectomy and peeling of epiretinal membrane. Clinical & Experimental Ophthalmology. 2005; **33**(4):373-378

[37] Gupta OP, Brown GC, Brown MM. A value-based medicine cost-utility analysis of idiopathic epiretinal membrane surgery. American Journal of Ophthalmology. 2008; **145**(5):923-928

[38] Kinoshita T, Imaizumi H, Okushiba U, Miyamoto H, Ogino T, Mitamura Y. Time course of changes in metamorphopsia, visual acuity, and OCT parameters after successful epiretinal membrane surgery. Investigative Ophthalmology & Visual Science. 2012; **53**(7):3592-3597

[39] Kinoshita T, Imaizumi H, Miyamoto H, Katome T, Semba K, Mitamura Y. Two-year results of metamorphopsia, visual acuity, and optical coherence tomographic parameters after epiretinal membrane surgery. Graefe's Archive for Clinical and Experimental Ophthalmology. 2016;**254**(6):1041-1049

[40] Rahman R, Stephenson J. Early surgery for epiretinal membrane preserves more vision for patients. Eye (London, England). 2014;**28**(4):410-414

[41] Mitamura Y, Hirano K, Baba T, Yamamoto S. Correlation of visual recovery with presence of photoreceptor inner/outer segment junction in optical coherence images after epiretinal membrane surgery. The British Journal of Ophthalmology. 2009;**93**(2):171-175

[42] Jeon S, Jung B, Lee WK. Long-term prognostic factors for visual improvement after epiretinal membrane removal. Retina. 2018 May 14. DOI: 10.1097/IAE.0000000000002211

[43] Shimozono M, Oishi A, Hata M, Matsuki T, Ito S, Ishida K, Kurimoto Y. The significance of cone outer segment tips as a prognostic factor in epiretinal membrane surgery. American Journal of Ophthalmology. 2012;**153**(4):698-704

[44] Sugiura Y, Okamoto F, Okamoto Y, Hiraoka T, Oshika T. Contrast sensitivity and foveal microstructure following vitrectomy for epiretinal membrane. Investigative Ophthalmology & Visual Science. 2014;**55**(11):7594-7600

[45] Inoue M, Morita S, Watanabe Y, et al. Preoperative inner segment/outer segment junction in spectral-domain optical coherence tomography as a prognostic factor in epiretinal membrane surgery. Retina. 2011;**31**(7):1366-1372

[46] Itoh Y, Inoue M, Rii T, Hirota K, Hirakata A. Correlation between foveal cone outer segment tips line and visual recovery after epiretinal membrane surgery. Investigative Ophthalmology & Visual Science. 2013;**54**(12):7302-7308

[47] Kim JH, Kang SW, Kong MG, Ha HS. Assessment of retinal layers and visual rehabilitation after epiretinal membrane removal. Graefe's Archive for Clinical and Experimental Ophthalmology. 2013;**251**(4):1055-1064

[48] Cobos E, Arias L, Ruiz-Moreno J, et al. Preoperative study of the inner segment/outer segment junction of photoreceptors by spectral-domain optical coherence tomography as a prognostic factor in patients with epiretinal membranes. Clinical Ophthalmology. 2013;**7**:1467-1470

[49] Kim HJ, Kang JW, Chung H, Kim HC. Correlation of foveal photoreceptor integrity with visual outcome in idiopathic epiretinal membrane. Current Eye Research. 2014; **39**(6):626-633

[50] Theodossiadis PG, Theodossiadis GP, Charonis A, Emfietzoglou I, Grigoropoulos VG, Liarakos VS. The photoreceptor layer as a prognostic factor for visual acuity in the secondary epiretinal membrane after retinal detachment surgery: Imaging analysis by spectral-domain optical coherence tomography. American Journal of Ophthalmology. 2011;**151**(6):973-980

4

OCT Application Before and After Cataract Surgery

Xiaogang Wang, Jing Dong, Suhua Zhang and
Bin Sun

Abstract

Optical coherence tomography (OCT), especially anterior segment OCT (AS-OCT), plays an important role in ophthalmology. With the technology evolving from time-domain to spectral-domain, more and more detailed ocular information has become available. Anterior segment OCT provides particularly useful information for cataract surgeons. This chapter focuses mainly on AS-OCT evaluation of eyes before and after cataract surgery. Four aspects including: (1) anterior lens capsule and lens epithelium evaluation using spectral-domain OCT (SD-OCT); (2) investigation of clear corneal incision in femtosecond laser assisted cataract surgery using SD-OCT; (3) capsular block syndrome evaluation before and after treatment using SD-OCT; (4) IOL power calculation in post-myopic excimer laser eyes using SD-OCT, will be discussed in this chapter.

Keywords: OCT, anterior lens capsule, clear corneal incision, capsular block syndrome, Fuchs heterochromic cyclitis, intraocular lens

1. Introduction

Since the introduction of ophthalmic optical coherence tomography (OCT) in 1991, it has been widely used in ophthalmology over the years [1]. The OCT interferometer detects and measures the echo delay time of light, which is projected from a super-luminescent diode and then reflected from different ocular structures. Compared with the 100-μm image resolution of ultrasonography, OCT can, in a non-invasive, non-contact procedure, provide detailed cross-sectional images of the eye on a 10-μm scale. Compared to conventional time-domain anterior segment OCT (AS-OCT) system (1300 nm), a shorter-wavelength infrared light beam (820 nm) is used for the spectral-domain AS-OCT system. This chapter will mainly focus on anterior segment time-domain and spectral-domain OCT applications before and after cataract surgery. Four aspects will be discussed in this chapter:

- Anterior lens capsule and lens epithelium evaluation in senile cataract and Fuchs' heterochromic cyclitis using spectral-domain anterior segment OCT (SD-OCT);
- Investigation of clear corneal incision in manual phacoemulsification and femtosecond laser assisted cataract surgery using SD-OCT;
- Capsular block syndrome evaluation before and after treatment using SD-OCT;
- IOL power calculation (true net power measurement) in post-myopic excimer laser eyes using SD-OCT.

2. Anterior lens capsule complex measurement using SD-OCT

The lens, as a transparent structure, is a very important refractive element of the human eye. It consists of three major components: capsule, epithelium, and lens substance [2]. The lens epithelial cells and fibers keep the balance of molecules moving into and out of the lens. Previous histological studies have demonstrated that the lens capsule thickness varies by location and that the posterior capsule is the thinnest. The lens epithelium, a single layer of cuboidal cells beneath the anterior capsule, extends to the equatorial lens bow. The lens substance consists of densely packed cells with little extracellular space. With the development of time-domain

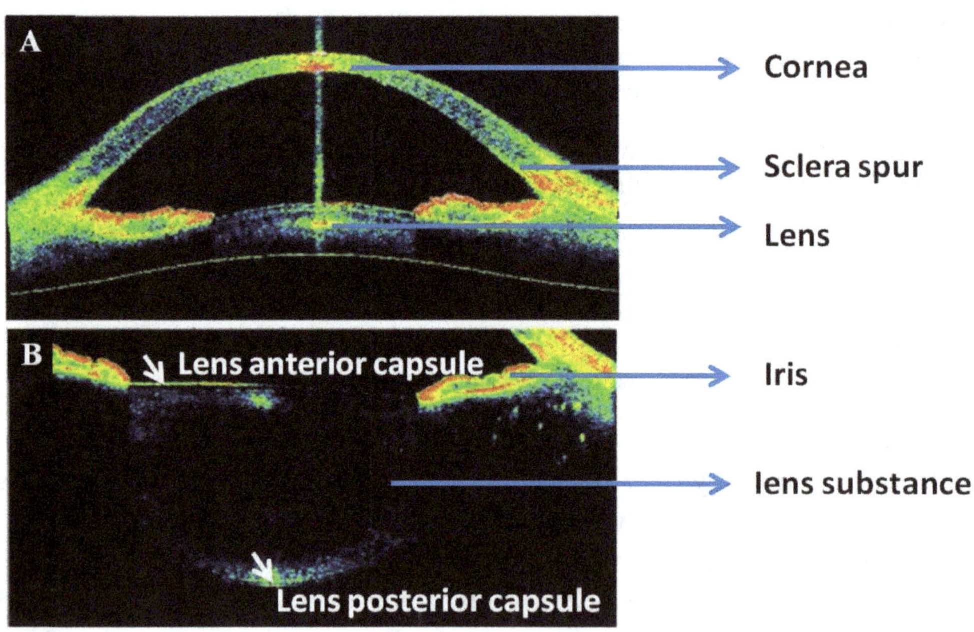

Figure 1. The entire anterior chamber and lens cross-sectional images using OSE-1200 time-domain anterior segment optical coherence tomography (software version 2013.1.1.90; Moptim, Inc., Shenzhen, Guangdong, China). Panel A shows the anterior segment structure: cornea, sclera spur, iris and lens; panel B shows the lens anterior capsule, lens posterior capsule, and lens substance.

OCT, it became possible to image the entire anterior chamber and lens in vivo (**Figure 1**) [3]. Due to the limited resolution (around 15-μm), it was not possible to measure the thickness of the lens capsule or the epithelium.

A previous study manually measured and constructed an anterior lens capsule thickness map across the entire field of view using a femtosecond laser OCT system, which has a central wave length of 780 nm with an axial resolution of 2.3 μm [4]. In a study conducted by Szkulmowski et al., it was reported that the anterior lens capsule and epithelium could be clearly imaged using a SD-OCT system with a central wavelength of 820 nm and axial resolution of 4.2 μm with the help of the speckle contrast reduction technique [5]. The commercial Avanti RTVue XR spectral-domain OCT system provides a high-resolution anterior segment scanning protocol with a scan length of 8 mm and an axial resolution of 5 μm. It can show a substantially clearer delineation after the two highly reflective layers, the anterior lens capsule and the subcapsular epithelium, are combined (**Figure 2**).

We defined the combination of anterior lens capsule and the subcapsular epithelium as the anterior lens capsular complex (ALCC) in a previous study [6]. One hundred thirty-four normal eyes (age range: 5–86 years) were investigated using the Avanti RTVue XR OCT system. The results indicated that the manual measurement of ALCC was both reproducible and reliable. The mean thickness of the central ALCC was approximately 33 μm, which is approximately 15 μm thicker than the anterior lens capsule values calculated using time-domain OCT and other imaging modalities [4, 7]. Therefore, we hypothesized that the subcapsular epithelium was approximately 15 μm thick in vivo. Moreover, a positive correlation between age and ALCC was noted in our study. A 10-year increase in age resulted in a 0.74–1.4 μm increase in the ALCC thickness. From a certain point of view, these findings were consistent

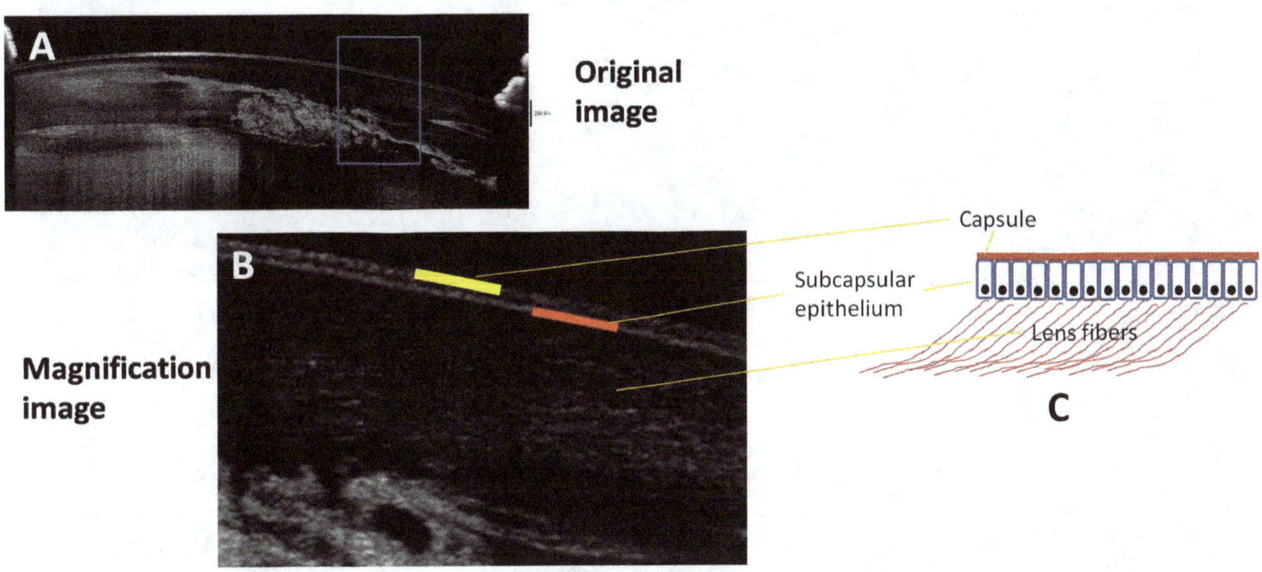

Figure 2. A horizontal anterior segment scanning image of the central part of the lens and the dilated pupil margin in a 34-year-old female using the Avanti RTVue XR spectral-domain optical coherence tomograph (panel A). Panel B shows a magnification of the selected area in panel A (blue frame). Panel C demonstrates the schematic diagram of the anterior lens capsule (corresponding to the yellow reflective layer in panel B), the subcapsular epithelium (corresponding to the red reflective layer in panel B), and the lens fibers.

with previous findings regarding the positive correlation between age and lens capsule or total lens thickness [8, 9].

With the help of anterior segment SD-OCT, researchers also can obtain more detailed useful information regarding accommodation, presbyopia, Fuchs' heterochromic iridocyclitis (**Figure 3**), posterior capsule opacification, and pseudoexfoliation syndrome [10–13]. Moreover, with the OCT technology development, the respective measurement of anterior capsule, posterior capsule and epithelium layer thickness, even plotting corresponding topography in specific regions will be available in the future.

2.1. Summary

In summary, anterior segment SD-OCT can be used to visualize anterior and posterior lens capsule, lens epithelium, keratic precipitates, iris stroma atrophy. The use of anterior segment SD-OCT will enable us to better investigate changes in lens structure of patients with Fuchs' heterochromic iridocyclitis or other lens related conditions.

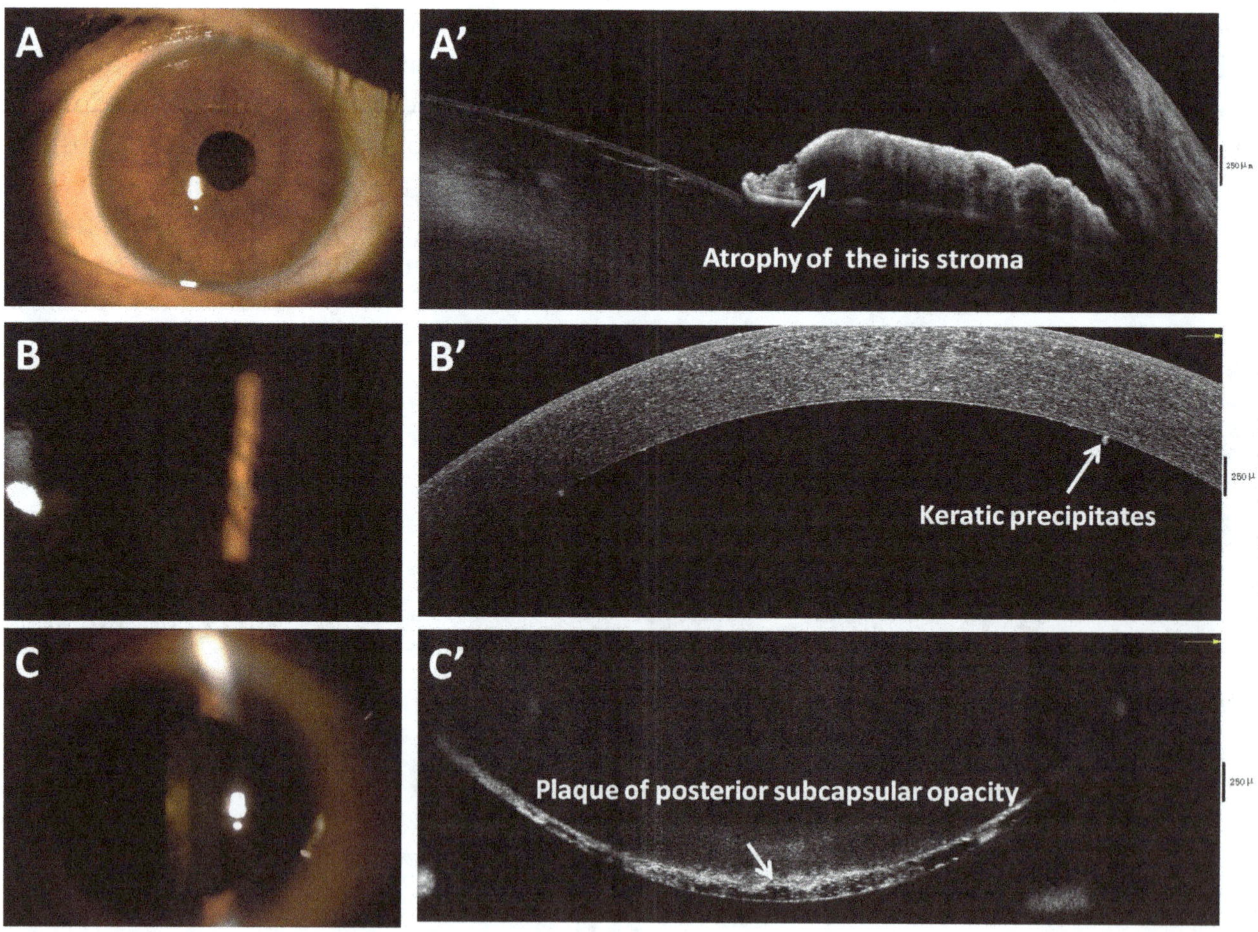

Figure 3. Color images and optical coherence tomography cross-sectional images of a 60-year-old female with Fuchs' heterochromic iridocyclitis. The anterior color slit-lamp photos and corresponding anterior segment OCT cross-sectional images show atrophy of the iris stroma (panel A, A'), small keratic precipitates scattered over the entire corneal endothelium (panel B, B'), and plaque of posterior subcapsular opacity (panel C, C').

3. Investigation of clear corneal incision using SD-OCT

In most industrialized countries, cataract surgery accounts for the largest proportion of surgical interventions in ophthalmology. The advent of minimal incision, phacoemulsification (introduced by Charles Kelman in the 1970s), and foldable intraocular lens, has made cataract surgery safer and more efficient [14]. Moreover, modern cataract surgery combined with new generation intraocular lens types, which can be designated refractive surgery, aims to provide optimal visual quality and render the visual function better [15]. As a significant part of the cataract surgery, the constructional architecture of proper clear corneal incisions (CCIs) is vital for a perfect outcome of phacoemulsification. Faulty CCI construction can lead to complications, such as wound leak, Descemet's membrane detachment, and excessive surgically-induced astigmatism, and is a situation every cataract surgeon attempts to avoid. However, it is not easy to predictably construct perfect manual single-plane, two-plane, or three-plane clear corneal tunnels using steel or diamond blades [16]. With the higher expectations of patients from modern cataract and refractive surgery and the advent of trifocal and accommodating IOLs, femtosecond laser was introduced into cataract surgery by Zoltan Nagy in 2009 [17]. Previous studies demonstrated that a femtosecond laser-assisted cataract surgery technique could provide repeatable, predictable clear corneal incisions, perfect capsulotomies, and safe nuclear fragmentation [18, 19]. Therefore, CCIs created using femtosecond laser have the advantage of predictable configuration and dimensions.

Clinical manual CCI parameters (incision location, angle of incision, incision length) and features (posterior wound gape, Descemet's membrane detachment, posterior wound retraction, loss of coaptation along the CCI tunnel) in the early postoperative period (up to 1 month) of standard cataract surgery have been reported [20–23]. Based on the above-mentioned studies, we evaluated the quantitative CCI parameters and features in subjects who underwent femtosecond laser-assisted cataract surgery [24]. Except for no sign of loss of coaptation along the CCI tunnel, all the other three CCI features were found in femtosecond laser CCI (**Figure 4**).

As expected, the femtosecond laser lens fragmentation ensures that the phacoemulsification energy (Femto group: 16 ± 13%; manual group: 20 ± 5%) and effective phacoemulsification time (Femto group: 17 ± 9 s; manual group: 32 ± 13 s) were dramatically lower in the Femto group than in the conventional manual group. Moreover, the femtosecond laser group had a lower incidence of Descemet's membrane detachment and posterior wound gape at each follow-up time-point. However, a higher incidence of posterior wound retraction was found in the femtosecond laser group.

Descemet's membrane detachment may potentially hinder the local endothelium pump mechanism and affect corneal wound healing. The routine procedure for CCI by femtosecond laser is from the anterior chamber (inner cornea) to the epithelium (outer cornea), which makes the Descemet's membrane detachment an unusual complication for this group. However, phacoemulsification probe manipulation through the CCI, the blunt dissection of the tunnel, and incision hydration probably contributed to the occurrence of Descemet's membrane detachment in the femtosecond group. For the difference in posterior wound gape incidence, we are inclined to implicate the difference in tunnel incision geometry between the two groups. Compared to 1-plane manual CCI, we mainly used a 2-plane CCI in femtosecond group. As previous studies have mentioned, a 2-plane CCI with a partial lamellar cut positioned parallel to the collagen lamellae may improve the shearing force effects of the stromal collagen lamellae across the entire depth of the cornea [25–27]. Posterior wound retraction, defined as an abrupt step-off or recession of the central edge of the posterior wound surface, was not observed in manual group in this study. This may be attributed to the relatively high incidence of posterior wound gape, in which the posterior wound margins were still separated. A high incidence of posterior wound retraction in the femtosecond group may indicate remodeling of the CCI resulting from endothelial cell necrosis, molecular dissociation, and biomechanical and thermal changes from the femtosecond laser [28]. A previous study, using transmission electron microscopy confirmed the difference between femtosecond laser corneal flap formation (necrotic keratocytes) and microkeratome corneal flap formation (keratocyte apoptosis), which may potentially explain the different incidence of posterior wound retraction in this study [29]. Moreover, the above-mentioned three CCI features may cause changes to posterior corneal curvature, corneal astigmatism, and total corneal power; these should be evaluated in future studies.

3.1. Summary

Anterior segment SD-OCT can highlight CCIs findings that are not as obvious by UBM, slit lamp. The ability to detect detailed postoperative corneal incision changes of standard or femtosecond laser-assisted cataract surgery is clinically important as it allows for the evaluation

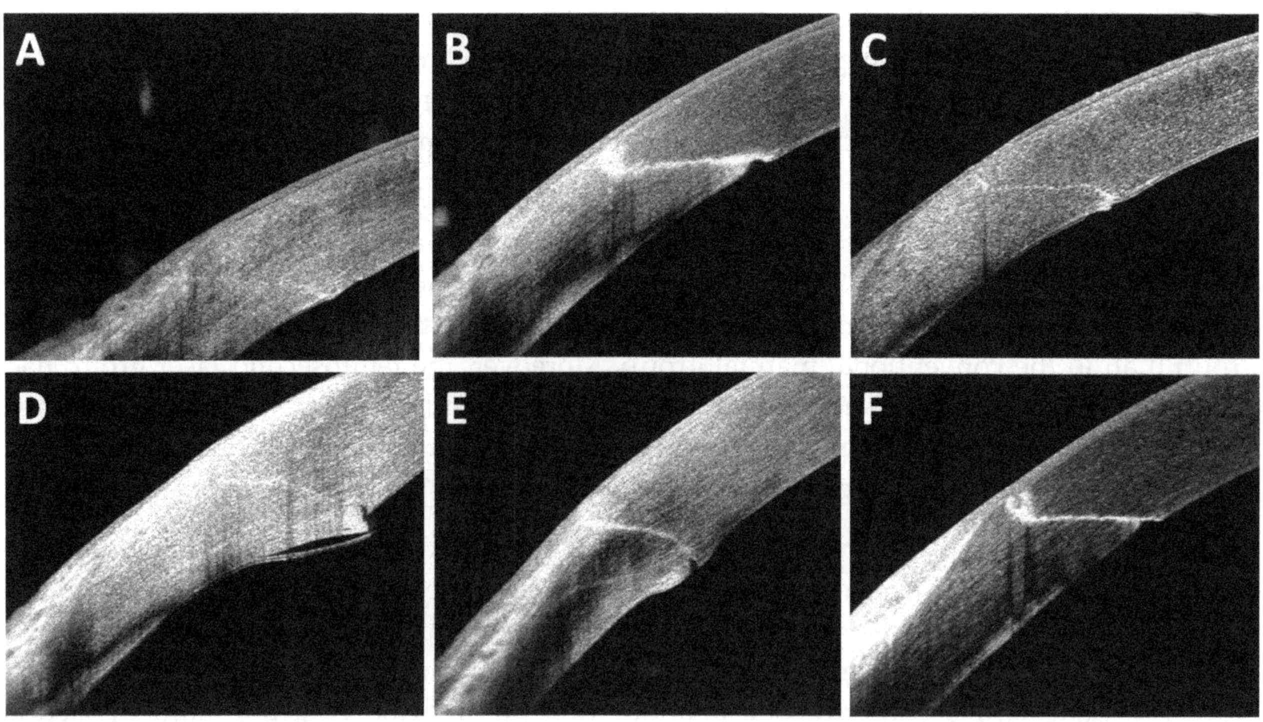

Figure 4. High-resolution anterior segment SD-OCT clear corneal incision images of femtosecond laser-assisted cataract surgery showing a 1-plane CCI (panel A), 2-plane CCI (panel B), 3-plane CCI (panel C), stripping of Descemet's membrane (panel D), posterior wound gape (panel E), and posterior wound retraction (panel F).

and comparison of surgical induced astigmatism and corneal remodeling by different surgical technology. In the future, clear corneal incision length, inner and outer corneal incision thickness, even the lens capsulotomy margin may be evaluated in traditional and femtosecond laser-assisted cataract surgery using OCT.

4. Capsular block syndrome evaluation before and after treatment using SD-OCT

Capsular block syndrome (CBS), as an uncommon complication of phacoemulsification, is characterized by the accumulation of liquid between the IOL and posterior capsule [30]. Davison and Holtz first described this syndrome in 1990 and 1992, respectively [31, 32]. In

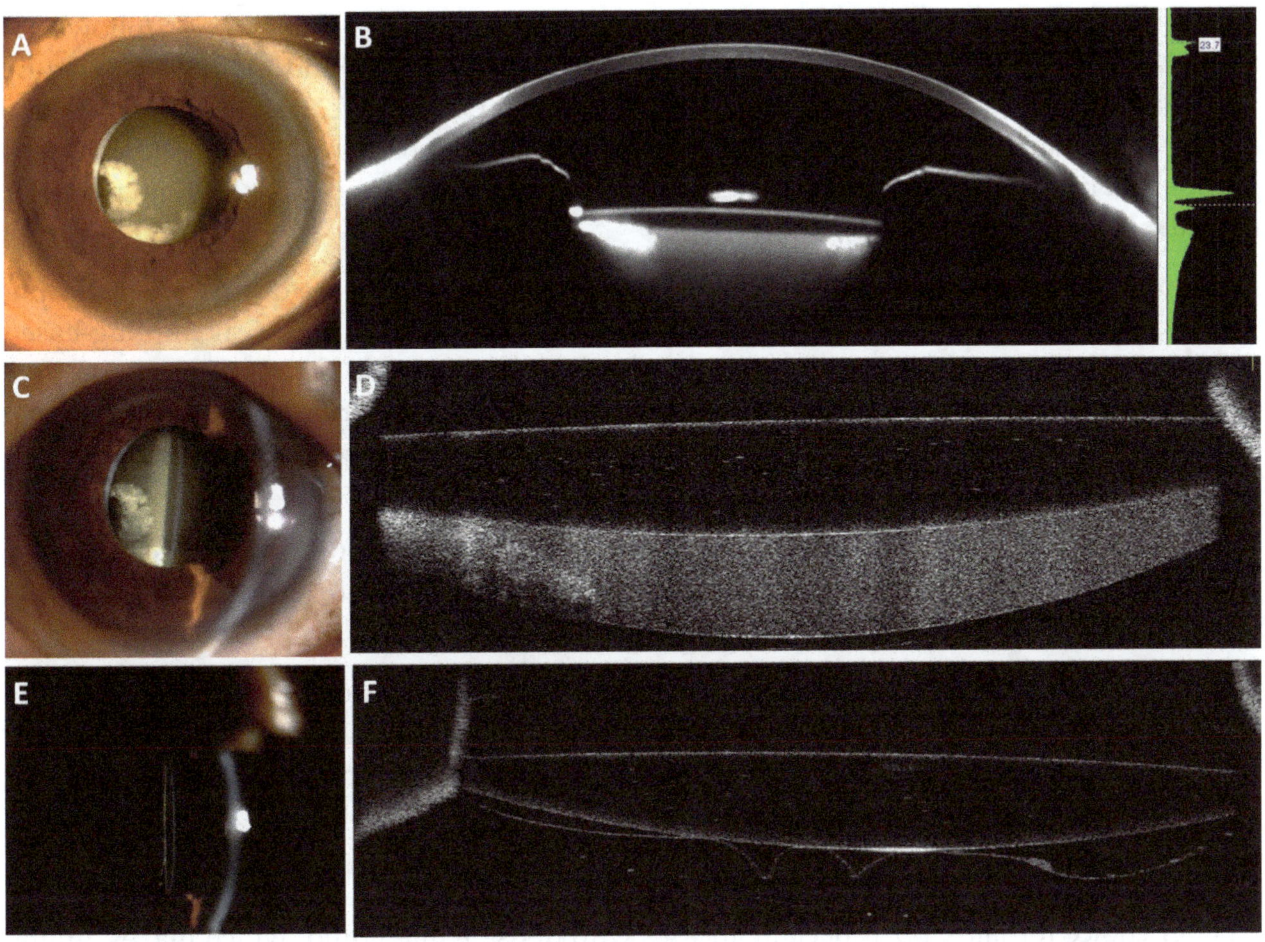

Figure 5. Slit lamp, Pentacam Scheimpflug, and AS-OCT images of an ultra-late capsular block syndrome before (panels A–D) and after surgery (panels E and F). Slit lamp photograph shows white proliferation tissue infero-nasally and nasal tight adhesion of anterior capsule opening fibrosis and IOL (panel A). Scheimpflug-based photography showing the contour of the IOL and the underlying milky-white fluid (panel B). Slit lamp photograph showing a large amount of white fluid trapped behind the IOL (panel C). AS-OCT showing a transparent IOL and accumulation of a milky-white liquefied substance between the posterior capsular bag and IOL (panel D). Slit lamp photograph showing posterior capsular folds and no milky-white liquid after surgery (panel E). AS-OCT shows that the capsular block syndrome is resolved after surgery, with parts of posterior capsule in contact with IOL and posterior capsule folds (panel F).

1993, Masket first used the term CBS to refer to this condition [33]. Due to a continuous capsulorhexis and adhesion of anterior capsule to the IOL, the exchange of aqueous between the anterior chamber and inner capsular bag gets blocked and fluid is retained behind the IOL [34]. Generally, CBS is related to IOL implantation in the capsular bag, but it has also be reported in cases with IOL implantation in the sulcus [35, 36]. Various manifestations of CBS, such as decreased visual acuity, ocular hypertension, closed angle glaucoma, and posterior capsule rupture have been reported. The two main reasons for vision loss include: (1) the effective position of IOL moves forward (myopic shift); (2) a white liquid accumulates behind the IOL (lacteocrumenasia) [30]. Based on time to development, CBS can be divided into three types: intraoperative capsular block, early postoperative CBS, and late postoperative CBS [37, 38]. Most intraoperative CBS occurs due to hydrodissection maneuvers in posterior polar or white cataract surgeries. Due to the block of capsulorhexis borders, liquid accumulates between the posterior nucleus and the posterior capsule. Increasing pressure in the capsular bag may cause posterior capsular rupture and even lens luxation into the vitreous [38]. Early postoperative CBS occurs 1–15 days after cataract surgery. The two main causes are as follows: (1) viscoelastic accumulation behind the IOL; (2) osmotic gradient behind the IOL induced by viscoelastic materials or trapped lens fragments [38, 39]. On average, late postoperative CBS occurs approximately 3.8 years after cataract surgery and deposition of a white fluid (proliferation and pseudo-metaplasia of the lens epithelium) is found between the IOL and posterior capsular bag [34, 40].

A simple, clinical examination can diagnose most CBS cases. With the development of ophthalmic imaging technology t, a definitive diagnosis can be achieved using Scheimpflug-based photography, AS-OCT, or anterior segment UBM. Compared with Scheimpflug-based photography, spectral domain AS-OCT fails to provide complete anterior chamber information but it can provide more details about the IOL and any fluid between the IOL and posterior capsular bag (**Figure 5**).

In some CBS cases with relatively transparent fluid behind the IOL and a large distance between IOL and posterior capsule, UBM, Scheimpflug-based photography or AS-OCT can just demonstrate a partial cross-sectional image (**Figure 6**).

Compared to surgical management, we may also choose anterior or posterior capsulotomy with a Nd:YAG laser to treat CBS, especially for early postoperative and non-cellular late postoperative cases [41]. Due to the relatively lower success rate and higher recurrence rate for anterior capsulotomy, some doctors may choose posterior capsulotomy [42]. In some cases, posterior capsulotomy may cause unexpected irregular posterior capsule rupture, which may cause the IOL to drop into the vitreous cavity (**Figure 7**). Therefore, surgical management is a better choice for late CBS, especially incases with dense white liquid, which makes aiming the Nd:YAG laser accurately almost impossible, and the capsulotomy may cause IOP increase or vitreous inflammation [43]. As an important imaging technology, with the imaging depth enhanced, more and more details about CBS and other posterior capsular related disease can be investigated using OCT.

4.1. Summary

While varying in cause and course, these CBS cases all consistently demonstrated the ability of anterior segment SD-OCT to clearly diagnose and delineate with impressive detail the onset and treatment follow-up. Anterior segment SD-OCT offers extraordinary anatomic details, the more accurate diagnosis, and the potential of quantitative measurement to improve the assessment of treatment efficacy.

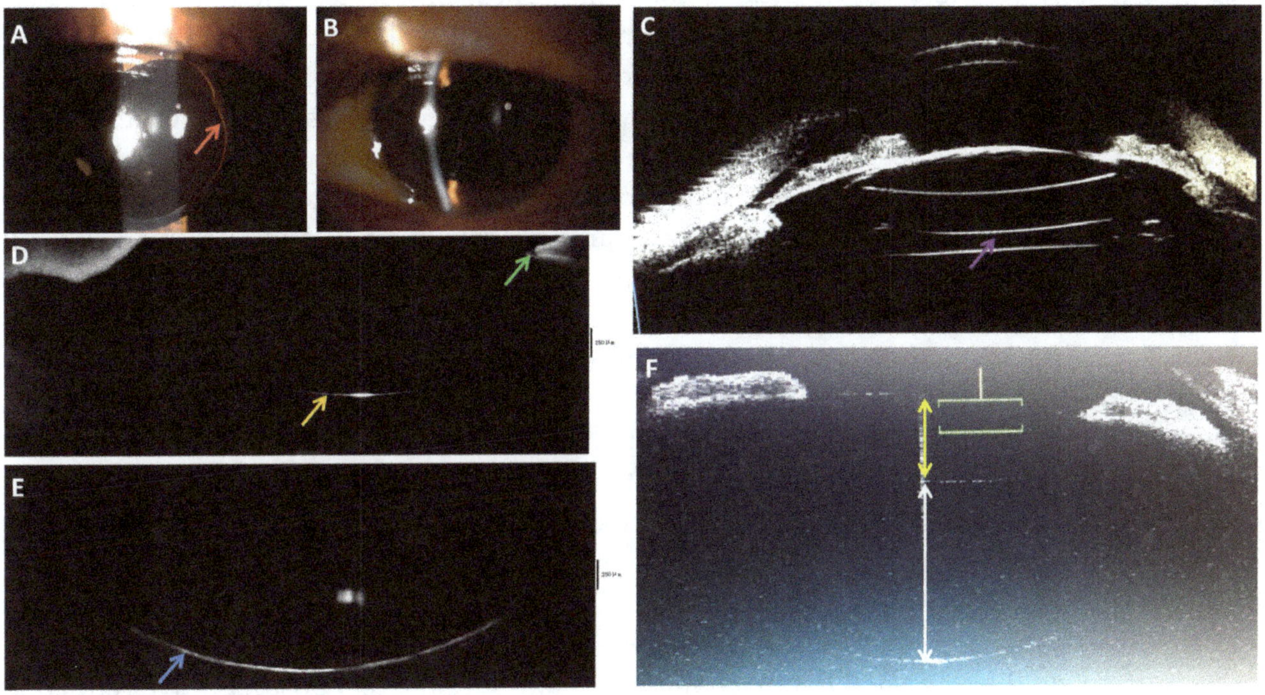

Figure 6. Slit lamp, UBM, and AS-OCT images of a late postoperative capsular block syndrome before Nd:YAG laser treatment. Slit lamp photograph showing capsulorhexis edge (red arrow), anterior IOL optic tightly in contact with the entire anterior capsule (panel A). Slit-lamp biomicroscopy showing transparent fluid behind the IOL (panel B). Due to the limited imaging penetration, UBM image showing artifacts (purple arrow) but not the posterior capsule (panel C). Due to limited imaging depth, spectral-domain AS-OCT fails to show posterior IOL surface (orange arrow), tight adhesion between anterior IOL surface and capsulorhexis edge (green arrow), and posterior capsule (panel E, blue arrow) in one cross-sectional image (panels D and E). Time-domain AS-OCT showing IOL thickness around 1.5 mm (yellow line segment) and the distance between IOL and posterior capsule of about 3.1 mm (white line segment) in one cross-sectional image (panel F).

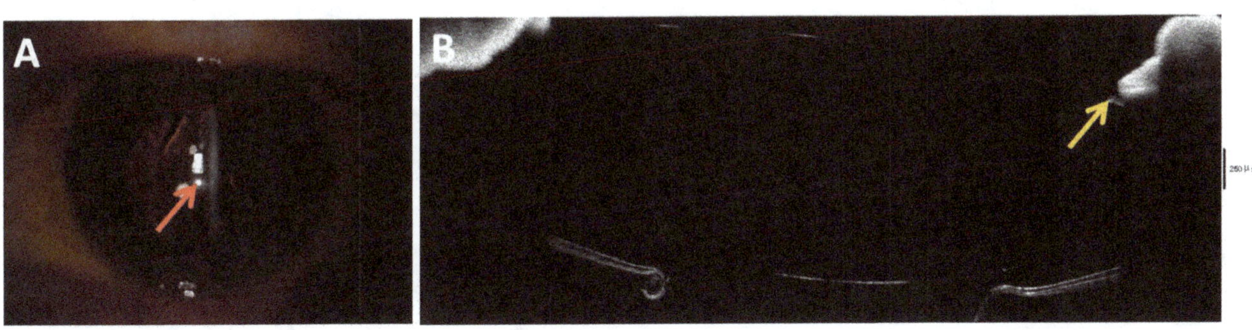

Figure 7. Slit-lamp and AS-OCT images of a late postoperative capsular block syndrome after Nd:YAG laser treatment. Slit-lamp photograph shows irregular posterior capsule rupture (red arrow) after ND:YAG laser treatment (panel A). Spectral-domain AS-OCT cross-sectional image showing posterior capsule breaks with capsular edge rolling and significant decrease in the distance between the IOL and posterior capsule (compared to **Figure 6** panel F). The tight adhesion between anterior IOL surface and anterior capsulorhexis edge (yellow arrow) may prevent the IOL from falling into the vitreous cavity through the big posterior capsule rupture (panel B).

5. IOL power calculation in post-myopic excimer laser eyes using SD-OCT

It is well known that correct IOL power calculation in patients undergoing cataract surgery depends mainly on the accurate measurement of corneal power, axial length, corneal keratometry, and the effective lens position after surgery [44, 45]. Due to index of refraction error, instrument error, and IOL formula error, precise prediction of IOL power is always a big challenge for cataract surgery in patients with previous corneal refractive surgery (PRK, LASIK, RK) [46–51]. For post corneal refractive surgery cataract patients, both, patient expectations of spectacle independence and reduction in the accuracy of conventional IOL power calculation formulas due to previous corneal surgery should be considered. To deal with these issues, many innovative post-corneal refractive surgery IOL power calculation formulas have been developed [52–58]. Compared to traditional keratometry, RTVue spectral-domain AS-OCT can measure anterior and posterior corneal curvature and then calculate the net corneal power, which in conjunction with IOLMaster biometry data (AL, ACD) provides the IOL power [59]. Previous studies have demonstrated that Fourier-domain AS-OCT can provide highly repeatable corneal power measurement and spectral-domain OCT-based IOL formulas have also provided promising results in post-refractive surgery IOL calculation in eyes undergoing cataract surgery; this is especially meaningful for patients for whom prior data are not available [59–61]. To avoid significant IOL power fluctuation between different formulas, surgeons can also use ASCRS online post-refractive IOL calculator (link: http://iolcalc.ascrs.org/) to get the average IOL power value to make sure the real postoperative refraction deviation from the target refraction is not large (**Figure 8**).

5.1. Summary

Anterior segment SD-OCT can noncontactly provide true net corneal power, which is essential for IOL power calculation after excimer laser corneal surgery. The SD-OCT-based IOL formulas enable to provide promising results in post-refractive surgery IOL calculation, especially meaningful for eyes whose prior data unavailable.

IOL calculation formulas used: Double-K Holladay 1[1], Shammas-PL[2], Haigis-L[3], OCT-based[4], & Barrett True K[5]

Using ΔMR		Using no prior data	
[1]Adjusted EffRP	--	[2]Wang-Koch-Maloney	--
[2]Adjusted Atlas 9000 (4mm zone)	--	[2]Shammas	20.59 D
[1]Adjusted Atlas Ring Values	--	[3]Haigis-L	20.97 D
Masket Formula	--	[1]Galilei	--
Modified-Masket	--	[2]Potvin-Hill Pentacam	19.87 D
[1]Adjusted ACCP/ACP/APP	--	[4]OCT	21.25 D
[5]Barrett True K	--	[5]Barrett True K No History	19.78 D

Average IOL Power (All Available Formulas): 20.49 D

Min: 19.78 D

Max: 21.25 D

Figure 8. Average IOL power information for all available formulas using ASCRS online post-refractive IOL calculator.

6. Conclusions

In conclusion, OCT, as a noninvasive and high-resolution imaging technology, can provide the ophthalmologist with clinically useful findings not only about the retina, but also for the cornea, lens, and anterior chamber. Anterior segment high-speed SD-OCT system offers efficient information about lens capsule evaluation, clear corneal incision investigation, capsular block syndrome management, and post-refractive surgery IOL power calculation. In the future, anterior segment SD-OCT may be a useful tool for detecting and monitoring more ocular disease progression and treatment response in clinic.

Grant information

This work was supported by the National Natural Science Foundation of China under Grant No. 81501544.

Financial interests

The authors have neither a conflict of interest nor commercial interest in the equipment mentioned in this paper.

Author details

Xiaogang Wang[1*], Jing Dong[2], Suhua Zhang[1] and Bin Sun[1]

*Address all correspondence to: movie6521@163.com

1 Department of Cataract, Shanxi Eye Hospital, Taiyuan, China

2 Department of Ophthalmology, The First Hospital of Shanxi Medical University, Shanxi, PR China

References

[1] Huang D, Swanson EA, Lin CP, Schuman JS, Stinson WG, Chang W, Hee MR, Flotte T, Gregory K, Puliafito CA, et al. Optical coherence tomography. Science. 1991;**254**:1178-1181

[2] Seland JH. Ultrastructural changes in the normal human lens capsule from birth to old age. Acta Ophthalmologica. 1974;**52**:688-706

[3] Radhakrishnan S, Rollins AM, Roth JE, Yazdanfar S, Westphal V, Bardenstein DS, Izatt JA. Real-time optical coherence tomography of the anterior segment at 1310 nm. Archives of Ophthalmology. 2001;**119**:1179-1185

[4] Kaluzny BJ, Gora M, Karnowski K, Grulkowski I, Kowalczyk A, Wojtkowski M. Imaging of the lens capsule with an ultrahigh-resolution spectral optical coherence tomography prototype based on a femtosecond laser. The British Journal of Ophthalmology. 2010;**94**:275-277

[5] Szkulmowski M, Gorczynska I, Szlag D, Sylwestrzak M, Kowalczyk A, Wojtkowski M. Efficient reduction of speckle noise in optical coherence tomography. Optics Express. 2012;**20**:1337-1359

[6] Dong J, Jia Y, Zhang Y, Zhang H, Jia Z, Zhang S, Wu Q, Hu Q, Zhang T, Wang X. Anterior lens capsule and epithelium thickness measurements using spectral-domain optical coherence tomography. BMC Ophthalmology. 2017;**17**:94

[7] Hawlina M, Stunf S, Hvala A. Ultrastructure of anterior lens capsule of intumescent white cataract. Acta Ophthalmologica. 2011;**89**:e367-e370

[8] Zeng Y, Liu X, Wang T, Zhong Y, Huang J, He M. Correlation between lens thickness and central anterior chamber depth. Eye Science. 2012;**27**:124-126

[9] Barraquer RI, Michael R, Abreu R, Lamarca J, Tresserra F. Human lens capsule thickness as a function of age and location along the sagittal lens perimeter. Investigative Ophthalmology & Visual Science. 2006;**47**:2053-2060

[10] Farouk MM, Naito T, Shinomiya K, Eguchi H, Sayed KM, Nagasawa T, Katome T, Mitamura Y. Optical coherence tomography reveals new insights into the accommodation mechanism. Journal of Ophthalmology. 2015;**2015**:510459

[11] Kim E, Ehrmann K, Uhlhorn S, Borja D, Arrieta-Quintero E, Parel JM. Semiautomated analysis of optical coherence tomography crystalline lens images under simulated accommodation. Journal of Biomedical Optics. 2011;**16**:056003

[12] Kaluzny BJ, Szkulmowska A, Kaluzny JJ, Bajraszewski T, Szkulmowski M, Kowalczyk A, Wojtkowski M. In vivo imaging of posterior capsule opacification using spectral optical coherence tomography. Journal of Cataract and Refractive Surgery. 2006;**32**:1892-1895

[13] Zheng X, Sakai H, Goto T, Namiguchi K, Mizoue S, Shiraishi A, Sawaguchi S, Ohashi Y. Anterior segment optical coherence tomography analysis of clinically unilateral pseudoexfoliation syndrome: Evidence of bilateral involvement and morphologic factors related to asymmetry. Investigative Ophthalmology & Visual Science. 2011;**52**:5679-5684

[14] Pandey SK, Milverton EJ, Maloof AJ. A tribute to Charles David Kelman MD: Ophthalmologist, inventor and pioneer of phacoemulsification surgery. Clinical & Experimental Ophthalmology. 2004;**32**:529-533

[15] Saraiva J, Neatrour K, Waring Iv GO. Emerging technology in refractive cataract surgery. Journal of Ophthalmology. 2016;**2016**:7309283

[16] Calladine D, Ward M, Packard R. Adherent ocular bandage for clear corneal incisions used in cataract surgery. Journal of Cataract and Refractive Surgery. 2010;**36**:1839-1848

[17] Nagy Z, Takacs A, Filkorn T, Sarayba M. Initial clinical evaluation of an intraocular femtosecond laser in cataract surgery. Journal of Refractive Surgery. 2009;**25**:1053-1060

[18] Bissen-Miyajima H, Hirasawa M, Nakamura K, Ota Y, Minami K. Safety and reliability of femtosecond laser-assisted cataract surgery for Japanese eyes. Japanese Journal of Ophthalmology. 2018;**62**:226-230

[19] Agarwal A, Jacob S. Current and effective advantages of femto phacoemulsification. Current Opinion in Ophthalmology. 2017;**28**:49-57

[20] Fine IH, Hoffman RS, Packer M. Profile of clear corneal cataract incisions demonstrated by ocular coherence tomography. Journal of Cataract and Refractive Surgery. 2007;**33**:94-97

[21] Schallhorn JM, Tang M, Li Y, Song JC, Huang D. Optical coherence tomography of clear corneal incisions for cataract surgery. Journal of Cataract and Refractive Surgery. 2008;**34**:1561-1565

[22] Wang L, Dixit L, Weikert MP, Jenkins RB, Koch DD. Healing changes in clear corneal cataract incisions evaluated using Fourier-domain optical coherence tomography. Journal of Cataract and Refractive Surgery. 2012;**38**:660-665

[23] Calladine D, Packard R. Clear corneal incision architecture in the immediate postoperative period evaluated using optical coherence tomography. Journal of Cataract and Refractive Surgery. 2007;**33**:1429-1435

[24] Wang X, Zhang Z, Li X, Xie L, Zhang H, Koch DD, Wang L, Zhang S. Evaluation of femtosecond laser versus manual clear corneal incisions in cataract surgery using spectral-domain optical coherence tomography. Journal of Refractive Surgery. 2018;**34**:17-22

[25] Smolek MK, McCarey BE. Interlamellar adhesive strength in human eyebank corneas. Investigative Ophthalmology & Visual Science. 1990;**31**:1087-1095

[26] Shin TJ, Vito RP, Johnson LW, McCarey BE. The distribution of strain in the human cornea. Journal of Biomechanics. 1997;**30**:497-503

[27] Serrao S, Lombardo G, Schiano-Lomoriello D, Ducoli P, Rosati M, Lombardo M. Effect of femtosecond laser-created clear corneal incision on corneal topography. Journal of Cataract and Refractive Surgery. 2014;**40**:531-537

[28] Schultz T, Tischoff I, Ezeanosike E, Dick HB. Histological sections of corneal incisions in OCT-guided femtosecond laser cataract surgery. Journal of Refractive Surgery. 2013;**29**:863-864

[29] Santhiago MR, Wilson SE. Cellular effects after laser in situ keratomileusis flap formation with femtosecond lasers: A review. Cornea. 2012;**31**:198-205

[30] Velez M, Velasquez LF, Rojas S, Montoya L, Zuluaga K, Balparda K. Capsular block syndrome: A case report and literature review. Clinical Ophthalmology. 2014;**8**:1507-1513

[31] Davison JA. Capsular bag distension after endophacoemulsification and posterior chamber intraocular lens implantation. Journal of Cataract and Refractive Surgery. 1990;**16**:99-108

[32] Holtz SJ. Postoperative capsular bag distension. Journal of Cataract and Refractive Surgery. 1992;**18**:310-317

[33] Masket S. Postoperative complications of capsulorhexis. Journal of Cataract and Refractive Surgery. 1993;**19**:721-724

[34] Miyake K, Ota I, Miyake S, Horiguchi M. Liquefied aftercataract: A complication of continuous curvilinear capsulorhexis and intraocular lens implantation in the lens capsule. American Journal of Ophthalmology. 1998;**125**:429-435

[35] Basti S, Nayak H, Mathur U. Capsular bag distension after optic capture of a sulcus-fixated intraocular lens. Journal of Cataract and Refractive Surgery. 1999;**25**:293-295

[36] Durak I, Ozbek Z, Ferliel ST, Oner FH, Soylev M. Early postoperative capsular block syndrome. Journal of Cataract and Refractive Surgery. 2001;**27**:555-559

[37] Kim HK, Shin JP. Capsular block syndrome after cataract surgery: Clinical analysis and classification. Journal of Cataract and Refractive Surgery. 2008;**34**:357-363

[38] Miyake K, Ota I, Ichihashi S, Miyake S, Tanaka Y, Terasaki H. New classification of capsular block syndrome. Journal of Cataract and Refractive Surgery. 1998;**24**:1230-1234

[39] Sugiura T, Miyauchi S, Eguchi S, Obata H, Nanba H, Fujino Y, Masuda K, Akura J. Analysis of liquid accumulated in the distended capsular bag in early postoperative capsular block syndrome. Journal of Cataract and Refractive Surgery. 2000;**26**:420-425

[40] Eifrig DE. Capsulorhexis-related lacteocrumenasia. Journal of Cataract and Refractive Surgery. 1997;**23**:450-454

[41] Pinsard L, Rougier MB, Colin J. Neodymium:YAG laser treatment of late capsular block syndrome. Journal of Cataract and Refractive Surgery. 2011;**37**:2079-2080

[42] Colakoglu A, Kucukakyuz N, Topcuoglu IE, Akar S. Intraocular pressure rise and recurrence of capsular block syndrome after neodymium:YAG laser anterior capsulotomy. Journal of Cataract and Refractive Surgery. 2007;**33**:1344-1346

[43] Qu J, Bao Y, Li M, Zhao M, Li X. Surgical management of late capsular block syndrome. Journal of Cataract and Refractive Surgery. 2010;**36**:1687-1691

[44] Findl O. Biometry and intraocular lens power calculation. Current Opinion in Ophthalmology. 2005;**16**:61-64

[45] Olsen T. Calculation of intraocular lens power: A review. Acta Ophthalmologica Scandinavica. 2007;**85**:472-485

[46] Hoffer KJ. Intraocular lens power calculation after previous laser refractive surgery. Journal of Cataract and Refractive Surgery. 2009;**35**:759-765

[47] Rosa N, Capasso L, Lanza M, Iaccarino G, Romano A. Reliability of a new correcting factor in calculating intraocular lens power after refractive corneal surgery. Journal of Cataract and Refractive Surgery. 2005;**31**:1020-1024

[48] Shammas HJ, Shammas MC. No-history method of intraocular lens power calculation for cataract surgery after myopic laser in situ keratomileusis. Journal of Cataract and Refractive Surgery. 2007;**33**:31-36

[49] Rosa N, De Bernardo M, Borrelli M, Lanza M. New factor to improve reliability of the clinical history method for intraocular lens power calculation after refractive surgery. Journal of Cataract and Refractive Surgery. 2010;**36**:2123-2128

[50] Abulafia A, Hill WE, Koch DD, Wang L, Barrett GD. Accuracy of the Barrett True-K formula for intraocular lens power prediction after laser in situ keratomileusis or photorefractive keratectomy for myopia. Journal of Cataract and Refractive Surgery. 2016;**42**:363-369

[51] Alio JL, Abdelghany AA, Fernandez-Buenaga R. Management of residual refractive error after cataract surgery. Current Opinion in Ophthalmology. 2014;**25**:291-297

[52] Aramberri J. Intraocular lens power calculation after corneal refractive surgery: Double-K method. Journal of Cataract and Refractive Surgery. 2003;**29**:2063-2068

[53] Saiki M, Negishi K, Kato N, Ogino R, Arai H, Toda I, Dogru M, Tsubota K. Modified double-K method for intraocular lens power calculation after excimer laser corneal refractive surgery. Journal of Cataract and Refractive Surgery. 2013;**39**:556-562

[54] Feiz V, Mannis MJ, Garcia-Ferrer F, Kandavel G, Darlington JK, Kim E, Caspar J, Wang JL, Wang W. Intraocular lens power calculation after laser in situ keratomileusis for myopia and hyperopia: A standardized approach. Cornea. 2001;**20**:792-797

[55] Latkany RA, Chokshi AR, Speaker MG, Abramson J, Soloway BD, Yu G. Intraocular lens calculations after refractive surgery. Journal of Cataract and Refractive Surgery. 2005;**31**:562-570

[56] Savini G, Barboni P, Zanini M. Intraocular lens power calculation after myopic refractive surgery: Theoretical comparison of different methods. Ophthalmology. 2006;**113**: 1271-1282

[57] Borasio E, Stevens J, Smith GT. Estimation of true corneal power after keratorefractive surgery in eyes requiring cataract surgery: BESSt formula. Journal of Cataract and Refractive Surgery. 2006;**32**:2004-2014

[58] Haigis W. Intraocular lens calculation after refractive surgery for myopia: Haigis-L formula. Journal of Cataract and Refractive Surgery. 2008;**34**:1658-1663

[59] Fram NR, Masket S, Wang L. Comparison of intraoperative aberrometry, OCT-based IOL formula, Haigis-L, and Masket formulae for IOL power calculation after laser vision correction. Ophthalmology. 2015;**122**:1096-1101

[60] Tang M, Chen A, Li Y, Huang D. Corneal power measurement with Fourier-domain optical coherence tomography. Journal of Cataract and Refractive Surgery. 2010;**36**:2115-2122

[61] Wang Q, Hua Y, Savini G, Chen H, Bao F, Lin S, Lu W, Huang J. Corneal power measurement obtained by Fourier-domain optical coherence tomography: Repeatability, reproducibility, and comparison with Scheimpflug and automated keratometry measurements. Cornea. 2015;**34**:1266-1271

5

Novelty Detection-Based Internal Fingerprint Segmentation in Optical Coherence Tomography Images

Rethabile Khutlang, Pheeha Machaka,
Ann Singh and Fulufhelo Nelwamondo

Abstract

Biometric fingerprint scanners scan the external skin's features onto a 2-D image. The performance of the automatic fingerprint identification system suffers first and foremost if the finger skin is wet, worn out or a fake fingerprint is used. We present an automatic segmentation of the papillary layer method, from images acquired using contact-less 3-D swept source optical coherence tomography (OCT). The papillary contour represents the internal fingerprint, which does not suffer from the external finger problems. It is embedded between the upper epidermis and papillary layers. Speckle noise is first reduced using non-linear filters from the slices composing the 3-D image. Subsequently, the stratum corneum is used to extract the epidermis. The epidermis, with its depth known, is used as the target class of the ensuing novelty detection. The outliers resulting from novelty detection represent the papillary layer. The contour of the papillary layer is segmented as the boundary between target and rejection classes. Using a mixture of Gaussian's novelty detection routine on images pre-processed with a regularized anisotropic diffusion filter, the papillary contours—internal fingerprints—are consistent with those segmented manually, with the modified Williams index above 0.9400.

Keywords: biometrics, novelty detection, segmentation, internal fingerprint, optical coherence tomography (OCT)

1. Introduction

Biometric identification uses identifiers unique to individuals; because of that, it edges out token-based and knowledge-based identification systems on safety and reliability. Individuals can be described using biometric identifiers provided that they are sufficiently different for a population. Usable biometric identifiers should be easy to acquire; the acquired measurement should be in a form conducive to the extraction of the descriptive features. Extraction should preferably not be intrusive to an individual. They should be extractable on the whole population using the identification system. Fingerprints are popular biometric identifiers for identifying and authenticating individuals. Of all identifiers, fingerprints perform competitively on the factors used in assessing the suitability of any trait [1].

The external skin of the palm finger consists of a series of ridges and furrows, whose pattern determines the fingerprint's uniqueness. Local ridge characteristics that occur at the ridge's bifurcation and ending contribute to this uniqueness. Old age, disease or manual labour can depreciate the fingerprint's uniqueness if the ridges are worn out.

The external finger skin is the interface between an individual and a fingerprint recognition system. The performance of such systems depends on the conditions of the external finger skin. It suffers if the skin is scarred, wet, worn out or if a fake fingerprint is used [2]. Furthermore, standard 2-D readers capture the fingerprint onto a glass surface or a fingerprint paper card in the case of ink-based offline methods. To obtain the 2-D fingerprint image, the subject has to press their finger against a surface. The performance of a fingerprint recognition system using such contact-based acquisition is again negatively affected by the pressure exerted by the finger when making contact with the surface [3]. The pressure is usually non-uniform and results in captured 2-D images that have non-linear distortions. Lastly, 2-D imaging and signal processing of surface topology of a finger do not protect bypassing such systems by a fake fingerprint, which has the third dimension in depth [4].

The internal structure of a finger, the papillary layer, can be used to represent a fingerprint to alleviate the problems associated with the external skin's ridges and valleys. Actually, the papillary layer is the source of the fingerprint structure. It is the blueprint of the visible fingerprint undulations. During development, the basal layer of the epidermis grows faster than the two layers beneath and on top of it, the dermis and upper epidermis layers [5]. Pressure causes the basal layer to deform into the folds pattern that stays with an individual forever. That folds pattern forms an internal fingerprint; it is protected because it is inside the skin, and hence, it cannot be destroyed by superficial skin cuts. The fingerprint recognition system that uses such a fingerprint cannot be fooled by fake fingerprints as fake fingerprints are superficial to finger skin whereas the fingerprint at the papillary layer is beneath the epidermis. Manapuram et al. [6] proposed using optical coherence tomography (OCT) to image the three-dimensional structure of a finger to a depth that reaches the papillary layer of the finger. The internal fingerprint embedded between the upper epidermis and papillary layers is used for identification, instead of the surface fingerprint. Additionally, since OCT is contact-less, that fingerprint does not suffer distortions caused by the finger when making contact with the scanner.

A typical fingerprint recognition system is made up of sensing and acquisition, image enhancement, feature extraction, matching and decision-making components. Since the internal fingerprint is the blueprint to the external skin ridges and folds, the same recognition pipeline is applied. This chapter is focused on segmentation of the internal fingerprint, the papillary layer, from swept source optical coherence tomography (SS-OCT) 3-D images. The tissue beneath the surface has been imaged using time domain OCT for biometrics before [4, 6], while in the Fourier domain OCT, swept source OCT is preferred over spectral domain OCT as it minimizes dispersion and speckle effects better [7, 8]. In Ref. [9], spectral domain OCT was used to extract intricate biometric details such as the distribution of sweat pores and the pattern of the capillary bed and on the other hand, Zam et al. [10] used correlation mapping OCT.

Over a pre-determined depth range, Refs. [8] and [9] averaged XY cross-sectional images to project a 3-D image to 2-D image to segment the internal fingerprint. The fingertip curvature is removed by detecting points at the boundary between air and tissue in Ref. [10]. The points are then aligned to a straight line and concatenated to form a 2-D fingerprint. Akbari and Sadr [11] used vertical gradient thresholding to segment the external fingerprint from an artificial dummy covering it; this was an implicit segmentation of the internal fingerprint. Column accumulation functions are used to segment the internal fingerprint in Ref. [12]; they actually sample the three-dimensional contour of the papillary layer.

This chapter presents the pipeline to segment the internal fingerprint. The method preserves the curvature of the papillary layer. First, the cross-sectional images of the 3-D OCT image are filtered to reduce the effects of speckle noise. Then, the multilevel image thresholds the Otsu segmentation method [13], which is used to detect the outermost skin layer from each filtered slice. The stratum corneum, the outermost skin layer, is used to estimate the extent of the epidermis. The epidermis forms the target data of the ensuing novelty detection, which is applied to image slices, and the boundary to the outlier objects is the contour of the papillary layer—the internal fingerprint. The segmented internal fingerprint has the 3-D profile features that 2-D fingerprints' pattern loses [14]. OCT does not suffer the problem of typical 2-D acquisitions, where variance in pressure exerted to acquire 2-D fingerprints results in deviations in the features extracted from each acquisition on the same finger.

2. Materials and methods

A swept source OCT system (OCS1300SS, Thorlabs, USA) was used to capture the internal finger structure. The central wavelength of 1325 nm and spectral bandwidth of 100 nm were parameters of the swept laser optical source with an average power output of 10.0 mW. The source had an axial scan rate of 16 kHz. The OCT system had a maximum imaging depth of 3 mm. Scattering properties of a sample as a function of depth are contained in an A-scan for a fixed position of the scanned beam. A collection of A-scans results in a cross-sectional image (B-scan). The collection of B-scans results in a volumetric image as shown in **Figure 1**.

2.1. 3-D internal fingerprint segmentation

We use novelty detection machine learning techniques to separate the papillary junction from the upper epidermis. As can be seen in **Figure 1**, the human finger skin shows distinct regions when imaged with OCT. Corneum stratum is clearly visible as a high-pixel intensity

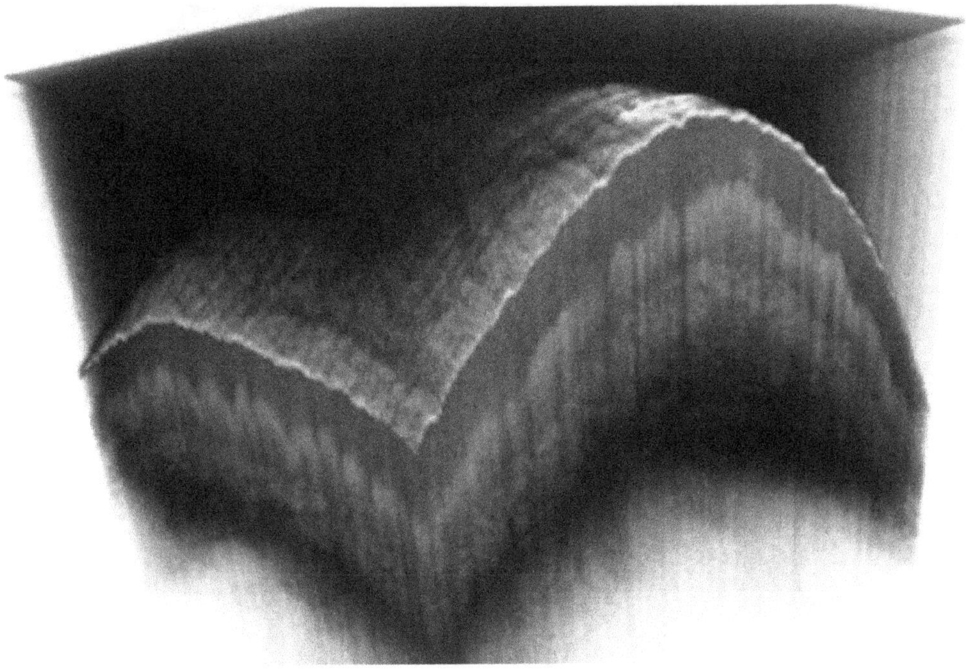

Figure 1. 3-D OCT scan made of 512 cross-sectional images at a human fingertip.

region due to its tissue scattering properties. The rest of the epidermis forms a different class altogether (hereupon referred to as the upper epidermis), with its low and uniform intensity pixels sandwiched between the stratum corneum and the papillary junction. The papillary junction is a distinct region with high-pixel intensity and internal fingerprint undulations clearly visible. We use the stratum corneum, Section 2.2, just to locate the extent of the low-pixel intensity epidermis region—the upper epidermis. This upper epidermis forms the one class in novelty detection that can be characterized and learnt, the target class. Our hypothesis is that the papillary junction pixels, being different in texture, will be classified as an outlier by a novelty detection routine trained using this low-pixel intensity upper epidermis region. The routines are trained using only such low-intensity pixel values but are expected to classify all pixels at a height lower than the low pixel's intensity region used for training. **Figure 2** shows such a low-pixel intensity upper epidermis region used as a training set for novelty detection routines for a single cross-sectional image. This band of training data pixels is located using the stratum corneum edge. Pixels below this band (annotated by a green colour) are sent to novelty detection routines to classify as the target or the outlier.

A 3-D OCT scan is processed on a cross-sectional basis to segment the internal fingerprint. First, the cross sections are filtered to reduce speckle noise. Then, a threshold is applied to detect the stratum corneum. The stratum corneum is used to locate the upper epidermis, which in turn is used to train novelty detection routines to find the undulations of the papillary junction. The undulations of the papillary junction are the internal fingerprints; a 3-D fingerprint is found by concatenating the 2-D cross-sectional images. The workflow is illustrated in **Figure 3**. Below is the expansion of the speckle noise reduction, stratum corneum edge detection and the eventual novelty detection methods used as a papillary contour segmentation pipeline.

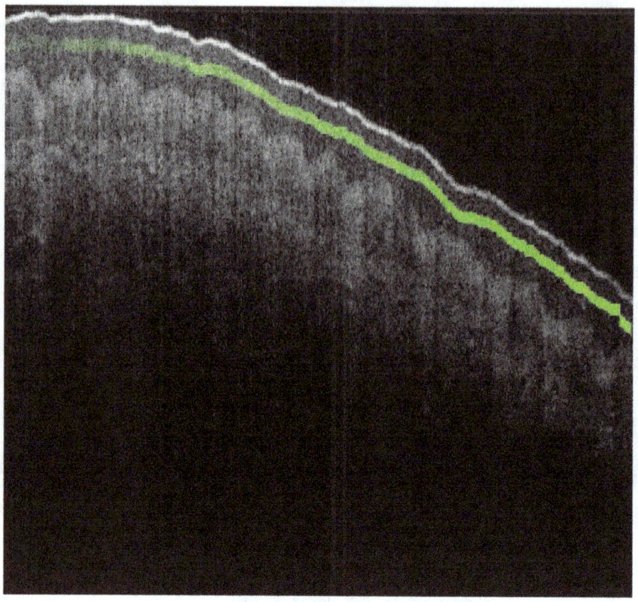

Figure 2. A band located using the corneum stratum edge and used as a training set for novelty detection routines.

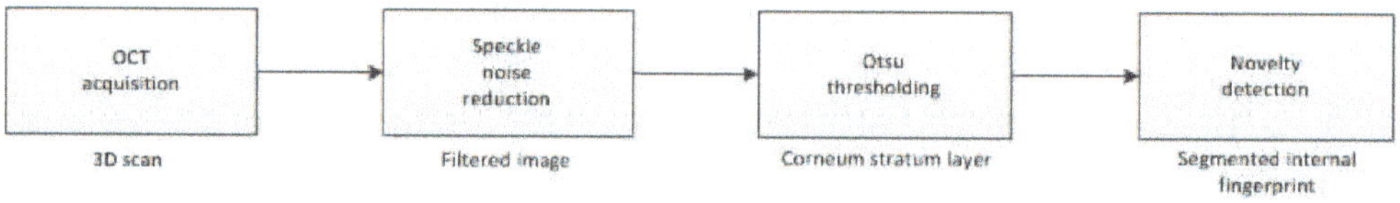

Figure 3. The internal fingerprint segmentation workflow.

2.2. Corneum stratum detection

As a pre-processing step, cross-sectional images of the 3-D OCT scan are filtered using the anisotropic diffusion - Perona and Malik's partial differential equations (PDE) - filter due to its soft-edge preservation characteristics [15]. The edges of the papillary junction undulations are soft. The heat equation (equivalent to the convolution of the signal with Gaussian's at each scale) with the signal as the initial datum u_0 is improved by the Perona and Malik filter by reformulating it as a non-linear equation of the porous medium type:

$$\frac{\partial u}{dt} = div\left(g(|\nabla u|)\nabla u\right), \ u(0) = u_0 \tag{1}$$

In this equation, g is a smooth non-increasing function. Its regularized version was also applied as it is stable in the presence of speckle noise [16]. The stability brought about by Catté et al. [16] is due to the replacement of the gradient $|\nabla u|$ by its estimate $|DG_\sigma * u|$ in the Perona and Malik model (1); G_σ is a Gaussian function.

The two filters were compared to the total variation denoising technique, which performs denoising as an infinite-dimensional minimization problem [17]. Speckle noise results from the coherent nature of laser radiation and the interferometric detection of the scattered light [11]. To minimize speckle noise, [14] applied rotating kernel transformation, while [12] employed parallel processing to speed up median filtering to suppress speckle noise.

After the pre-processing step, we then segment the cross-sectional images using the two-image thresholds of the Otsu method to detect the stratum corneum edge. The filtered cross-sectional image forms an input to a non-parametric method of threshold selection. The filtered image pixels can be represented in L gray levels [1, 2, ..., L], where we assume that there are two thresholds, $1 \leq k_1 < k_2 < L$, for separating an image into three classes. Otsu [13] introduced the discriminant criterion measures used in discriminant analysis to evaluate how strong a threshold is. In this case, segmentation is seen as an optimization problem to search for the two thresholds, k_1' and k_2', that maximize the discriminant criterion measure σB^2—a function of the two variables k_1 and k_2:

$$\sigma B^2(k'_1, k'_2) = \max_{1 \leq k_1 < k_2 < L} \sigma B^2(k_1, k_2) \quad (2)$$

Thresholds are selected in a sequential search by using cumulative probabilities of class occurrence and class mean levels [13]. The highest threshold extracts the stratum corneum. The stratum corneum edge is represented by the topmost pixels of its perimeter.

2.3. Novelty detection to segment papillary layer

Novelty detection is used as a segmentation method because the 3-D internal fingerprint is defined as the boundary between the upper epidermis pixels and the papillary layer pixels. Novelty detection is applied to cases where the class of objects that are not of interest, for example outliers, cannot be sufficiently modelled [18]. Only the upper epidermis pixels, the target class as shown by a green band in **Figure 2** can be sufficiently modelled in this case. Novelty detection routines are trained to recognize the upper epidermal layer. The upper epidermal layer is extracted using the detected stratum corneum edge. According to Ref. [8], the epidermis extends to an average of 0.34 mm at the palm finger region. Epidermal pixel values, from a depth of 10 to that of 20 pixels from the stratum corneum edge, are used as objects of novelty detection routines. An example training dataset extracted using this procedure is shown in **Figure 2** as a band of pixels annotated by a green colour. All pixels at a depth below the green band constitute the test set that is an input to a trained novelty detection routine. The aim is to train novelty detection techniques to recognize only the upper epidermis layer. The papillary layer would be the rejection region of this technique, with the papillary contour at the boundary between target and rejection (outlier) classes.

Gaussian, mixture of Gaussians (MoG), k-means and k nearest neighbour (kNN) routines are used. The target data are modelled as a Gaussian distribution when using a Gaussian routine. To create a more robust description of the target objects, MoG uses n Gaussians [19], where n is determined empirically. k-Means novelty detection technique describes the target dataset using k clusters. The cluster centres are placed using the standard k-means clustering procedure [19]. The kNN routine labels test objects by comparing them to target objects using the Euclidean distance [20].

Training novelty detection routines involve setting a percentage error a routine can make, that is, the number of target objects that may be misclassified as outliers on the training set. To train a Gaussian routine, the density estimate is avoided to minimize numerical instabilities, and just the Mahalanobis distance is used:

$$f(x) = (x - \mu)^T \sum^{-1} (x - \mu) \tag{3}$$

The distance $f(x)$ of a test object x from the mean of the target data; the novelty detection routine is defined as:

$$h(x) = \begin{cases} target \;\; if \;\; f(x) \leq \theta \\ outlier \; if \; f(x) > \theta \end{cases} \tag{4}$$

The mean μ and covariance matrix $\sum$ are just training set estimates, and the threshold θ is based on the percentage error a routine is allowed to make [21]. An object is labelled a target object if its distance from mean is less than the set threshold and labelled an outlier otherwise. Training MoG and k-means routines involve determining the number of Gaussians and clusters, respectively, to optimally represent the training data. The leave-one-out cross-validation error is used to optimize k for the kNN routine on the training dataset.

The same percentage error is set during the training of different routines to compare performance on a test set. The function derived using the set percentage error is used to map pixels (extracted at a depth higher than the section used for training) as a target or an outlier on each cross section of the 3-D image. For each cross-sectional image of a 3-D OCT scan, pixels below the green band, as in **Figure 2**, are objects to be classified as either the target or the outlier. Objects/pixels classified as target objects are labelled one and as outliers, labelled zero. The labels are translated back to the object/pixel coordinates; and the papillary contour is an edge between the zero- and the one-labelled regions of an image. The papillary layer contour is the boundary between the target (upper epidermis) and rejection (papillary layer) classes. The 3-D papillary contour is obtained by concatenating the detected 2-D contours together. The procedure is shown in Algorithm 1.

Algorithm 1. Algorithm to segment an internal fingerprint

Input = 512 cross sections

output = []

for all *i* in length(*input*) **do**

this_cross_sec = input(i)

denoised_im = filter*(this_cross_sec)*

c_s = corneum-stratum-detect*(denoised_im)*

train_data = denoised_im(c_s +10: c_s + 20)

trained_routine = novelty-detection-routine*(train_data, fraction_reject)*

test_im = denoised_im(c_s + 21: length*(denoised_im))*

test_im_labels = map-labels(*test_im* * *trained_routine)*

papillary_contour = perimeter-rejection-class(*test_im_labels*)

output = concatenate(*output, papillary_contour)*

end for

2.4. Evaluation of the segmented papillary contour

Papillary contours were outlined manually from the slices composing the 3-D image. The manual outlines represented the gold standard used in assessing the performance of different routines. The agreement between the gold standard papillary contours and those segmented automatically was assessed using the Hausdorff distance [22] and the modified Williams index (MWI) [23]. The MWI specifies whether the contour outlined by routine 0 agrees with the set of n manual contours as much as a manual contour agrees with another contour from the manual set; it is defined as:

$$MWI = \frac{\frac{1}{n}\sum_{j=1}^{n}\frac{1}{D_{0j}}}{\frac{2}{n(n-1)}\sum_{j=1}^{n-1}\sum_{j'=j+1}^{n}\frac{1}{D_{jj'}}} \tag{5}$$

where

$$D_{jj'} = \frac{1}{N}\sum_{i=1}^{N} H(x_{ij}, x_{ij'}) \tag{6}$$

$D_{jj'}$ denotes the agreement between two observers j and j'. x_{ij} denotes observer j outlining image i and $H(x,y)$ is the Hausdorff distance between images contours x and y.

3. Results

The two-image thresholds of the Otsu method were determined automatically for each cross section. The input to the two-image thresholds Otsu segmentation method was the denoised cross-sectional image. The output was the exterior edge of the stratum corneum. Each denoising technique pronounced pixel intensities of the stratum corneum layer differently; the Otsu method was able to detect the change in the gradient between the stratum corneum layer and air. **Figure 4** shows the detected edge for the three denoising routines that were used.

The objects used to train novelty detection routines had one feature, pixel intensity value of the unit 8 cross-sectional image. The pixels were extracted at 10 pixel depth from the stratum corneum contour detected using the two image thresholds Otsu method. A set of 50 YZ cross-sectional scans was used to study the agreement between papillary contours segmented by two researchers and the novelty detection routines. The comparisons were made using the Hausdorff distance. T11 and T12 represent the first observer, outlining the papillary contours

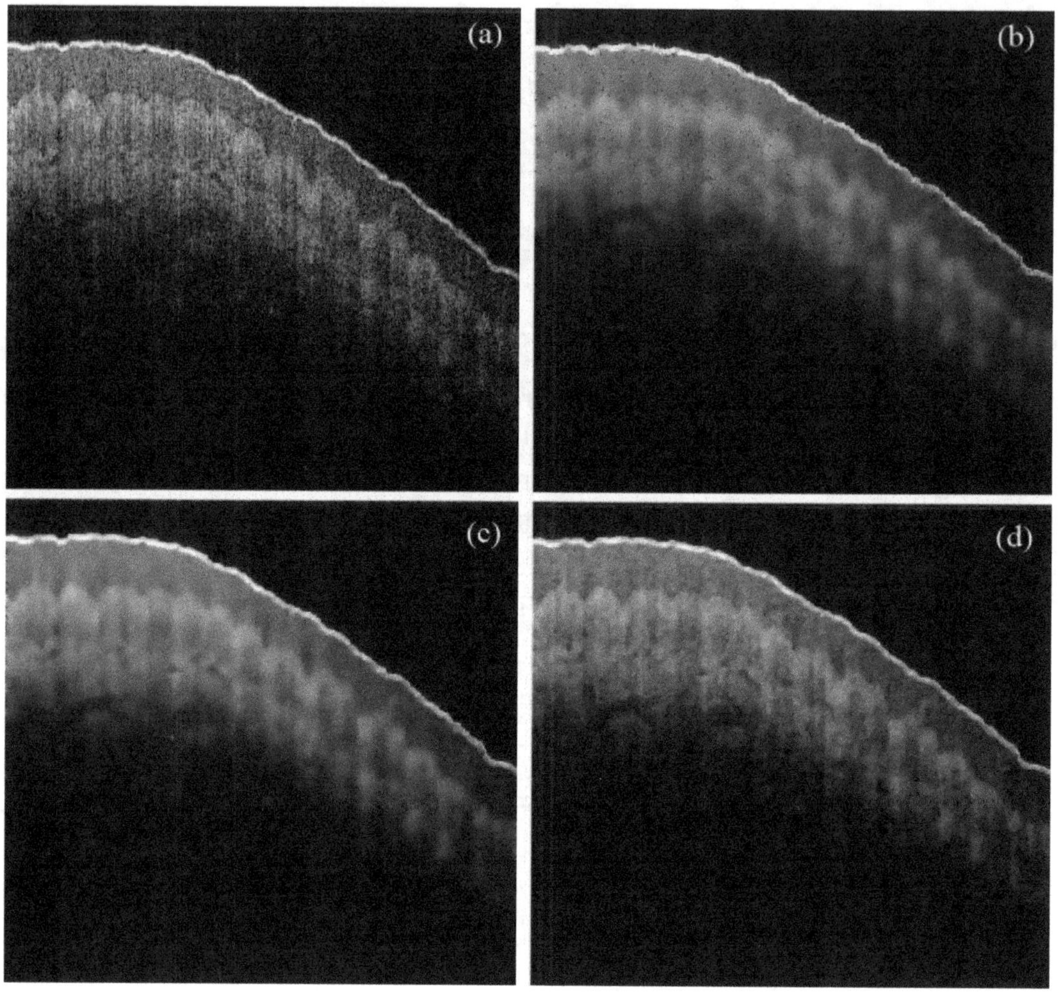

Figure 4. A raw cross-sectional image (a) together with the corneum stratum edge overlaid on its filtered version using anisotropic diffusion (b), its regularized version (c) and the total variation denoising technique (d).

for the first and second time. T2 represents the second observer, while Gau, MoG, KM and *k*NN represent Gaussian, mixture of Gaussians, k-means and *k* nearest neighbour routines respectively. The agreement between contours outlined by an observer and between observers is shown in **Table 1**.

The Hausdorff distance was used to determine both the number of Gaussians and clusters to use from the 50 scans. A plot of the Hausdorff distance as a function of the number of Gaussians or clusters is shown in **Figure 5**. Three Gaussians were used with the mixture of Gaussians, and three clusters were used with the k-means routine. *k* was optimized using the leave-one-out cross-validation for each cross-sectional image segmentation using the *k*NN routine.

The Hausdorff distance was used to obtain the MWI for comparing computer-generated contours to hand-drawn ones. The MWI is the ratio between the average computer-observer

	T11 and T12	T21 and T22	T11 and T21	T12 and T22
Mean ± Std	4.5424 ± 0.4363	4.4313 ± 0.3823	4.5054 ± 0.4062	4.4993 ± 0.4240

Table 1. Comparison of manual papillary segmentation between two observers.

agreement and the average observer-observer agreement. Contours outlined by two volunteers constituted four manual observations per object. **Table 2** shows the agreement between the volunteers and novelty detection routines in segmenting anisotropic diffusion filtered scans and the MWI of the routines, together with the 95% confidence interval estimate for the MWI, assuming a standard normal distribution. **Table 3** shows the evaluation of the novelty

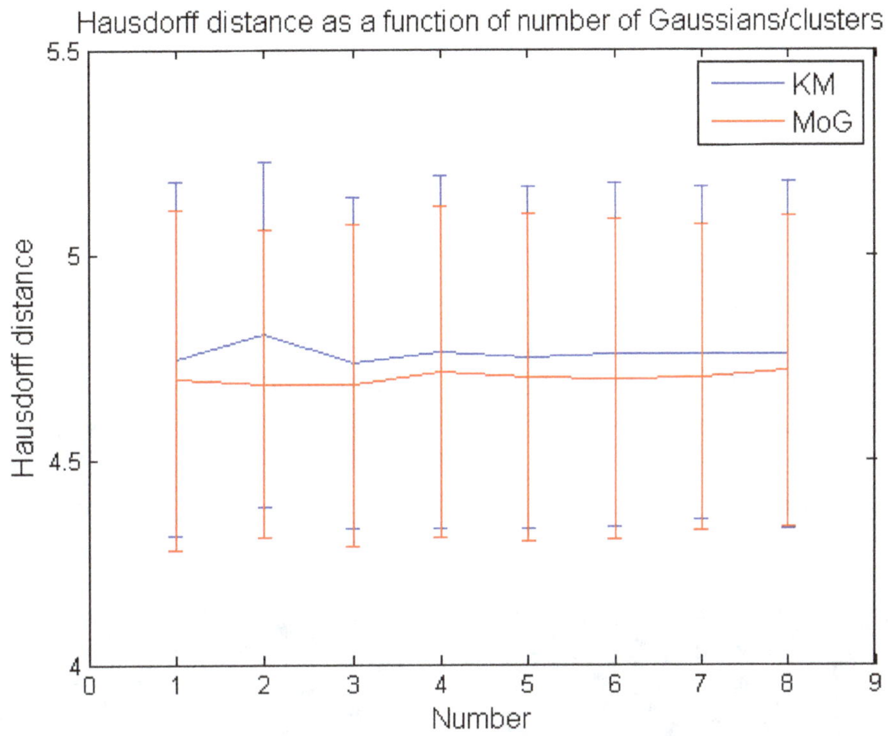

Figure 5. Hausdorff distance as a function of the number of Gaussians for MoG and clusters for k-means.

	T11 and AL	T21 and Al	MWI	Confidence interval
Gau	4.7554 ± 0.4355	4.7282 ± 0.3832	0.9450	(0.9416, 0.9485)
MoG	4.7262 ± 0.3823	4.7111 ± 0.4111	0.9498	(0.9465, 0.9530)
KM	4.7627 ± 0.4917	4.7920 ± 0.4914	0.9386	(0.9353, 0.9420)
*k*NN	4.7664 ± 0.4053	4.7118 ± 0.4271	0.9455	(0.9421, 0.9489)

Table 2. Comparison between manual papillary segmentation and segmentation using novelty detection techniques on anisotropic filtered images.

	T11 and AL	T21 and Al	MWI	Confidence interval
Gau	4.7113 ± 0.4091	4.7302 ± 0.4106	0.9504	(0.9474, 0.9535)
MoG	4.680 ± 60.3934	4.7088 ± 0.3598	0.9548	(0.9518, 0.9578)
KM	4.7350 ± 0.4038	4.7435 ± 0.4028	0.9473	(0.9442, 0.9505)
*k*NN	4.7295 ± 0.3667	4.7631 ± 0.3678	0.9474	(0.9445, 0.9502)

Table 3. Comparison between manual papillary segmentation and segmentation using novelty detection techniques on regularized anisotropic filtered images.

detection segmentation techniques with the regularized anisotropic diffusion filtered images as the input, while **Table 4** shows that of total variation filtered images as input.

	T11 and AL	T21 and Al	MWI	Confidence interval
Gau	4.9777 ± 0.4550	5.0235 ± 0.4336	0.8967	(0.8937, 0.8997)
MoG	5.0263 ± 0.3451	5.0317 ± 0.3532	0.8902	(0.8874, 0.8931)
KM	5.1393 ± 0.4133	5.1580 ± 0.4228	0.8703	(0.8674, 0.8733)
*k*NN	4.9324 ± 0.3660	4.8878 ± 0.3632	0.9138	(0.9109, 0.9167)

Table 4. Comparison between manual papillary segmentation and segmentation using novelty detection techniques on total variation filtered images.

Mixture of Gaussians had the best overall performance in segmenting the papillary contour across the three denoising techniques. For each denoising technique, the papillary contour segmented using the MoG has been overlaid and compared with a manual papillary outline for that cross section in **Figure 6**. Novelty detection techniques generally struggled to segment the papillary contour from scans pre-processed using the total variation denoising technique. The 3-D papillary contour segmented using the worst performing novelty detection routine, k-means, on total variation denoised scans is shown in **Figure 7**, side by side with the same

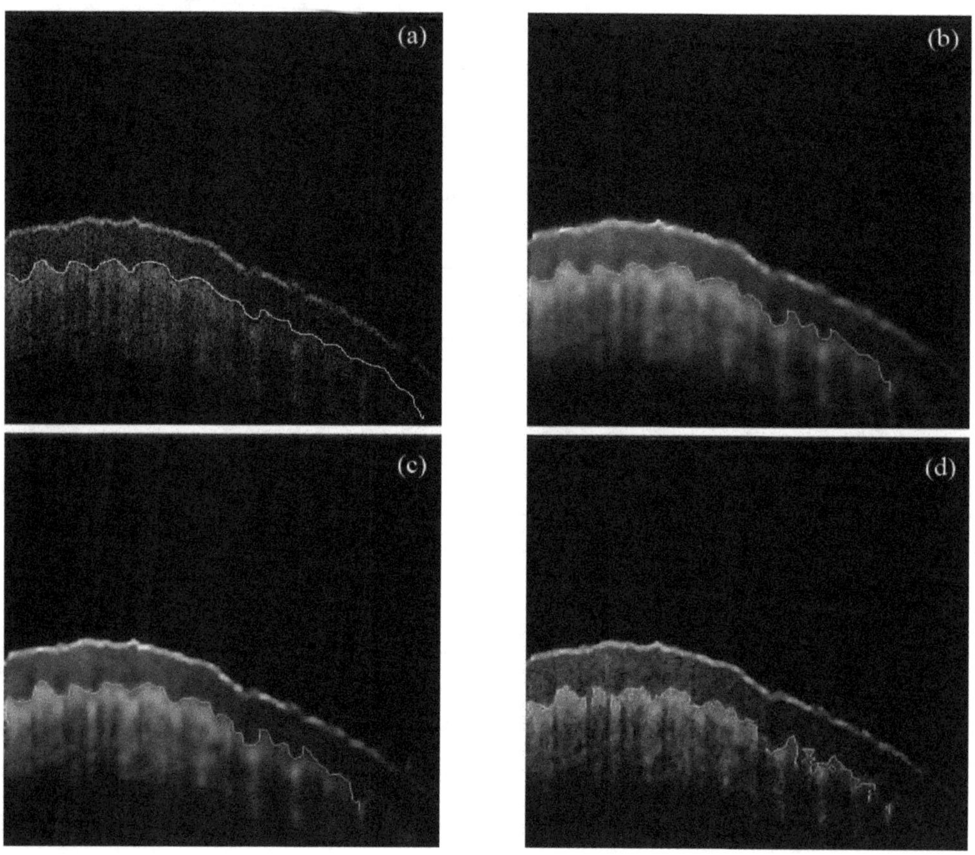

Figure 6. A raw cross-sectional image with papillary contour manually outlined (a) together with the overlaid papillary contour segmented using the MoG routine when that cross section is pre-processed using anisotropic diffusion (b), its regularized version (c) and the total variation denoising technique (d).

scan segmented using the MoG routine when pre-processed using the regularized anisotropic diffusion filter, the best performing workflow.

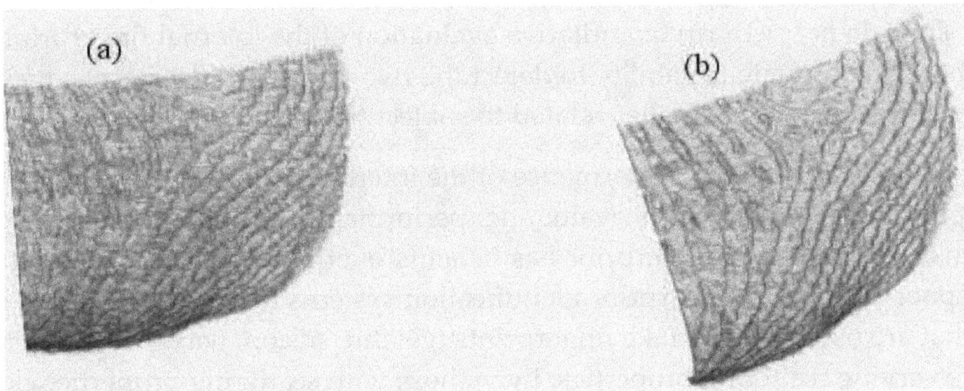

Figure 7. A 3-D papillary contour segmented using the k-means routine on a scan pre-processed using the total variation technique (a), side by side with the same scan pre-processed with regularized anisotropic diffusion and segmented using MoG.

4. Discussion

The aim of our chapter was to segment the internal fingerprint from swept source optical coherence tomography 3-D scans. This forms one component of the internal fingerprint recognition system that uses an OCT scanner as a contact-less acquisition device. The system is composed of the following components: sensing, 3-D internal fingerprint segmentation, feature extraction, matching and decision-making components. We use an SS-OCT system as a sensing component. The feature extraction and subsequent components have not been implemented.

No evaluation of internal fingerprint segmentation was found in the literature for direct comparison with our results. An edge-based segmentation technique was applied to detect an artificial layer glued to a fingertip in Ref. [11]. They used vertical gradient edge detection technique, where the dummy fingerprint was glued to the fingertip and the method marked out the border between the real skin and the artificial layer. However, the segmented border was subjectively evaluated.

Both Refs. [8] and [9] averaged XY cross-sectional images of a 3-D OCT scan to obtain the 2-D internal fingerprint image. Lui and Buma [9] had removed the overall fingertip curvature without affecting the fine-scale undulation of the friction ridge by fitting a third-order polynomial to the stratum corneum edge. We deduce that their resultant 2-D internal fingerprint was more accurate than that of Ref. [8] because the rectangle selected to average across cut more evenly across the papillary region for the straightened fingertip rather than the fingertip retaining the original curvature. They both did not perform quantitative evaluation of their XY averaging segmentation technique.

Sousedik et al. [12] segment an OCT scan of a fingertip into two 3-D fingerprint layers—the surface fingerprint and an internal one embedded between the upper epidermis and the papillary layers. However, they do not produce a continuous 3-D internal fingerprint layer but rather a scattered point cloud. This is the fundamental difference between their method and the one presented in this chapter, which produces a continuous 3-D surface of the internal fingerprint. They do not perform quantitative evaluation of the internal fingerprint segmentation but rather they evaluate the ability to detect the two layers of fingerprints; they got a 90% ability in the scans without anomalies related to subject finger motion.

We quantitatively evaluated the performance of the internal fingerprint segmentation method that is proposed [24]. Aside from evaluating performance of the proposed segmentation procedure, using the internal fingerprint has benefits over the surface fingerprint. It is more difficult to spoof automated fingerprint identification systems that use an internal fingerprint. Substrates that are used to make fake fingerprints (gelatin, silicon, waxes of difference concentration) have varying scattering properties. Even those with scattering properties close to those of human fingers (polydimethylsiloxane mixed with titanium oxide [9]) have a problem in that the OCT will reveal a stratum corneum layer of abnormal thickness. The proposed segmentation method uses the fact that the epidermis extends to an average of 0.34 mm at the palm finger region [9]; it can be adapted to raise an alert if an internal fingerprint is not detected within an expected range. Furthermore, using the internal fingerprint minimizes the impact of fingerprint surface cuts, but deep cuts will still present a problem.

An advantage of extracting features from a 3-D internal fingerprint is that the 2-D (flat) fingerprint pattern loses the 3-D profile features that also provide information that can be used to uniquely identify an individual [14]. The automated fingerprint identification system that uses OCT as a sensor includes all of the 2-D morphological features, along with the 3-D profile which will increase discrimination performance. Performance comparisons will be made by using extended 2-D minutiae features in the 3-D space to include height and angle information and by using finger surface codes as 3-D features [25]. **Figure 8** shows the internal and external fingerprint of the same finger—the external one is a conventional 2-D optical scan that is cropped to correspond to the OCT-scanned internal one. We propose that an eventual recognition performance of the system being developed will be an improvement over conventional

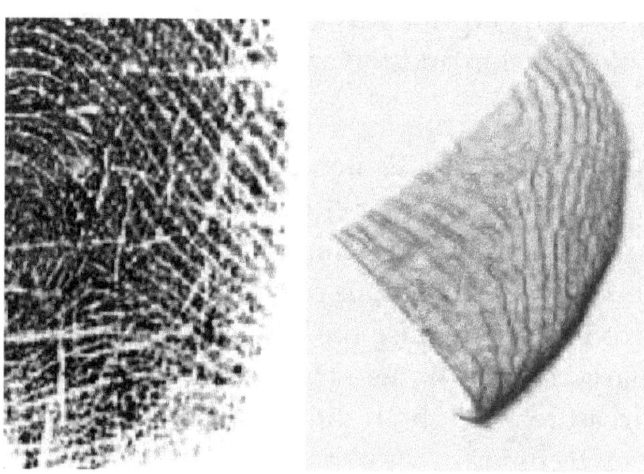

Figure 8. The image on the left is a conventional 2-D external fingerprint that has been cropped to an area corresponding to that scanned by the OCT, right image, of the same finger.

systems as physical deterioration of an external fingerprint will be countered by using the internal fingerprint.

Sousedik et al. [12] used a support vector machine to detect the layer that corresponds to a fake fingerprint glued to a fingertip, using the overall energy of the layers as a feature vector. They did not use machine learning for matching different fingertips but rather for detecting artefacts glued to fingertips. Kumar and Kwong [25] implemented matching the 3-D surface fingerprints obtained using a single camera, using both the finger surface code and 3-D minutiae as features. They got a better matching performance when combining 3-D features with 2-D features than using just 2-D features. This suggests that 3-D fingerprint features will be effective in the matching and the decision-making component of the internal fingerprint-based identification system.

With human observers used as a gold standard, mixture of Gaussians performed best in segmenting the 3-D papillary contour—internal fingerprint—according to the Hausdorff distance. On the selected pre-processing technique, the regularized anisotropic diffusion filter, the average Hausdorff distance was the lowest. The standard deviation was the lowest, which suggests that the mixture of Gaussians stably produces contours consistent with those of human volunteers. The average Hausdorff distance of the method is higher than that among human volunteers as the method does not outperform humans. To train novelty detection techniques that are compared, they were set at the same percentage error that they can make on the target data.

Other novelty detection routines can be used in the proposed segmentation workflow. There is little difference in the segmentation performance between the routines that were tested. We have not implemented 3-D internal fingerprint recognition routines to assess the impact of the difference in segmentation performance on the eventual recognition performance of the entire system. The impact of segmentation performance of different novelty detection routines on the overall system recognition performance might not be significant, in which case the novelty detection routines could be ranked by other desirable aspects, for instance speed.

Novelty detection techniques had the poorest performance segmenting OCT scans pre-processed with the total variation denoising filter, according to the Hausdorff distance. Such filtered cross-sectional images had high- and low-intensity specks across the epidermal and papillary layers observed visually. The specks negatively affected the performance of novelty detection routines. The *k*NN routine, which computes the distance to the optimized *k* nearest neighbours, had the best performance of these routines. Scans pre-processed with the anisotropic diffusion filter also had such specks, be it on a level less than that observed with the total variation denoising filter. That might explain why superior performance was obtained when using its regularized version. Quantitative performance evaluation of different filtering techniques was not explicitly done, and if done it will definitely order the different OCT speckle noise reduction techniques according to performance.

When the upper limit of the MWI confidence interval is greater than one, it demonstrates that an automatically detected contour agrees with the set of manual contours at least as well as manual segmentations are in agreement. The upper limit obtained with the best segmentation pipeline—using a regularized anisotropic diffusion filter and a mixture of Gaussians routine—was not greater that one. To improve novelty detection, texture features could be explored. The epidermis and the dermis layers have different textures. Moreover, neighbourhood information was not incorporated in novelty detection as individual pixel values were used as features. A nine-pixel neighbourhood can be used as a feature set instead of a single pixel. This might better represent spatial information. Even though the computer-observer agreement was not at least as well as observer-observer agreement, the confidence interval was narrow suggesting that the variability was not erratic and that the method is stable.

Unrolling algorithms can be used to convert the segmented 3-D internal fingerprints to their 2-D equivalent fingerprints. The 2-D equivalent fingerprints will not have the distortions caused by pressure exerted when capturing conventional 2-D fingerprints. Alternatively, 3-D profile features can be extracted from the segmented 3-D internal fingerprints. Such features can be used for matching instead of features extracted from traditional contact-based scanners that often suffer non-linear distortions.

5. Conclusion

The proposed workflow automatically segments the contours of the papillary layer—the internal fingerprint. The 3-D OCT scan is processed on a per cross-sectional image basis. First, the slices are filtered by a regularized anisotropic diffusion filter to reduce the effects of speckle noise. Then, the Otsu method is used to detect the stratum corneum, and multilevel image thresholds are determined automatically for each slice. The stratum corneum is used as a marker to extract a set of epidermal layer pixels to be used as the training data in the ensuing novelty detection. The mixture of Gaussians mapping is used to label pixels at a depth higher than the depth used to extract the training pixels on each cross section. The contour of the papillary layer is the internal fingerprint. The 3-D internal fingerprint image is obtained by concatenating the 2-D papillary contours together.

Laser radiation loses focus towards the extremes of a fingertip because of the fingertip's curvature. The result is that skin penetration weakens and the weak reflected light translates into low-pixel intensity values. This affects stratum corneum detection, and at times, the Otsu segmentation method returns a non-continuous stratum corneum edge. Corneum stratum edge detection will be improved using regression methods. The left topmost and right topmost extreme pixels of the returned connected components constituting the stratum corneum can be stitched together. Vertically sweeping an image from left to right, the right topmost extreme point will be connected to the closest, Euclidean distance-wise, left topmost extreme pixel using regression methods. A linear least squares fitting technique will not always give the output as a single connected object when fed with two disjointed edges in an image; hence, non-linear regression routines will be investigated.

The epidermis extends to an average of 0.34 mm at the finger region [8]. The 10-pixels depth from which the extraction of the epidermis layer began was empirically determined. The aim was to exclude the stratum corneum was extracting pixels that forms the training set of novelty detection routines. The routines were given pixel values at a depth higher than the extracted training pixel dataset to classify, with the undulations of the papillary contour expected to be the border between the target and rejection regions.

An automated segmentation workflow has been established for the 3-D internal fingerprint. The segmented internal fingerprint does not suffer problems associated with the external fingerprint. The method preserves the 3-D profile features that are lost with the 2-D fingerprints' pattern. It has the potential to segment the papillary contours as well as a manual segmentation, with post-processing improvements.

Author details

Rethabile Khutlang[1*], Pheeha Machaka[2], Ann Singh[3] and Fulufhelo Nelwamondo[4]

*Address all correspondence to: rkhutlang@csir.co.za

1 Biometrics Research Group, Identity Authentication, CSIR Modelling and Digital Science, Pretoria, South Africa

2 Network Security, Network and Data Security, CSIR Modelling and Digital Science, Pretoria, South Africa

3 Laser Sources Group, CSIR National Laser Centre, Pretoria, South Africa

4 CSIR Modelling and Digital Science, Pretoria, South Africa

References

[1] Jain, A., Ross, A., Prabhakar, S.: An introduction to biometric recognition. IEEE Transactions on Circuits and Systems for Video Technology, 2004; **14**(1): 4–20

[2] Shiratsuki, A., Sano, E., Shikai, M., et al.: Novel optical fingerprint sensor utilizing optical characteristics of skin tissue under fingerprints. Biomedical Optics, International Society for Optics and Photonics, 2005; 80–87

[3] Maltoni, D., Cappelli, R.: Advances in fingerprint modeling. Image and Vision Computing, 2009; **27**(3): 258–268

[4] Cheng, Y., Larin, K. V.: In vivo two-and three-dimensional imaging of artificial and real fingerprints with optical coherence tomography. IEEE Photonics Technology Letters, 2007; **19**(20): 1634–1636

[5] Kücken, M., Newell, A. C.: A model for fingerprint formation. EPL (Europhysics Letters), 2004; **68**(1): 141

[6] Manapuram, R. K., Ghosn, M., Larin, K. V.: Identification of artificial fingerprints using optical coherence tomography technique. Asian Journal of Physics, 2006; 15: 15–27

[7] Dubey, S. K., Mehta, D. S., Anand, A., et al.: Simultaneous topography and tomography of latent fingerprints using full-field swept-source optical coherence tomography. Journal of Optics A: Pure and Applied Optics, 2008; **10**(1): 015307

[8] Bossen, A., Lehmann, R., Meier, C.: Internal fingerprint identification with optical coherence tomography. IEEE Photonics Technology Letters, 2010; **22**(7): 507–509

[9] Liu, M., Buma, T.: Biometric mapping of fingertip eccrine glands with optical coherence tomography. IEEE Photonics Technology Letters, 2010; **22**(22): 1677–1679

[10] Zam, A., Dsouza, R., Subhash, H. M., et al.: Feasibility of correlation mapping optical coherence tomography (cmOCT) for anti-spoof sub-surface fingerprinting. Journal of Biophotonics, 2013; **6**(9): 663–667

[11] Akbari, N., Sadr, A.: Automation of fingerprint recognition using OCT fingerprint images. Journal of Signal and Information Processing, 2012; **3**: 117

[12] Sousedik, C., Breithaupt, R., Busch, C.: Volumetric fingerprint data analysis using optical coherence tomography. In Proceeding of the Biometrics Special Interest Group (BIOSIG), Darmstadt, September 2013, pp. 1–6

[13] Otsu, N.: A threshold selection method from gray-level histograms. Automatica, 1975; **11** (285–296): 23–27

[14] Chang, S., Flueraru, C., Larin, K., et al.: Fingerprint spoof detection by NIR optical analysis. INTECH Open Access Publisher, Ottawa, 2011

[15] Perona, P., Malik, J.: Scale-space and edge detection using anisotropic diffusion. IEEE Transactions on Pattern Analysis and Machine Intelligence, 1990; **12**(7): 629–639

[16] Catté, F., Lions, P. L., Morel, J. M., et al.: Image selective smoothing and edge detection by nonlinear diffusion. SIAM Journal on Numerical Analysis, 1992; **29**(1): 182–193

[17] Getreuer, P.: Rudin-Osher-Fatemi total variation denoising using split Bregman. Image Processing On Line, 2012; **10**: 74–95

[18] Bishop, C. M.: Novelty detection and neural network validation. IEE Proceedings of Vision, Image and Signal Processing, 1994; **141**(4): 217–222

[19] Bishop, C. M.: Neural networks for pattern recognition. Oxford University Press, Oxford, 1995

[20] Duda, R. O., Hart, P. E., Stork, D. G.: Pattern classification. John Wiley & Sons, 2012

[21] Tax, D. M. J. (ed.).: Ddtools, the data description toolbox for matlab. Delft University of Technology, Delft, 2005

[22] Huttenlocher, D. P., Klanderman, G., Rucklidge, W. J.: Comparing images using the Hausdorff distance. IEEE Transactions on Pattern Analysis and Machine Intelligence, 1993; **15**(9): 850–863

[23] Chalana, V., Kim, Y.: A methodology for evaluation of boundary detection algorithms on medical images. IEEE Transactions on Medical Imaging, 1997; **16**(5): 642–652

[24] Khutlang, R., Nelwamondo, F. V.: Novelty detection-based internal fingerprint segmentation in optical coherence tomography images. In 2014 Second International Symposium on Computing and Networking (CANDAR), Shizuoka, December 2014, pp. 556–559

[25] Kumar, A., Kwong, C.: Towards contactless, low-cost and accurate 3D fingerprint identification. IEEE Transactions on Pattern Analysis and Machine Intelligence, 2015; **37**(3): 681–696

6

OCT in Glaucoma Diagnosis, Detection and Screening

Aydin Yildiz

Abstract

Glaucoma is a chronic and progressive optic neuropathy in which increased intraocular pressure is the most important risk factor in the etiopathogenesis. The basic pathology is the progressive loss of retinal ganglion cells (RGCs) especially the death of the axons of ganglion cells initially (apoptosis), followed by peripapillary retinal nerve fiber layer (RNFL) defects. Since optical coherence tomography (OCT)'s first demonstration in 1991 by Huang et al. and introduction commercially in 1996, it began gaining popularity in 2000s for retinal evaluation and the detection, diagnosis, and follow-up of glaucoma. Previously available OCT instruments used a technique referred to as time-domain (TD-) OCT, followed by spectral-domain (SD-) OCT, which has an increased scan acquisition rate, allowing for a more detailed sampling of the area of interest. Recently, swept-source OCT (SS-OCT), a newer generation of OCT, has been introduced. Clinical assessment using multiple parameters, including peripapillary RNFL, ganglion cells, optic nerve head, and macular parameters, has proven useful for managing and diagnosing glaucoma as well as for evaluating risk in glaucoma suspects. In this chapter, we aim to evaluate the use of OCT and its modalities in diagnosis, screening, and progression of glaucoma.

Keywords: OCT, glaucoma, retinal nerve fiber layer, ganglion cell, optic nerve

1. Introduction

Glaucoma is a progressive optic neuropathy where intraocular pressure is considered to be the most significant risk factor in its etiopathogenesis. The fundamental pathology of the disease is the progressive loss of the ganglion cells. Glaucoma predominantly affects the inner macular retinal layers: the macular RNFL (mRNFL), ganglion cell layer (GCL) and inner plexiform layer (IPL) where ganglion cell complex (GCC) consists of RNFL, GCL and IPL thickness [1]. The ganglion cell damage occurs at the lamina cribrosa level in the optic disc; first, the axons get damaged, then the ganglion cells which these axons are connected to disappear through a programmed cell death called apoptosis. This loss of axons and ganglion cells cannot be identified with any clinical diagnosis methods before it exceeds a certain critical threshold [2–5]. Research in this area shows that the earliest symptom that can be detected clinically in glaucoma is the loss or thinning of the retinal nerve fiber layer (RNFL). The loss or thinning of the neuroretinal tissue is usually detected later on [6–8].

Circumpapillary RNFL (cpRNFL) and GCC thickness measurements are the parameters that have high performance in detecting glaucoma-detecting ability and are comparable to cpRNFL thickness [9–11].

OCT is an imaging method that obtains high-resolution sections of biological tissues, and it is possible to simply define this mechanism as the conversion of the light that is reflected from the tissue to an image [12–14].

Commonly used in the area of ophthalmology especially in the past 20 years, the optical coherence tomography (OCT) has provided significant contributions for the early diagnosis of the glaucoma disease and monitoring and analysis of the glaucoma patients [14–18].

2. OCT from past to present

OCT is first developed by Huang et al. in 1991, at the Massachusetts Institute of Technology in Boston [19]. Studies of Dr. Fujimoto who was an important member of the team who developed OCT, on femtosecond lasers and interferometers that can release energy in very short periods of time have been defining in terms of the development of the device [20]. The first OCT device known as the OCT-1 has been introduced by a company called Humprey, which was acquired by Carl Zeiss in 1991. In the following years, OCT-2, which had an increased resolution, and finally OCT-3 (Stratus OCT) were developed. All three devices are referred to as time domains [21–24].

This term is used more commonly, especially after the spectral domain (Fournier domain) OCT technology became available in 2002, in order to clarify the difference between the two technologies. OCT-3 is the last manufactured product with the time domain technology, which provides a significant increase in resolution compared to OCT-1 and OCT-2 [25, 26].

Today, all OCT devices that are manufactured have the spectral domain technology. Simply put, while the operating principle of time domain OCT is associated with the delay in the reflection time of light, the actual variable in spectral domain OCT is the change in the optic frequency. The important differences between these devices that demonstrate themselves on clinical basis are the high axial resolution, being affected by eye movements at a minimum level and low artifacts. To date, axial resolution obtained through spectral domain OCT devices has reached up to a value of 3 microns, and these devices are rightfully referred to as OCTs with very high speeds and very high resolutions [27, 28].

As also mentioned earlier, the OCT calculates the delay in the reflection of light from different layers of the tissue. Light reflected from the deep layers of the tissue would exhibit a longer period of delay, compared to that of the light reflected from the surface. The distribution of the intensity of the reflected light according to this period of delay is demonstrated as the axial A-mode scan. Many A-mode scans are obtained through scans across the sample, and these are converted into gray or colored scales indicating the signal intensity [29, 30].

The most critical issue for the formation of the image in OCT systems is the measurement of the time difference of the lights reflecting from different tissues, that is, the reflection delay. A reference mirror which provides the time difference is available in time domain OCTs. This mobile mirror system is a factor that limits the speed of obtaining an image in OCT. In the spectral domain OCT system on the other hand, the mirror is fixed. Thanks to this feature, the mirror movement which limits the speed is avoided [31].

In all OCT systems manufactured since the clinical use of the OCT technology, super luminescent diodes (SLDs) have been used as sources of light. In time domain OCT-3 whose axial resolution in the tissue is the highest, the resolution value is approximately 8–10 microns. Super luminescent diode lasers that could be different from each other but similar to each other in terms of the range of wave light emissions are also used in spectral domain OCT devices. Axial resolution in these devices has been lowered up to 3 microns [14].

Thanks to the development of the spectral domain OCT technology, the speed for obtaining images has also increased and risen up to 70,000 A-mode scans per second from 400 A-mode scans (OCT-3) per second. The increase in the scan speed has lowered the amount of the artifact in the image even further [32].

3. OCT use in glaucoma and some basic protocols

There are several OCT devices working with similar principles but vary in diagnostic ability, acquisition speed and resolution. In this section, three commonly used SD-OCTs that are the Spectralis (Heidelberg Engineering, Dossenheim, Germany), the Cirrus (Carl Zeiss Meditec, Dublin, CA) and the RTVue (Optovue Inc., Fremont, CA) and their features are discussed. Several studies have addressed the diagnostic accuracy of the SD-OCTs one by one or compared them to time-domain technology [1, 14, 32–42].

Since RNFL is, without a doubt one of the most important factors which is also discussed extensively in the literature, a comparison between the protocols through this value will be made and the diagnostic accuracy of this value will be examined [27].

However, in recent studies comparing protocols on the capability of OCT in the diagnosis of glaucoma, no significant differences were observed between the protocols [14, 31, 32].

4. A-Cirrus Zeiss glaucoma scanning protocol

Cirrus TM High Definition (HD)-OCT Spectral Domain (Carl Zeiss Meditec, Dublin; CA) used for the analysis of glaucoma.

At present, Cirrus high-definition (HD)-OCT is a widely used device to evaluate circumpapillary RNFL (cp-RNFL) thickness in clinical practice similarly as RTVue-100.

It is possible for us to find the necessary quantitative and qualitative data for a good management of glaucoma in this OCT device. It allows us to study the morphology and manometry of the optic disc and the peripapillary nerve fibers [37].

Even the first generation of these devices was able to display the retinal layers for us in vivo during the RNFL thickness measurement. In fact, many studies have shown the similarity between the OCT measurements and the histological sections. For this reason, the thickness of the RNFL is crucial for the early diagnosis of glaucoma and for being able to have an opinion on its progression [27, 29].

Cirrus Zeiss TM HD-OCT is an advanced technology in glaucoma research which is easy to use. It is possible for us to obtain precise and thorough information about the peripapillary area and the RNFL with this system [38, 39]. Main scanning models are provided below.

4.1. Optic disc scanning

Optic disc is recorded by Cirrus Zeiss TM HD-OCT within a 6x6 mm cube consisting of 200-B mode scans, each of which consists of 200-A mode scans. This area is divided into sections for analysis. (**Figure 1**).

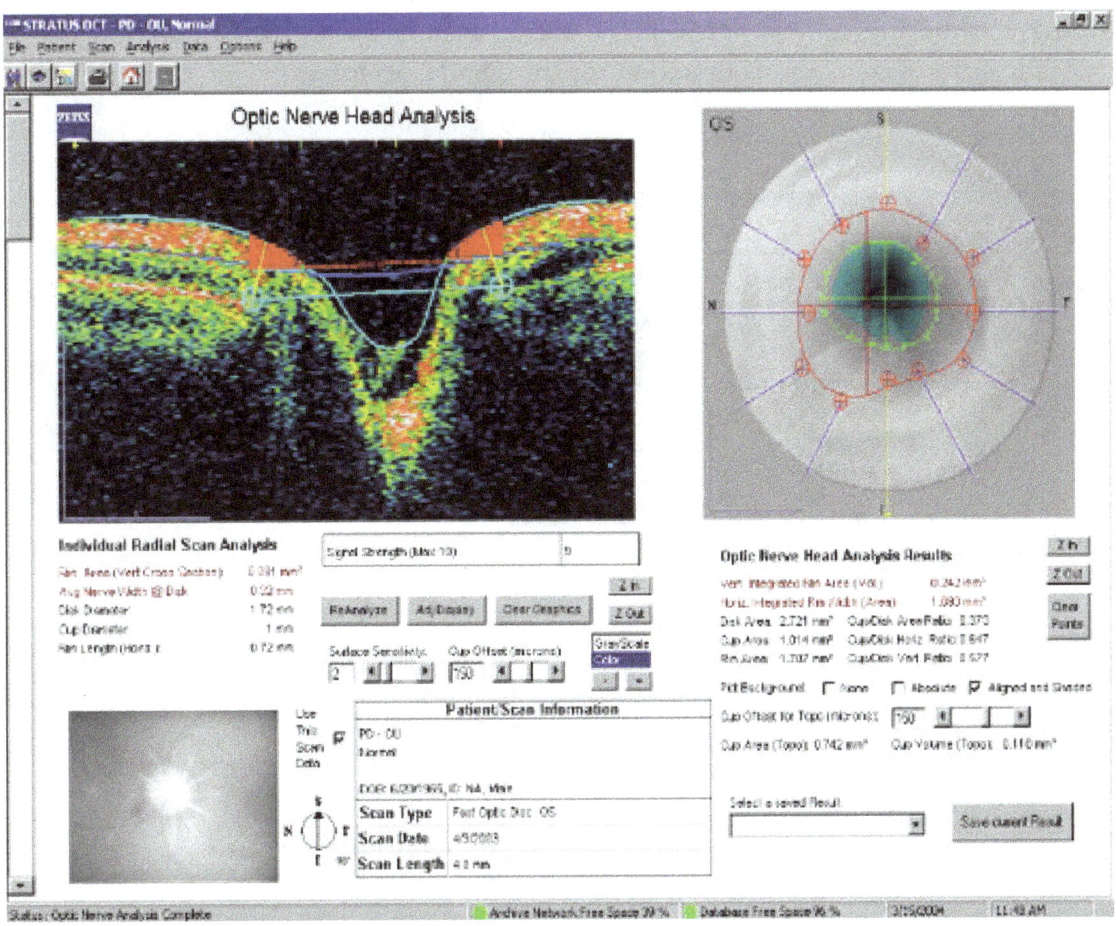

Figure 1. Optic disc scanning in Cirrus Zeiss.

The device automatically identifies the center of the optic disc through data in this cube and forms a 3.46 mm circle around the disc, which enables the RNFL thickness around the peripapillary ring to be analyzed and compared with normative data. The most important point here is the ability to perform RNFL analysis with a reliable level of precision repetitively, even though the optic disc is not placed in the center during the scan.

Signal Power.

The value of the signal power is a value between 0 and 10 for the entire scan, with 10 being the maximum value. The threshold value is 5 and signal power values lower than that represent the values that are below the acceptable threshold value. In some patients, it may not be possible to obtain high signal power. In such cases, the clinician should assess whether the signal obtained for scan analyses are acceptable or not.

4.2. Fundus image

While the fundus image is being created, the fundus image obtained through scanning laser ophthalmoscopy and the OCT fundus image are superimposed. This image appears on the upper section of the RNFL analysis screen. (**Figure 2**) The location of the calculation ring for the temporal, superior, nasal, inferior and temporal (TSNIT) section analyses is displayed in red. The operator can adjust the location of this ring following the shot if she/he likes to; however, that is often not necessary since this task is usually performed accurately through the automatic centering functionality. The B-mode scan image is the calculation ring generated from the cube of data and is flattened for the TSNIT orientation.

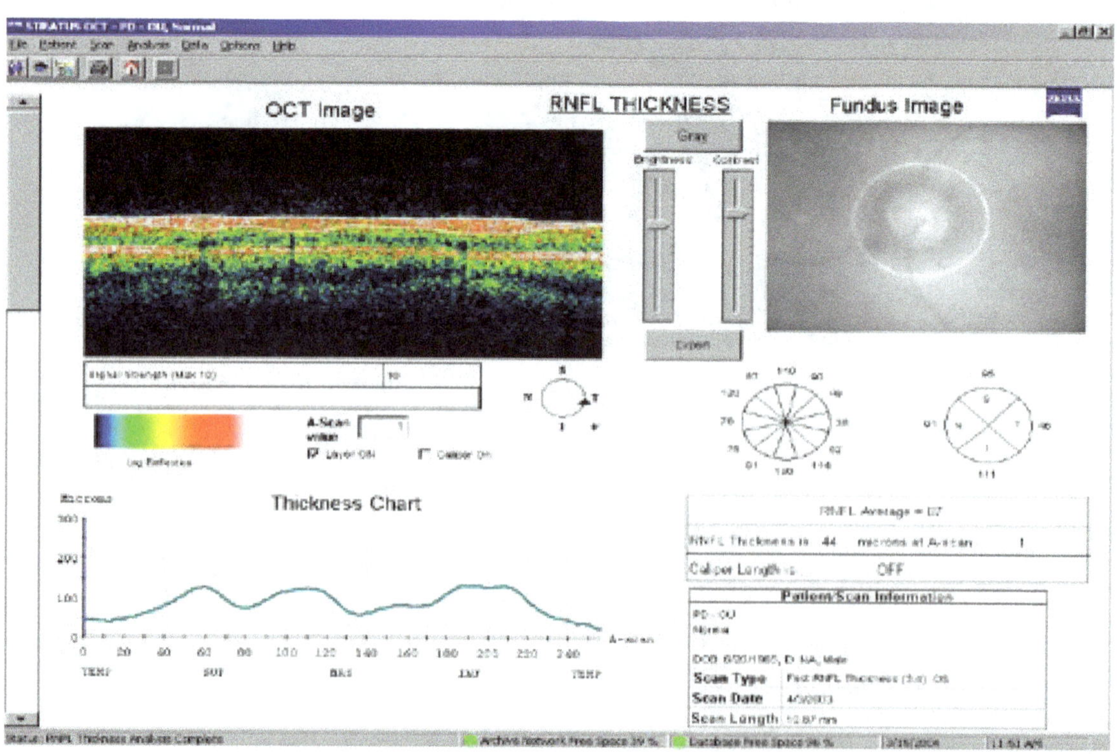

Figure 2. RNFL analysis screen in Cirrus Zeiss.

4.3. RNFL thickness map

The RNFL thickness map is calculated based on all the data of the scanned cube. The color scale used here is similar to that of a topographic map, where cold colors represent thinned areas while hot colors represent thick areas. In this way, the RNFL thickness at all points of the 6 × 6 mm area can be seen. The map excludes the optic disc displayed in dark blue. (**Figure 3**).

In the color scale used to demonstrate the normal and defective areas in the RNFL, thickness of the nerve fiber layers ranging from zero (blue) to 350 μm (white) are indicated using color codes.

4.4. Average thickness values

The RNFL thickness across the TSNIT calculation ring is also displayed in a numerical chart format. In this chart, the average thickness of each point across the calculation is demonstrated for both eyes. (**Figure 3**) In addition, average thickness for each quadrant is also demonstrated separately and in time zones. Ultimately, in all these charts, the values of the patient are compared to normative data.

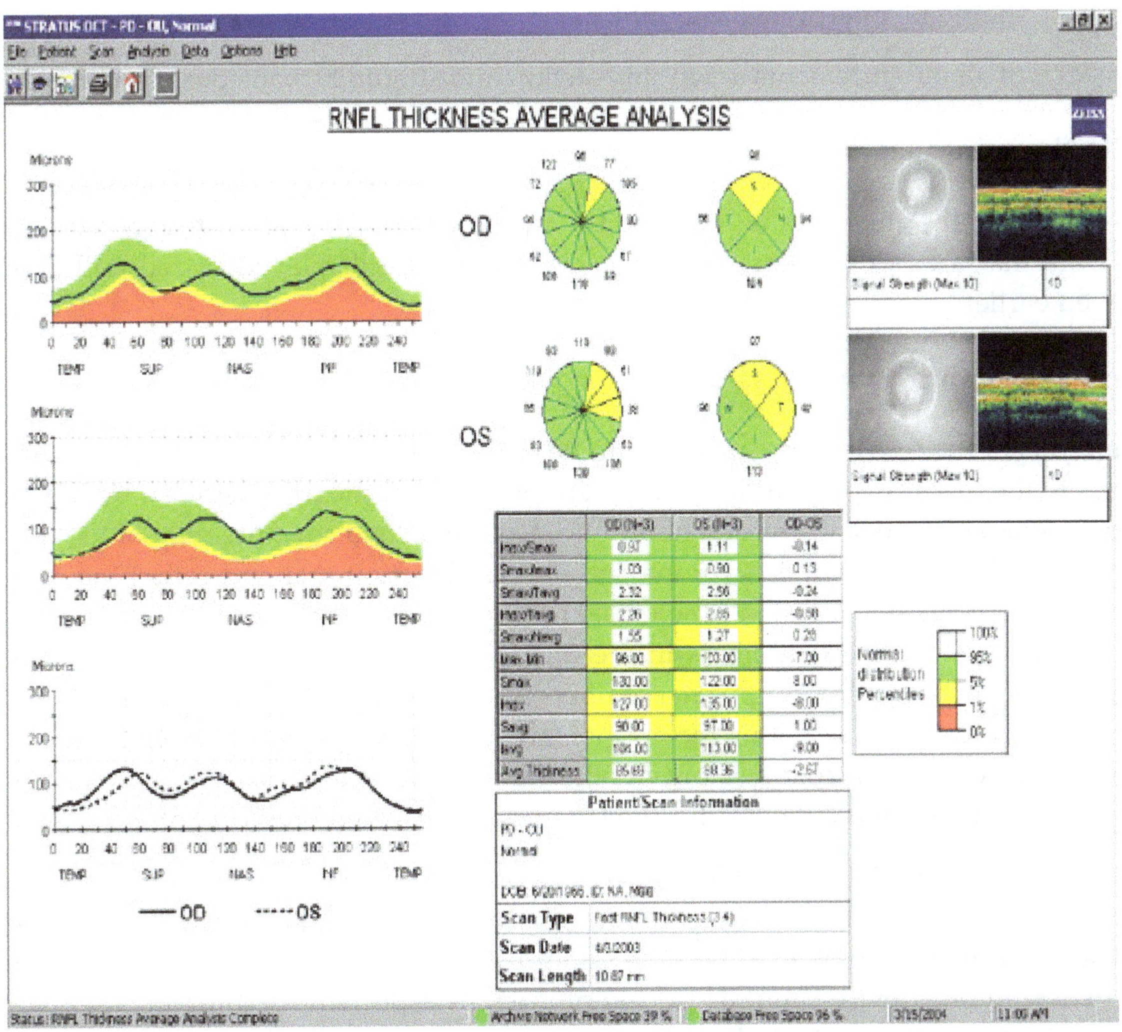

Figure 3. RNFL thickness map in Cirrus Zeiss.

4.5. TSNIT thickness profile

The TSNIT thickness profile demonstrates the RNFL thickness for each point across the peripapillary ring and compares these values to the normative database. In these comparisons of patients in the same age group, color codes (white, green, yellow and red) are used. (**Figure 3**).

4.6. The normative database for RNFL

The RNFL normative database is used for glaucoma patients who are older than 18. This database allows us to compare the patient's data in the area that we are clinically interested in, with the data of other individuals in the same age group.

In order to demonstrate the normal distribution percentages of the individuals in the same age group, the RNFL normative database uses the colors as below:

Red: The lowest portion of 1% with regard to all measurements is in the red zone and these indicators must be considered as abnormal.

Yellow: In case the measurements are within the lowest portion of 5%, they are displayed in yellow and should be interpreted as doubtful.

Green: 90% of all measurements are in this section and should be considered as normal.

4.7. The deviation map

The patient's RNFL thickness is compared with the normative data through the deviation map. Data that are out of the range of normal values are displayed in red and yellow as described earlier.

4.8. Analysis of the results

The analysis of the results for glaucoma can be easily performed at a single glance with this device. On the first row, the fundus images are provided at the top, followed by the B-mode images of the peripapillary area neighborhood. On the second row, the map of the thickness of the nerve fibers is provided, accompanied by the deviation map indicating the difference between the normal thickness and the measured thickness. On the third row, rings indicating the thickness of the nerve fibers in the quadrants are provided. On the fourth row, a colored table where the thickness of nerve fibers is indicated in microns and that allows us to understand if the values are within the normal (green), doubtful (yellow) or pathological (red) range, thanks to different colors, is provided. In the resulting analysis, data for the right eye are provided on the left, while data for the left eye are provided on the right.

In conclusion, Cirrus Zeiss TM HD-OCT device offers us good qualitative and quantitative information about the glaucomatous damage in patients [42–44]. However, the diagnosis and follow-up of glaucoma can be quite complicated at times. Therefore, since making a diagnosis with one device can mislead the physicians especially in difficult cases, comprehensive clinical exam data including the patient's visual field must be gathered while making a diagnosis.

5. Optovue-RTVue 100 glaucoma scanning protocol

In glaucoma research, four scanning models for the Optovue-RTVue spectral domain OCT (RTVue Optovue Inc. Fremont, CA) device are used.

5.1. Optic disc scanning

The optic disc is calculated through a 6 × 6 mm cube consisting of 101 lines. 3D optic disc scanning is used especially for the formation of reference lines and the determination of optic disc veins. The 3D reference line represents the optic disc limits created automatically by a software that uses the 3D optic disc scan.

5.2. Map of the optic disc head

In this protocol, 13 circular and 9 radial scans with 1.3–4.9 mm diameters around the optic disc head are performed. These scans limit the area between the retinal pigment epithelium and the optic disc head. Here, the device automatically calculates the center of the optic disc and not the center of the scan itself. The same calculation is also automatically used in progression maps (**Figure 4**).

The map of the optic disc head provides significant information about the morphology of the optic disc. It provides insight, especially on the cup-to-disc ratio of the optic disc, the 3.45 mm

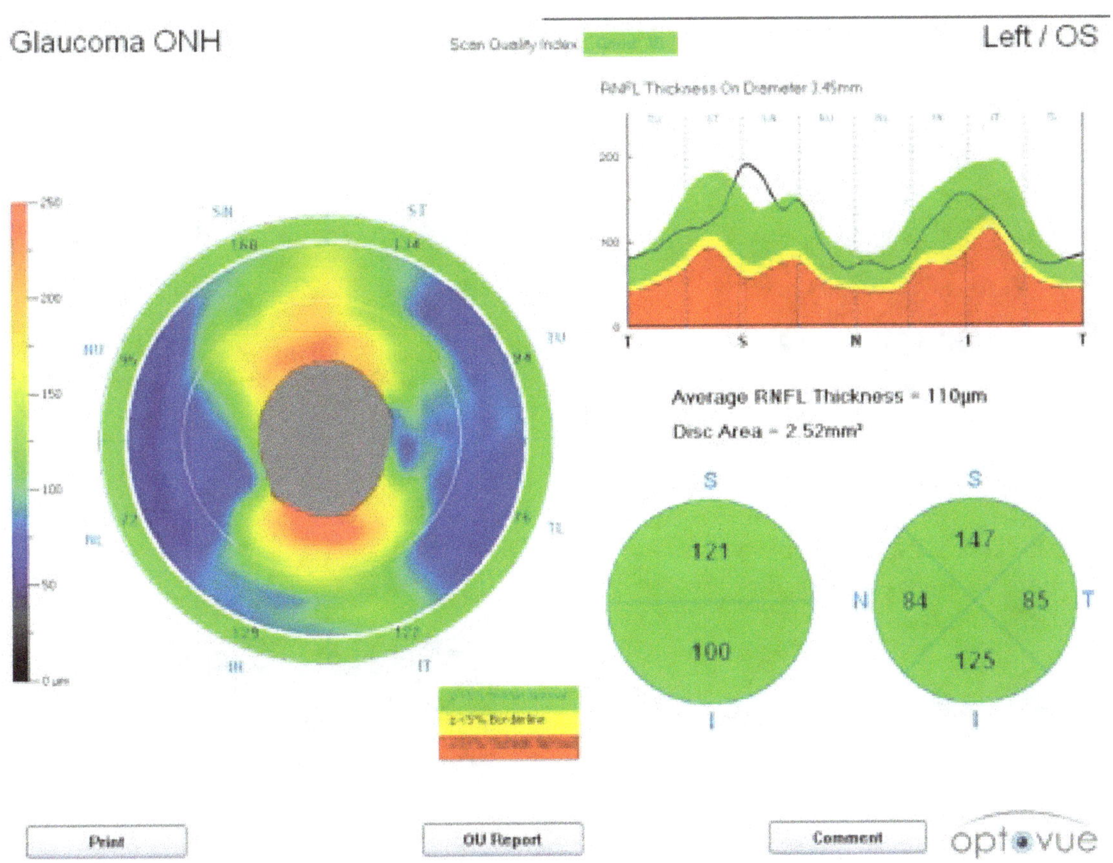

Figure 4. Optic disc head map in RTVue.

circular RNFL area whose center is the optic disc head and the RNFL area located at the rim of the optic disc, 2 mm away.

5.3. RNFL scan

This scan is used to analyze the RNFL and it has shown that RNFL parameters of the RTVue-100°CT has good specificity for the detection of glaucoma [45]. The RNFL scanning pattern completes four circular scans with diameters of 3.45 mm in 0.16 s by aiming for the optic disc head. The average of these four scans is calculated and the result is presented with normative parameters.

The RNFL thickness profile at the optic disc head is the circular RNFL thickness with a diameter of 3.45 mm, which is the central optic disc and not the center of the scan itself. Ultimately, cases where the optic disc is decentralized do not affect the measurements. The RNFL thickness map is exhibited at the lower right area and the areas that are measured to be thin have a darker color while areas that are measured to be thick have a lighter color (**Figure 5**).

In the lower right section, there is the thickness profile. Here, the RNFL thickness profile is charted temporally, superiorly, nasally, inferiorly and temporally again, in that order, beginning from around the optic disc. This thickness profile is charted as a black line by being superimposed on normative data (so that values within the normal range remain in the green-shaded area, while values outside of the normal range remain in the red-shaded area). The RNFL and the optic disc head parameters are located at the left section.

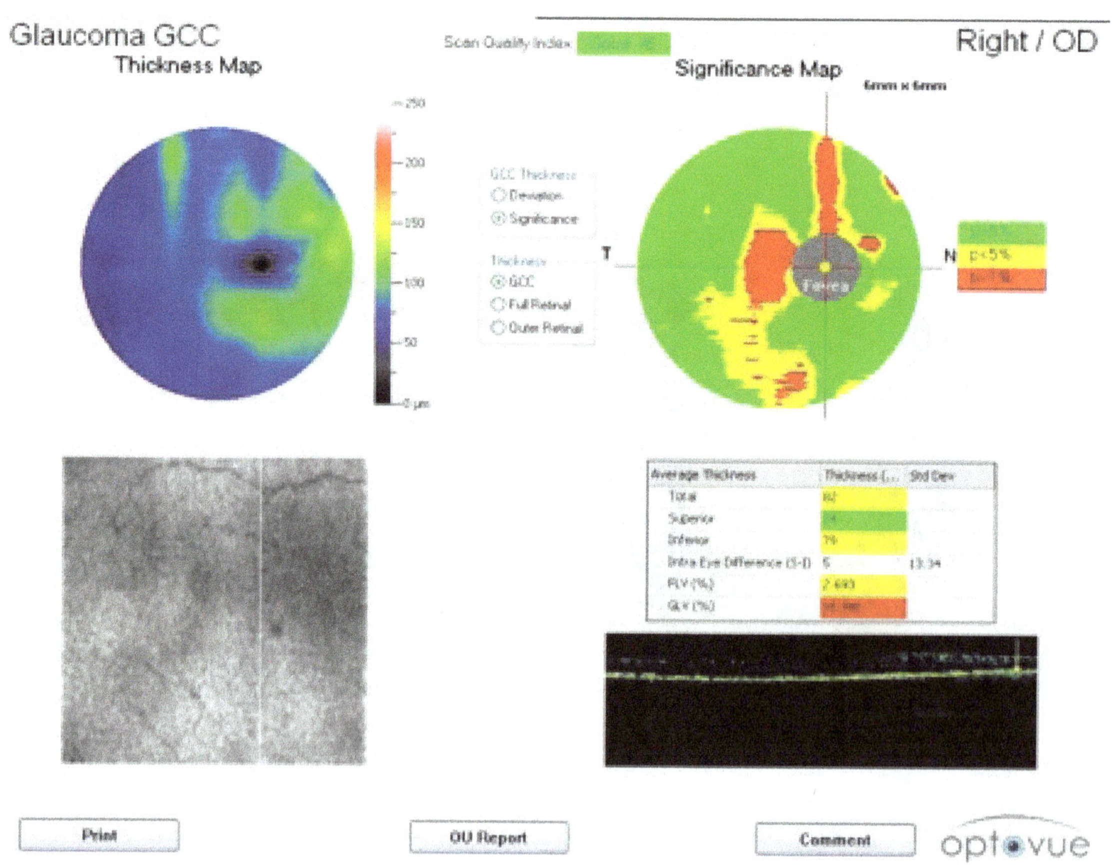

Figure 5. RNFL scan in RTVue.

5.4. RNFL glaucoma progression report

The RNFL 3.45 protocol identifies the RNFL thickness of the peripapillary area by performing circular scans with a diameter of 3.45 mm around the optic disc. What is important here is the sum of four 1024-A scans performed in 0.15 s, that is, the data of 4096 scans in total.

The RNFL output is divided into three sections. In the first section, regional RNFL thickness results are demonstrated with basal RNFL values and RNFL values of each subsequent check. The second section demonstrates the comparative TSNIT chart of RNFL, which is defined by a double hump pattern. The third section includes the value chart for average, superior and inferior RNFL. In addition, it illustrates the scans for each follow-up as a table including the changes between the basal scan and the last scan calculated in microns.

5.5. The map of the ganglion cell complex (GCC)

The GCC scan has provided new parameters for the diagnosis of glaucoma. The nerve fiber layer (NFL), the ganglion cell layer and the inner plexiform layer (IPL) make up the GCC in the macular area. Today, more emphasis is placed on GCC rather than the thickness of the whole retina in the diagnosis of glaucoma [44]. In studies regarding this issue, it has been shown that glaucoma mostly thins the nerve fibers, the ganglion cells and the IPL; and the inner nuclear layer at an intermediate level and that it does not affect the outer layers [44]. The GCC study is quite useful for the early diagnosis of glaucoma and the determination of the disease's progression, since the loss of ganglion cells occur before the visual pathway lesions and thinning of the nerve fibers [13]. RTVue, by having a mapping protocol of macular ganglion cell complex, exhibits a positive value in detecting glaucoma.

The GCC thickness is defined as the distance consisting of three inner retinal layers (nerve fiber layer, ganglion cell layer and the inner plexiform layer) beginning from the inner limiting membrane and ending at the inner plexiform layer. (**Figure 6**) All three layers are affected in glaucoma [44].

When the ganglion cells die, the ganglion cell layer gets thinner and when the axon nerve fiber layer which is a part of this cell is damaged, the nerve fiber layer gets thinner. The dendrites

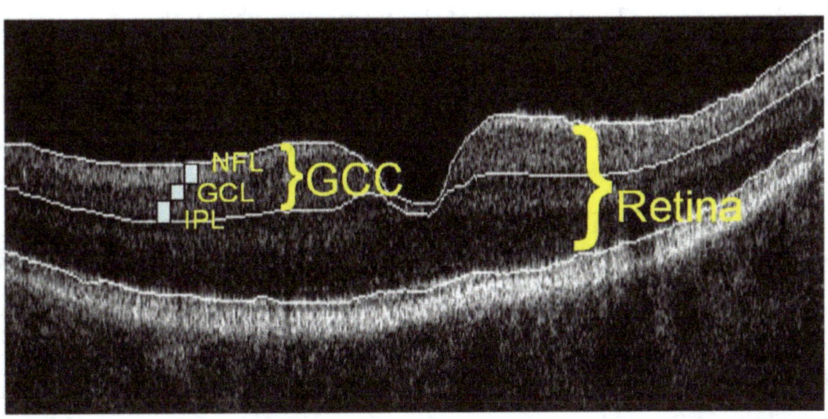

Figure 6. Anatomy of ganglion cell complex (GCC).

of the same cell are located at the inner plexiform layer and as this layer is affected, the inner plexiform layer gets thinner. So, the GCC scan measures the thickness of each of these three layers which are affected by the glaucoma [46].

Another advantage of the GCC thickness analysis is the macula's inclusion of the 50% of the ganglion cells in the retina. However, NFL is very thin in the macula and since NFLs change places to form a foveal cup there are none of them in the foveola. In the perifoveal region, the NFL is very thin but the ganglion cell layer and the IPL are much thicker [47, 48].

The scan includes 12 vertical lines and 1 horizontal line with a length of 7 mm. These lines are placed 0.5 mm away from each other and are focused on the temporal of the 1 mm fovea so that they include as many ganglion cells as possible. With this scan, the thickness map and the abnormal changes in the inner retina can be demonstrated.

The deviation map illustrates the deviations of normal values for different ages and races that are available in the normative database. The significance map reports the findings for the patient by comparing them with the normal values in the normative database on the basis of race. Red, yellow and green colors are used to note the differences in the follow-ups. It demonstrates the significance level or the statistical significance of the deviation when compared with a normal value. In short, the significance map demonstrates how significant the difference is compared to the normal value.

Another parameter here is the focal loss volume (FLV), which gives us the significant loss of GCC numerically. FLV is the sum of the significant loss of GCC topography, in terms of volume and is expressed as a percentage. At the same time, FLV is the most sensitive parameter which provides the difference between normal eyes and glaucomatous eyes (it is more sensitive than the GCC thickness parameters).

As it can be seen, while RTVue provides an excellent assessment of the ganglion cell layer it also allows a comparison to be made with the normal values, based on age and race. In follow-ups, progression analysis by RTVue compares the RNFL thickness measurements and the GCC map over time and thus, determines whether statistically significant changes have occurred or not [1, 26, 49].

5.6. GCC glaucoma progression report

The GCC progression report displays a total of four scans at the same time for both eyes, one of which is basal and the remaining three are for follow-ups. The output is divided into four sections. The first three sections are the GCC thickness map, the deviation map and the significance map. The GCC thickness map is the one coded with colors indicating the GCC thickness of the macular region. The deviation map is the one coded with colors indicating the loss percentages that the device determined according to the normal values based on the normative database. The significance map is the one demonstrating the statistically significant changes in comparison to the normal values by coding them in green, yellow and red colors. Finally, the fourth section includes the average, superior and inferior GCC chart. In this scan, the GCC thickness of the lower and upper hemisphere of the entire retina is scanned by excluding the foveal ring. Scan data are presented as changes between the basal scan and the last scan, calculated in microns.

5.7. RTVue OCT normative database

The normative database of RTVue OCT is the largest OCT normative database. As mentioned earlier, these databases allow to distinguish between normal cases and pathological ones. In this database, there are a total of 1600 eyes, 600 of which are from the USA and 1000 of which are from around the world. The data allow us to compare the measurements of the patients with measurements of other patients in the same age group. In the display coded with colors, green (normal), yellow (doubtful) and red (abnormal) are used.

It must be noted that comparisons with normative databases are only for statistical purposes and there may be normal people with values that are outside the normal range.

6. Heidelberg spectral glaucoma scanning protocol

Heidelberg Spectral Domain OCT (Spectralis, Heidelberg Engineering, Dossenheim, Germany) is an OCT device with a high scanning speed and axial resolution, allowing better reproducibility for image acquisition compared to time-domain OCT (TD-OCT) [31]. It is possible to obtain a very high-quality optic disc head image and perform peripapillary RNFL thickness analysis with this device.

In scans performed circularly, the scanned areas are automatically divided into sections while the RNFL thickness is measured and compared with the values in the normative database.

6.1. RNFL thickness profile

The OCT output in this device displays the peripapillary RNFL thickness classification by six standard pie charts:

1. Temporal (T)
2. Temporal Superior (TS)
3. Temporal Inferior (TI)
4. Nasal (N)
5. Nasal Superior (NS)
6. Nasal Inferior (NI)

In the ring which is in the middle of the pie chart, the average of the circular scan (G) is provided.

The chart in the lower right corner of the window demonstrates the RNFL thickness profile that has been measured through the circular scan and its comparison with the normal ranges. The black curve represents the RNFL thickness of the patient. In both charts, three colors are available where green represents the normal RNFL thickness, yellow represents the limit value and red represents the abnormal RNFL thickness (**Figure 7**).

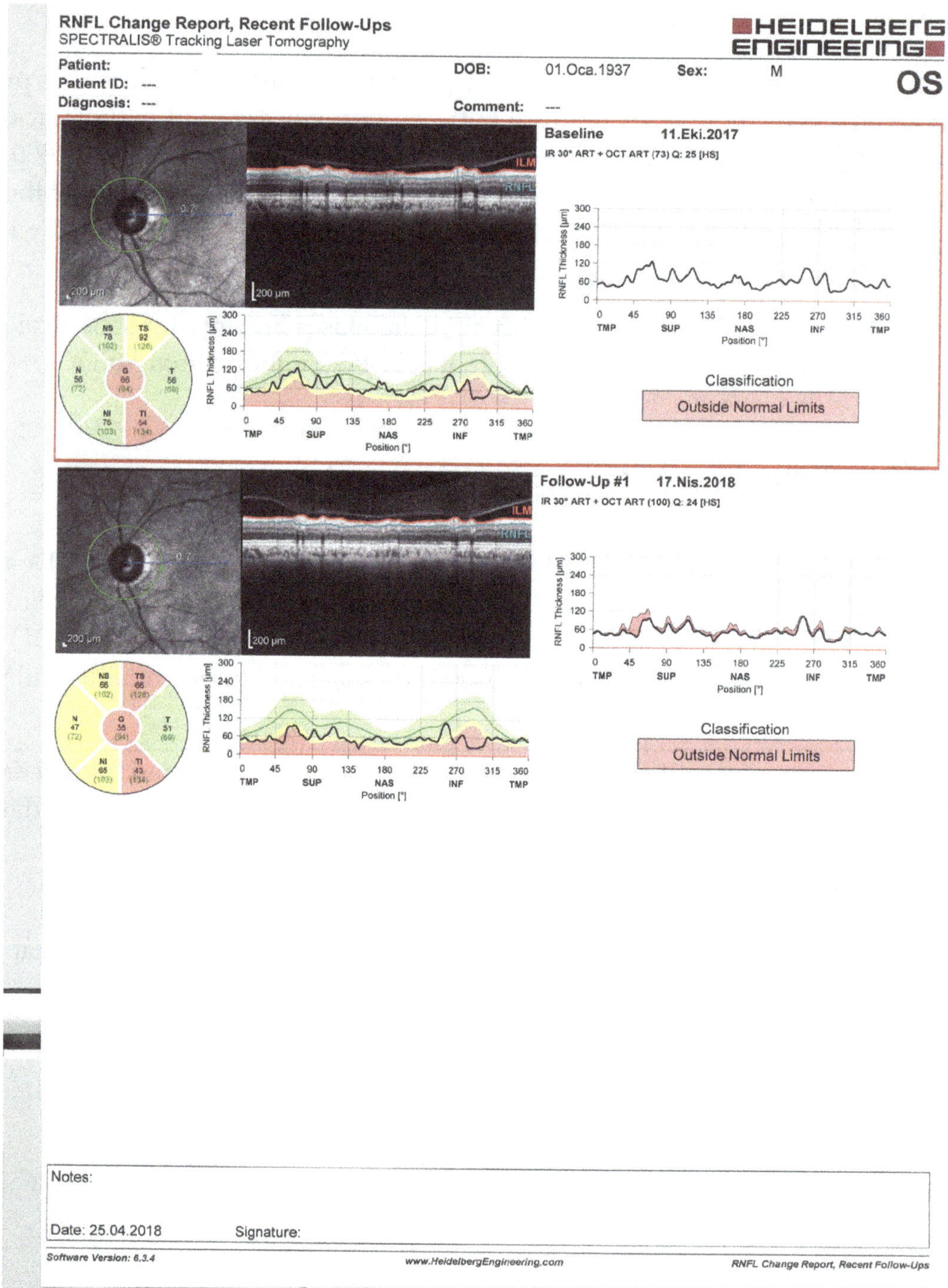

Figure 7. RNFL thickness map in Heidelberg.

On top of the output, the optic disc head scan and the real scan image of the optic disc head surroundings are provided, while the scanned image corresponding to the RNFL thickness chart is provided on the right side.

6.2. RNFL monitoring

Heidelberg spectral OCT obtains the changes in RNFL through time by using a special software formula and uses them for monitoring the patient. This software displays the rate of difference between the average measured thickness values for each section and the normal thickness values as a chart of change. Thanks to these software, changes that occur in the RNFL profile or the deterioration that occurs in the thickness over time can be detected at an early stage [50, 51].

6.3. The normative database of Heidelberg spectra OCT

There are 201 individuals registered in the normative database of this device, all of whom are Caucasian. Ages of these individuals range from 18 to 78, and 111 of them are male while 90 are female. The criteria for these people to be included in the database are naturally, their lack of a glaucoma history and the fact that they have normal intraocular pressure, visual field and optic disc appearance. The results have been organized as a normative database.

6.4. Posterior pole analysis

A new software called Posterior Pole Analysis is offered by the Heidelberg spectral OCT [33, 52]. Thickness of the entire posterior pole retina can be measured through this software. The posterior pole is scanned point by point, and the thickness asymmetry between the two eyes and the intraocular hemispheres are analyzed. Furthermore, the GCC loss is also assessed and findings for glaucoma at an early stage are analyzed through this software [53, 54].

OCT output for the analysis provides two basic maps. The first one is the map of hemisphere asymmetry while the second one is the map of RNFL thickness. The map of hemisphere asymmetry is in the form a grid where the average thicknesses of the upper and lower hemisphere are compared. Here, the squares that vertically have the same distance from the axe between the fovea and the optic disc are compared. While the squares in the upper half of the grid represent the differences between the RNFL thickness values in the superior and inferior regions, squares in the lower half represent the differences between the RNFL thickness values in the inferior and superior regions. If the difference between these values is zero or a positive value, the colored area looks white. If the area is dark gray or black, this refers to a local asymmetry in terms of RNFL thickness values.

In the literature, there are several studies evaluating the diagnostic ability of abovementioned devices with some minor differences in the results [1, 2, 6, 10, 16–21, 23–41].

Leung et al. reported that, in Spectralis, the global thickness parameter had the largest area under curve (AUC) in eyes with severe glaucoma [34]. Leite et al. reported that in Spectralis, superior quadrant RNFL followed by global RNFL, had the largest AUC and in Cirrus, global thickness was the parameter that has the largest AUC, with superior and inferior RNFL quadrants being the second and the third [54]. Park et al. and Leung et al. reported similar results with inferior, average and superior quadrant RNFL's having the best diagnostic performance for device Cirrus as Sehi et al. [29, 30, 34].

In their study, Leite et al. also showed that the diagnostic ability of all three devices for the nasal and temporal quadrants for glaucoma diagnosis was lower than the results received from the other quadrants [54]. This finding may be associated with the optic nerve damage profile in the early glaucoma where inferior and superior quadrants damaged earlier than in the nasal and temporal quadrants.

Although all these three devices represent difference in axial resolution and in time of acquisition, the final diagnostic performance for detection of glaucomatous defect generally reported to be similar.

Different results may of course be obtained due to different clinical settings, race differences, age and the severity of the disease.

In conclusion, since glaucoma is a condition that shows variations over time, it is crucial that it should be closely monitored. Especially, the change of the RNFL thickness values and the values of variation for the first and last exam of the patient must be analyzed carefully.

Acknowledgements

None.

Author details

Aydin Yildiz

Address all correspondence to: aydinyildiz@comu.edu.tr

Department of Ophthalmology, Canakkale Onsekiz Mart University, School of Medicine, Canakkale, Turkey

References

[1] Akashi A, Kanamori A, Nakamura M, Fujihara M, Yamada Y, Negi A. Comparative assessment for the ability of Cirrus, RTVue, and 3D-OCT to diagnose glaucoma. Investigative Ophthalmology & Visual Science. 2013;**54**:4478-4484

[2] Basic and Clinical Science Course (BCSC). Section 10: Glaucoma. San Francisco, CA: American Academy of Ophthalmology; 2016. pp. 20-38

[3] Weinreb RN, Aung T, Medeiros FA. The pathophysiology and treatment of glaucoma: A review. JAMA. 2014;**311**:1901-1911

[4] Medeiros FA, Alencar LM, Zangwill LM, Sample PA, Weinreb RN. The relationship between intraocular pressure and progressive retinal nerve fiber layer loss in glaucoma. Ophthalmology. 2009;**116**:1125-33 e1-3

[5] Hood DC, Kardon RH. A framework for comparing structural and functional measures of glaucomatous damage. Progress in Retinal and Eye Research. 2007;**26**:688-710

[6] Medeiros FA, Lisboa R, Weinreb RN, Liebmann JM, Girkin C, Zangwill LM. Retinal ganglion cell count estimates associated with early development of visual field defects in glaucoma. Ophthalmology. 2013;**120**:736-744

[7] Johnson CA, Sample PA, Zangwill LM, et al. Structure and function evaluation (SAFE): II. Comparison of optic disk and visual field characteristics. American Journal of Ophthalmology. 2003;**135**:148-154

[8] Jonas JB, Fernandez MC, Sturmer J. Pattern of glaucomatous neuroretinal rim loss. Ophthalmology. 1993;**100**:63-68

[9] Tan O, Chopra V, Lu AT. Detection of macular ganglion cell loss in glaucoma by Fourier-domain optical coherence tomography. Ophthalmology. 2009;**116**:2305-2314

[10] Schulze A, Lamparter J, Pfeiffer N, Berisha F, Schmidtmann I, Hoffmann EM. Diagnostic ability of retinal ganglion cell complex, retinal nerve fiber layer, and optic nerve head measurements by Fourier-domain optical coherence tomography. Graefe's Archive for Clinical and Experimental Ophthalmology. 2011;**249**:1039-1045

[11] Garas A, Vargha P, Hollo G. Diagnostic accuracy of nerve fibre layer, macular thickness and optic disc measurements made with the RTVue-100 optical coherence tomograph to detect glaucoma. Eye (London, England). 2011;**25**:57-65

[12] Pederson JE, Anderson DR. The mode of progressive disc cupping in ocular hypertension and glaucoma. Archives of Ophthalmology. 1980;**98**:490-495

[13] Hood DC, Raza AS, de Moraes CG, Liebmann JM, Ritch R. Glaucomatous damage of the macula. Progress in Retinal and Eye Research. 2013;**32**:1-211

[14] Leung CK, Cheung CY, Weinreb RN, et al. Evaluation of retinal nerve fiber layer progression in glaucoma: A study on optical coherence tomography guided progression analysis. Investigative Ophthalmology & Visual Science. 2010;**51**:217-222

[15] Medeiros FA, Alencar LM, Zangwill LM, Bowd C, Sample PA, Weinreb RN. Prediction of functional loss in glaucoma from progressive optic disc damage. Archives of Ophthalmology. 2009;**127**:1250-1256

[16] Wollstein G, Schuman JS, Price LL, et al. Optical coherence tomography longitudinal evaluation of retinal nerve fiber layer thickness in glaucoma. Archives of Ophthalmology. 2005;**123**:464-470

[17] Jaffe GJ, Caprioli J. Optical coherence tomography to detect and manage retinal disease and glaucoma. American Journal of Ophthalmology. 2004;**137**:156-169

[18] Manassakorn A, Nouri-Mahdavi K, Caprioli J. Comparison of retinal nerve fiber layer thickness and optic disk algorithms with optical coherence tomography to detect glaucoma. American Journal of Ophthalmology. 2006;**141**:105-115

[19] Huang D, Swanson EA, Lin CP, Schuman JS, Stinson WG, Chang W, Hee MR, Flotte T, Gregory K, Puliafito CA, et al. Optical coherence tomography. Science. 1991;**254**:1178-1181

[20] Fujimoto JG, Pitris C, Boppart SA, Brezinski ME. Optical coherence tomography: An emerging technology for biomedical imaging and optical biopsy. Neoplasia. 2000;**2**:9-25

[21] Hougaard JL, Heijl A, Bengtsson B. Glaucoma detection by stratus OCT. Journal of Glaucoma. 2007;**16**:302-306

[22] Parikh RS, Parikh S, Sekhar GC, et al. Diagnostic capability of optical coherence tomography (Stratus OCT 3) in early glaucoma. Ophthalmology. 2007;**114**:2238-2243

[23] Nouri-Mahdavi K, Nikkhou K, Hoffman DC, Law SK, Caprioli J. Detection of early glaucoma with optical coherence tomography (Stratus OCT). Journal of Glaucoma. 2008;**17**:183-188

[24] Lee EJ, Kim TW, Park KH, Seong M, Kim H, Kim DM. Ability of stratus OCT to detect progressive retinal nerve fiber layer atrophy in glaucoma. Investigative Ophthalmology & Visual Science. 2009;**50**:662-668

[25] Medeiros FA, Zangwill LM, Alencar LM, et al. Detection of glaucoma progression with stratus OCT retinal nerve fiber layer, optic nerve head, and macular thickness measurements. Investigative Ophthalmology & Visual Science. 2009;**50**:5741-5748

[26] Gonzalez-Garcia AO, Vizzeri G, Bowd C, et al. Reproducibility of RTVue retinal nerve fiber layer thickness and optic disc measurements and agreement with stratus optical coherence tomography measurements. American Journal of Ophthalmology. 2009;**147**: 1067-74, 74 e1

[27] Sull AC, Vuong LN, Price LL, et al. Comparison of spectral/Fourier domain optical coherence tomography instruments for assessment of normal macular thickness. Retina. 2010;**30**:235-245

[28] Medeiros FA, Zangwill LM, Bowd C, Vessani RM, Susanna R Jr, Weinreb RN. Evaluation of retinal nerve fiber layer, optic nerve head, and macular thickness measurements for glaucoma detection using optical coherence tomography. American Journal of Ophthalmology. 2005;**139**:44-55

[29] Park SB, Sung KR, Kang SY, Kim KR, Kook MS. Comparison of glaucoma diagnostic capabilities of Cirrus HD and stratus optical coherence tomography. Archives of Ophthalmology. 2009;**127**:1603-1609

[30] Sehi M, Grewal DS, Sheets CW, Greenfield DS. Diagnostic ability of Fourier-domain vs time-domain optical coherence tomography for glaucoma detection. American Journal of Ophthalmology. 2009;**148**:597-605

[31] Kim JS, Ishikawa H, Gabriele ML, et al. Retinal nerve fiber layer thickness measurement comparability between time domain optical coherence tomography (OCT) and spectral domain OCT. Investigative Ophthalmology & Visual Science. 2010;**51**:896-902

[32] Johnson DE, El-Defrawy SR, Almeida DR, Campbell RJ. Comparison of retinal nerve fibre layer measurements from time domain and spectral domain optical coherence tomography systems. Canadian Journal of Ophthalmology. 2009;**44**:562-566

[33] Knight OJ, Chang RT, Feuer WJ, Budenz DL. Comparison of retinal nerve fiber layer measurements using time domain and spectral domain optical coherent tomography. Ophthalmology. 2009;**116**(7):1271-1277. [PubMed: 19395086]

[34] Leung CK, Cheung CY, Weinreb RN, et al. Retinal nerve fiber layer imaging with spectral-domain optical coherence tomography: A variability and diagnostic performance study. Ophthalmology. 2009;**116**(7):1257-1263. 63, e1-2. [PubMed: 19464061]

[35] Sung KR, Kim DY, Park SB, Kook MS. Comparison of retinal nerve fiber layer thickness measured by Cirrus HD and stratus optical coherence tomography. Ophthalmology. 2009;**116**(7):1264-1270. 70, e1. [PubMed: 19427696]

[36] Vizzeri G, Weinreb RN, Gonzalez-Garcia AO, et al. Agreement between spectral-domain and timedomain OCT for measuring RNFL thickness. The British Journal of Ophthalmology. 2009;**93**(6):775-781. [PubMed: 19304586]

[37] Hwang YH, Kim YY, Kim HK, Sohn YH. Ability of Cirrus high- definition spectral-domain optical coherence tomography clock- hour, deviation, and thickness maps in detecting photographic retinal nerve fiber layer abnormalities. Ophthalmology. 2013;**120**:1380-1387

[38] Kotowski J, Folio LS, Wollstein G, et al. Glaucoma discrimination of segmented Cirrus spectral domain optical coherence tomography (SD-OCT) macular scans. The British Journal of Ophthalmology. 2012;**96**:1420-1425

[39] Sung KR, Na JH, Lee Y. Glaucoma diagnostic capabilities of optic nerve head parameters as determined by Cirrus HD optical coherence tomography. Journal of Glaucoma. 2012;**21**:498-504

[40] Bengtsson B, Andersson S, Heijl A. Performance of time-domain and spectral-domain optical coherence tomography for glaucoma screening. Acta Ophthalmologica. 2012;**90**: 310-315

[41] Leite MT, Zangwill LM, Weinreb RN, et al. Effect of disease severity on the performance of Cirrus spectral-domain OCT for glaucoma diagnosis. Investigative Ophthalmology & Visual Science. 2010;**51**:4104-4109

[42] Curcio CA, Allen KA. Topography of ganglion cells in human retina. The Journal of Comparative Neurology. 1990;**300**:5-25

[43] Arintawati P, Sone T, Akita T, Tanaka J, Kiuchi Y. The applicability of ganglion cell complex parameters determined from SD-OCT images to detect glaucomatous eyes. Journal of Glaucoma. 2013;**22**:713-718

[44] Zhang C, Tatham AJ, Weinreb RN, et al. Relationship between ganglion cell layer thickness and estimated retinal ganglion cell counts in the glaucomatous macula. Ophthalmology. 2014;**121**:2371-2379

[45] Paul C. To assess the glaucoma diagnostic ability of Fourier domain optical coherence tomography. American Journal of Engineering Research. 2013;**2**(11):104-110

[46] Mwanza JC, Durbin MK, Budenz DL, et al. Glaucoma diagnostic accuracy of ganglion cell-inner plexiform layer thickness: Comparison with nerve fiber layer and optic nerve head. Ophthalmology. 2012;**119**:1151-1158

[47] Kim NR, Lee ES, Seong GJ, Kim JH, An HG, Kim CY. Structure- function relationship and diagnostic value of macular ganglion cell complex measurement using Fourier-domain OCT in glaucoma. Investigative Ophthalmology & Visual Science. 2010;**51**:4646-4651

[48] Mansouri K, Leite MT, Medeiros FA, Leung CK, Weinreb RN. Assessment of rates of structural change in glaucoma using imaging technologies. Eye. 2011;**25**:269-277

[49] Cho JW, Sung KR, Lee S, et al. Relationship between visual field sensitivity and macular ganglion cell complex thickness as measured by spectral-domain optical coherence tomography. Investigative Ophthalmology & Visual Science. 2010;**51**:6401-6407

[50] Naithani P, Sihota R, Sony P, et al. Evaluation of optical coherence tomography and Heidelberg retinal tomography parameters in detecting early and moderate glaucoma. Investigative Ophthalmology & Visual Science. 2007;**48**:3138-3145

[51] Kim NR, Lee ES, Seong GJ, Choi EH, Hong S, Kim CY. Spectral-domain optical coherence tomography for detection of localized retinal nerve fiber layer defects in patients with open-angle glaucoma. Archives of Ophthalmology. 2010;**128**:1121-1128

[52] Rao HL, Zangwill LM, Weinreb RN, Sample PA, Alencar LM, Medeiros FA. Comparison of different spectral domain optical coherence tomography scanning areas for glaucoma diagnosis. Ophthalmology. 2010;**117**:1692-9, 9 e1

[53] Grewal DS, Tanna AP. Diagnosis of glaucoma and detection of glaucoma progression using spectral domain optical coherence tomography. Current Opinion in Ophthalmology. 2013;**24**:150-161

[54] Leite MT, Rao HL, Zangwill LM, Weinreb RN, Medeiros FA. Comparison of the diagnostic accuracies of spectralis, Cirrus and RTVue optical coherence tomography devices in glaucoma. Ophthalmology. 2011 July;**118**(7):1334-1309

7

Optic Nerve Changes in Diabetic Retinopathy

Andi Arus Victor

Abstract

Diabetic retinopathy (DR) is a devastating sight-threatening complication of diabetes mellitus (DM). Besides damaging the vascular system of the retina, DM will also destruct the tissue surrounding the retina, including the optic nerve. DR impairs the optic nerve by damaging its conduction and integrity. There are few clinical manifestations of optic nerve changes in DR such as diabetic papillopathy, neovascularization of optic disc, and optic nerve atrophy. These involve metabolic alterations related to DM, production of advanced glycation end products (AGEs), oxidative stress, and hemodynamic changes. Diagnostic tests including visual evoked potential (VEP) and optical coherence tomography (OCT) can detect functional and structural changes. This finding is important as it may reflect the early loss of retinal ganglion cell axons. As the neuronal loss is irreversible, it is pivotal to be able to screen these nervous system changes in the early stage of DR and prevent further deterioration.

Keywords: diabetes mellitus, diabetic papillopathy, diabetic retinopathy, neovascularization of optic disc, optical coherence tomography, optic nerve, optic atrophy, visual evoked potential

1. Introduction

Diabetic retinopathy (DR), a devastating sight-threatening complication of diabetes mellitus (DM), is one of the most prevalent health diseases worldwide with an incidence of 6.9% [1–3]. The number of people with diabetes is estimated to rise from 171 million in 2000 to 366 million in 2030. A study by Jin et al. in DM type 2 population showed that within 5 years, the cumulative incidence of DR was 46.9% with 13.9% population suffering from severe nonproliferative DR (NPDR) and 4.6% from proliferative DR (PDR). Hence, more people will be at risk of developing DR and in danger of losing their sight [4, 5].

DM endangers sight by damaging the neurovascular system of the eye, including the optic nerve [6, 7]. The damages include changes in angioarchitecture, blood flow and degenerative loss of neural tissue, morphological changes, changed protein expression, and changed neurotransmission and neurotransmitters [6–9]. Recently, not so many studies have been conducted to elucidate damage due to DM and DR in the optic nerve and central visual pathway. We hypothesize that optic nerve damage occurs due to few processes in DM. Such processes are metabolic alteration, oxidative stress, and ischemia [10]. These changes could be detected via modalities such as visual evoked potential, biomicroscopy, and fundus photography [11–13]. These changes usually occur after persistent metabolic alterations, which may lead to late detection [2, 14]. Therefore, early detection of optic nerve involvement in DR may be beneficial to provide timely recognition and management for patients at greater risk of DR progression [14].

2. Pathophysiology

There are few processes in DR affecting the optic nerve. Such processes are metabolic alterations related to DM, production of advanced glycation end products (AGEs), oxidative stress, and hemodynamic changes. These processes will be discussed in detail below.

2.1. Metabolic alterations

Findings from animal studies suggest that neurodegeneration in DR is caused by both diminished insulin receptor signaling and systemic hyperglycemia [15–17]. Insulin plays an important role, as insulin receptors in the retina stimulate neuronal development, growth, and anabolic synthesis [18, 19]. Therefore, a defect in insulin function either due to a low level of insulin or impaired sensitivity would hamper neuroretinal cells' survival. As diabetes progresses, retinal neurons start to degenerate by apoptosis within weeks after the onset [20, 21]. Metabolic alteration and hormonal factors might affect balance of some mediators including growth factors, cytokines, inflammatory, and adhesion molecules [22]. These alterations result in abnormal capillary permeability, apoptosis of capillary cells, and angiogenesis [23].

Metabolic alteration also damages neural conduction in the postretinal central visual pathway [10]. A recent study in diabetic rats showed that there is reduction of Na^+/K^+/ATPase enzyme in the optic nerve [24]. This enzyme is important for maintaining sodium potassium gradient within cells and controls the membrane axon depolarization/repolarization. When impaired, it suggests that the neuronal conduction and integrity are damaged.

2.2. Advanced glycation end products

Hyperglycemia induces reaction of sugar and protein via Maillard reaction and produces advanced glycation end products (AGEs) [25, 26]. AGEs play a huge role in complications of DM as it triggers further oxidative stress and vascular cross-linking and activates pro-inflammatory cytokines [20, 21]. Neriyanuri et al. reported that AGEs were independent predictors of development of DR in addition to blood glucose and glycated hemoglobin [14].

AGEs are long-lasting, irreversible products that can modify blood vessel elasticity [25]. High-level AGEs in the optic disc affect elasticity of lamina cribrosa. As the intraocular pressure increases, cribriform plates become unable to bear the strain. This condition may develop into glaucoma in DR [27].

2.3. Oxidative stress

Hyperglycemia stimulates increased flux through the glycolytic and tricarboxylic acid cycle pathways, hence resulting in excessive electrons within mitochondria [28]. These electrons would react with oxygen and form reactive oxygen species (ROS). Since mitochondria as cells' powerhouse also generate ROS on their own, they are also the first ones to be damaged by increased ROS. This results in reduced mitochondrial energy production, later causing loss of cellular and tissue function [29].

Oxidative stress also contributes to neural retinal ganglion cell and optic nerve injury through the impairment of L-glutamate/L-aspartate transporter (GLAST), which increases extracellular accumulation of glutamate and promotes excitotoxicity [30–32]. Glutamate is a neurotransmitter that plays a role in the regulation of neurohormonal activity and is found in high levels in the central nervous system. Upon stimulation of nerve cells, glutamate molecules are released from the glutamatergic synaptic vesicles and cause depolarization of the postsynaptic neuronal membrane, which generates signal. Accumulated glutamate in the synaptic space is then collected by adjacent astrocytes, afterward being broken down into glutamine [21].

In patients with DR, glutamate accumulates in extracellular space due to the following mechanisms: (1) reduction of Müller cell–specific enzyme glutamine synthetase, which converts glutamate to glutamine; (2) decrease in the retinal ability to oxidize glutamate to α-ketoglutarate; and (3) impairment of glutamate uptake by the glial cells [29]. The accumulation of glutamate results in overactivity of ionotropic glutamate receptors, such as α-amino-3-hydroxyl-5-methyl-4-isoxazole-propionate (AMPA) and N-methyl-D-aspartate (NMDA) receptors, which later causes uncontrolled intracellular calcium response in postsynaptic neurons and eventually cell death [33, 34]. Recent studies suggest that glutamate excitotoxicity results in apoptotic degenerative lesions [25]. Glutamate toxicity also causes depletion of glutathione, which is an antioxidant, thus contributing to oxidative stress [35].

A recent study in diabetic rats also showed marked increase in oxidative stress level shown by malondialdehyde (MDA) level in the optic nerve and visual cortex. In addition, they also found reduced antioxidant, glutathione (GSH), in both the optic nerve and visual cortex [24]. These results suggest significant oxidative stress in the optic nerve and visual cortex along with impairment in neuronal conduction and integrity. Other studies have also found similar result, showing impaired retrograde and anterograde axonal transport in the optic nerve of diabetic rats along with retinal ganglion cell axonopathy [36, 37]. A study by Sokol et al. showed that when induced with ischemia, myelinated axons degenerated and became disordered [38]. Further changes are swollen and collapsed axons, and by 90th minute, myelin sheaths were fragmented. Joachim et al. found axonal damage and gliosis of the optic nerve after ocular ischemia. Renner et al. found damaged optic nerve in an ischemic rat model. Histologic examination revealed demyelination and subsequent loss of myelin sheaths after ischemia [39]. In addition, they also found marked microglia activation, upregulation of astrocytes, reduction of myelin basic protein and myelin oligodendrocyte glycoprotein (MOG), as well as the reduction in oligodendrocytes [40]. The optic nerve structure was also affected as neurofilament was found to be distorted after 21 days of ischemia/reperfusion induction. Ischemia also seemed to impair neuronal immune system as the study found destroyed astroglia structure, hence leaving the nerve tissue susceptible to insults, i.e., oxidative stress [40].

2.4. Hemodynamic changes

Chronic hyperglycemia damages the retinal blood vessels and causes pericyte loss due to elevated sorbitol level. These result in involution of the vascular changes in microcirculation and loss of normal capillary exchange [12–14]. Microvascular anomalies and chronic inflammation may develop dysfunctional barriers permitting leakage of inflammatory molecules and immune cells from systemic circulation and cause further deterioration of the tissue [12, 41].

Another process that plays a major part in DR is capillary degeneration due to weakness and dilation of capillary walls' saccular outpouching, commonly known as microaneurysms. Rupture of these microaneurysms leads to leakage of endovascular products, including blood [9]. In DR, blood viscosity was significantly higher, thus resulting in reductions in blood flow. Persistent uncorrected blood flow causes chronic mild hypoperfusion, which might lead to ischemia and a rise in waste products [42, 43].

Accumulation of these molecules and cells leads to retinal occlusion, which later progresses into hypoxia [44]. Hypoxia results in upregulation of vascular endothelial growth factor (VEGF) platelet adhesiveness, erythrocyte aggregation, serum lipids, and fibrinolysis [45, 46]. VEGF promotes new blood vessel growth resulting in abnormal neovascularization [47].

3. Clinical manifestation

There are few clinical manifestations of optic nerve damage related to DM and DR that can be observed. Those are diabetic papillopathy, neovascularization of optic disc, and optic nerve atrophy [48]. Those will be discussed further below.

3.1. Diabetic papillopathy

3.1.1. Definition

Diabetic papillopathy (DP) is an ocular manifestation of both type 1 and type 2 DM characterized by unilateral or bilateral hyperemic disc swelling with minimal or no optic nerve dysfunction, which generally resolves without medical intervention [49, 50]. Patients with DP are often asymptomatic, but may sometimes experience transient decrease in visual acuity [50]. It is usually self-limiting and tends to resolve over a period of 2–10 months with the average time of 3.7 months, leaving minimal sequelae [51, 52]. Visual acuity generally recovers to better than 20/30 in most patients [53].

DP typically affects young people with type 1 DM, but it has also been reported to occur in elderly patients with type 2 DM. The prevalence of DP in both types of DM is 0.5% and the percentage of DP patients presenting with nonproliferative diabetic retinopathy (NPDR) is higher than in the proliferative diabetic retinopathy (PDR) [49].

3.1.2. Pathophysiology

The pathophysiology of diabetic papillopathy remains poorly understood and several theories have been suggested [49]. Some researchers suggest that DP is a subtype of anterior ischemic optic neuropathy (AION), but there are different features between DP and AION that others argue that it is a completely different pathological process [49, 50]. For instance, DP is an asymptomatic optic disc edema, whereas AION is an acute optic disc infarction [54, 55]. Researchers support the argument that the pathophysiology of DP is distinguishable from AION [50]. A study evaluating fluroangiographic aspects by Brancato et al. showed robust leakage of fluorescein, suggesting that DP is a local nonhypotensive vasculopathy [56]. These findings are supported by Bayraktar et al. and Regillo et al., who showed notable telangiectatic vasculature and fluroangiographic hyperfluorescence [54, 57]. Meanwhile, case studies of AION by Hayreh et al. and Shin et al. demonstrated notable filling defects in fluroangiography [55, 58]. These findings of AION contrast with the hyperfluorescence that has been noted in cases of DP.

In patients with DP, the degree of DR tends to be mild. Regillo et al. observed that DP might be a separate entity rather than extension of DR [57]. Otherwise, a case series by Ostri et al. reported that three out of four patients with DP who already had DR before proceeded to develop high-risk PDR. This condition is called "early worsening phenomenon of DR " where progression of retinopathy and papillopathy was accelerated, while adaptation was remarkably slow in the very first year [59]. Bayraktar et al. also reported two cases of nonproliferative diabetic retinopathy (NPDR), which later on were also diagnosed as having DP. A 3-month follow-up showed that retinopathy worsened and developed into proliferative diabetic retinopathy (PDR) [54]. Lubow et al. found that two of three patients with DP subsequently developed PDR and vitreous hemorrhage [60]. Hayreh et al. reported similar findings and observed three patients with DP, who later on were also diagnosed as having PDR [55]. Hence, DP should be considered as a risk factor for progression to PDR and patients should be observed closely taking into account this possibility [54].

Early DP study by Appen et al. hypothesized that DP patients sustain a local vasculopathy of the optic disc, presumably in relation to diabetes [61]. This vasculopathy induces transient leakage of fluid, which results in disc edema. The authors also suggest that the presence of edema causes axoplasmic flow turmoil. An earlier study by Freund et al. showed that prolonged hyperglycemia and anoxia due to the failure of glucose utilization cause damages to the optic nerve [62]. Recent study by Slagle et al. suggested that clinically visible interstitial edema of the optic nerve head due to vascular hyperpermeability initiates the pathology of DP [50].

Slagle et al. elucidate that tissue perfusion depends on two main factors: (1) the ability of the blood to reach the tissue through patent vessels and (2) the dispersion of nutrients to the tissue via fluid movement through the capillary bed. There are four primary forces that determine perfusion: (1) capillary pressure, (2) interstitial fluid pressure, (3) plasma colloid osmotic pressure, and (4) interstitial fluid colloid osmotic pressure [50]. The authors hypothesized that impairment in the transportation and reabsorption of fluid through the capillary walls causes capillary vasostatic perfusion pathology. Diabetes causes damages to vascular endothelium, which leads to initial vasculopathy characterized by increased vascular permeability [53]. Along with loss of pericytes, this causes hemodynamics and autoregulation derangements [53, 63].

In the early stage of diabetic vasculopathy, the hyperpermeability of diabetic capillaries causes excessive protein to spill from the plasma into the interstitium. This leads to the offsets of physiological osmotic gradient, creating deficiency in fluid reabsorption on the venule end of the capillary bed. Edema occurs when the lymphatic system is unable to correct this imbalance [50]. The typical transient initial edematous course of DP suggests that optic nerve capillaries are susceptible to this vasculopathy. Edema compresses vessels leading to ischemia as well as stagnates and prolongs cellular exposure to toxic effects from free radicals and cellular waste. In addition, edema might also compress nerve fibers causing axoplasmic flow derangements [61, 62, 64]. These hypotheses would explain the reported fluroangiographic hyperfluorescence in DP, its relatively benign nature compared to AION, and its transient course [50].

In the later stage of DP, ischemia may result from leukostasis-derived capillary occlusion due to retinal leukostasis effect and thickened capillary basement membranes, which affect retinal capillary endothelial function, perfusion, angiogenesis, and vascular permeability [64]. This results in a clinical picture resembling more like traditional AION sequelae with optic atrophy [50].

3.1.3. Clinical features

The main features of DP are painless visual loss, macular edema, disc hyperfluorescence on fluroangiography, and significant visual improvement after treatment [49, 54]. Differential diagnoses include infection, inflammation, metastatic infiltration, hypertension, and papilledema [52, 57, 65].

3.1.4. Diagnostic studies

Certain diagnostic criteria have to be met in order to recognize diabetic papillopathy. The current accepted diagnostic criteria include (1) confirmed diagnosis of diabetes; (2) unilateral or bilateral presence of optic disc edema; (3) normal intracranial pressure; (4) absence of inflammation, infiltration, or infection in the optic disc; and (5) a lack of substantial optic nerve dysfunction [50, 51]. Supportive examination to confirm DP includes fluorescein angiography (FA), orbital magnetic resonance imaging (MRI), and blood tests ranging from serum angiotensin-converting enzyme (ACE), antinuclear antibody (ANA), vitamin B12, folate, erythrocyte sedimentation rate (ESR), C reactive protein (CRP) to fluorescent treponemal antibody test [49].

3.1.5. Treatment

There is no evidence that the resolution of DP and the prevention of permanent visual loss can be promoted by definitive treatment. As stated before, in most cases, the edema resolves within a few months (average of 3.7 months) to no visual impairment [49]. Because of its self-limiting nature, the most common management is serial examinations. However, due to potential visual sequelae noted in certain cases, more efforts have to be made to identify at-risk patients and effective treatment to prevent this sequela.

Although originally thought to be related to glycemic control, systemic glucose manipulation has not shown any benefits in DP [51]. Hence, how diabetes treatment should be titrated to protect visual function in DP remains uncertain [59]. Current treatment aims to reduce disc edema in DP, including intravitreal anti-VEGF, which has been shown to increase visual acuity and decrease disc edema, and also periocular corticosteroids, which stabilizes the blood-ocular barrier at the disc [65–69].

3.2. Neovascularization of optic disc

3.2.1. Definition

Diabetic retinopathy is often associated with neovascular proliferation due to ischemia in the retina and release of angiogenic factors. These conditions cause neovascularization of the optic disc (NVD), also neovascularization elsewhere (NVE) [70, 71]. Patients with NVD have a poor visual prognosis due to high incidence of complication, such as vitreous hemorrhage, fibrous proliferation, and traction retinal detachment. NVD occurring in DR can be accompanied by NVE and NVI (neovascularization of the iris), which later on may develop into neovascular glaucoma (NVG), which is an optic neuropathy defined by changes in the optic nerve and associated with visual field defects and elevated intraocular pressure [70]. Recent studies have shown that PDR is the leading cause of neovascular glaucoma [72].

3.2.2. Pathophysiology

In DR, capillary occlusion and reduced perfusion in retina provoke cascade events related to hypoxia and lead to angiogenesis. Normally, pro-angiogenic factors (VEGF and angiopoietin-2) and antiangiogenic factors (pigment epithelium-derived growth factor) are in equilibrium [71]. Imbalance between those factors might trigger activation, proliferation, and migration of endothelial cells and pericytes and lead to neovascularization [71–73]. VEGF is produced in a variety of neuroretinal cells and plays a major part in promoting intraocular neovascularization. Inflammatory cytokines interleukin-6 (IL-6) is also correlated with the degree of neovascularization patients. Other potential pro-angiogenic factors include basic fibroblast growth factor (bFGF), transforming growth factor-beta 1 and -beta 2, nitric oxide, and endothelin-1 [73].

The new vessels at the disc can bleed spontaneously or with minimal trauma. The blood spills into the retina and between the retina and vitreous causing vitreoretinal hemorrhage. This condition attracts fibroglial elements and finally resulting in separation between inner layers of the retina and the underlying retinal pigment epithelium, which is known as tractional retinal detachment [3]. NVD and NVI do not always develop into NVG, although neovascularization always develops prior to intraocular pressure increase. This is primarily due to fibrovascular membrane that develops on the iris and iridocorneal angle, which later causes anterior synechiae, angle closure, and intraocular pressure elevation [49, 74].

3.2.3. Clinical features

In early stages of neovascularization, patients may be asymptomatic or may present with low vision. Ocular findings can be subtle in early stage, so case history and complete ocular examination are important to make early diagnosis [71–73].

3.2.4. Diagnostic studies

Fundus examination might trace the new vessels of the optic disc and reveal glaucomatous optic nerve damage [73–75]. In fluorescein angiography (FA), leakage from damaged vessels could be detected before development of visible neovascularization. Even though FA can aid early detection, the test is not always available [73, 76]. Using OCT angiography (OCTA), neovascularization around the optic disc at the level of the vitreous cavity might be observed in a faster and safer way [75]. Electroretinography and retinal angiography can be necessary to determine the origin of neovascularization in the retina. Meanwhile, gonioscopy is a low-cost and fast test, which can reveal NVI [73, 76].

3.2.5. Treatment

Early diagnosis will enable early treatment and prevent blindness due to optic nerve neovascularization. Tight glycemic control is also important [75]. Medical intervention to prevent further visual loss related to NVG is associated with lowering the IOP levels using topical β-adrenergic antagonists, α-2 agonists, and carbonic anhydrase inhibitors. Topical corticosteroid can also be used to reduce inflammation [73]. The main treatment for preventing NVD and NVE in DR is laser photocoagulation. Panretinal photocoagulation laser therapy in early stages is beneficial by inhibiting and reversing neovascularization [74]. Use of anti-VEGF, cyclophotocoagulation, cryotherapy, and surgery are among other therapeutic options.

3.3. Optic nerve atrophy

3.3.1. Definition

Optic nerve atrophy is the end result of any disease that causes optic nerve damage anywhere along the path from the retina to the lateral geniculate. Degeneration of axon will manifest as changes in color and structure of the optic disc. It is associated with variable degrees of visual dysfunction, including congenital, vascular, metabolic, inflammatory condition, trauma, and neoplasm [77, 78].

3.3.2. Pathophysiology

Optic nerve atrophy could result from many processes related to DM and DR. Such processes include neurodegeneration, oxidative stress, and ischemia. It may also develop as a result of optic nerve abnormalities mentioned above. Further study should be carried out to distinguish whether optic nerve atrophy occurs as a result of DR or complications of laser photocoagulation [10, 24, 36].

3.3.3. Clinical features

The main symptom of optic atrophy is vision loss. In optic nerve atrophy, axon loss and myelin shrinkage will show the pallor-appearing disc, widening of the optic cup, and decreased Kestenbaum index (less than 6) [78].

3.3.4. Diagnostic studies

Optic nerve atrophy is easy to diagnose, but finding the etiology is challenging. Further diagnostic test is necessary to identify the etiology of optic atrophy. Imaging study, such as ultrasonography, CT, and MRI, is used depending on the disease process. Other diagnostic tests are visual acuity testing, color vision testing, contrast sensitivity test, visual field testing, electroretinography, optical coherence tomography, and visual evoked response [78].

3.3.5. Treatment

No proven treatment is able to return the function of atrophic optic nerve. Experts believe that treatment initiated before the development of optic nerve atrophy can be very useful to save the remaining function. The goal of primary intervention is to prevent axon degeneration by finding and treating the cause of optic atrophy. In diabetic patients, tight glycemic control and early detection of DR are very important. If the main problem is found and well-treated, further damage can be prevented [78].

4. Diagnostic approach for detecting optic nerve changes in diabetic retinopathy

Various examination methods have been used to detect functional and structural optic nerve changes in patients with diabetic retinopathy.

4.1. Visual functional test

4.1.1. Visual acuity

As has been known, neurodegeneration is a progressive loss of structure and function of neurons. The quality of visual acuity (VA) depends on the normal condition of visual pathway. Visual acuity test is the standard test of visual function. There are two commonly used tools for evaluating VA, including the Snellen VA chart and the Early Treatment Diabetic Retinopathy Study (ETDRS) VA chart. The Snellen VA chart is a frequently used chart for measuring VA. This consists of different type, size, and number of letters in each row. In contrast, ETDRS-VA chart has an equal number of characters per row with relatively uniform legibility. Some studies agree that ETDRS-VA chart has more advantages over the Snellen VA chart. Moreover, besides VA tests, some experts suggested that psychophysical tests, such as visual field and contrast sensitivity test, should also be evaluated in DR patients with optic nerve complication. They found that those examinations were more sensitive than VA test only [13].

4.1.2. Contrast sensitivity

Contrast sensitivity is a test of the inner retina, with different spatial frequencies in specific neural pathways [13]. There is no algorithm to define the pattern of contrast sensitivity alteration in the early stage of DR. Adachi, Jochim, and Renner. observed reduced contrast sensitivity only at single low spatial frequency in cases of non–insulin-dependent diabetes mellitus without DR [79–81]. Meanwhile, Joltikov et al. and Safi et al reported decline in contrast sensitivity at all spatial frequencies early in the course of diabetic retinal sensory neuropathy [14, 82]. Joltikov et al. suggested that contrast sensitivity might be the most sensitive test for detection of subtle functional impairment in diabetic patients with or without retinopathy. In addition, contrast sensitivity test is more practical than electroretinography [13]. However, longitudinal study showed that reduced contrast sensitivity in the earlier stage of the disease might be reversible [82].

4.1.3. Visual fields

Another visual function affected by neurodegeneration is visual fields. A common test for evaluating the visual field in diabetic retinopathy is perimetry. Various perimetry methods have been applied including white-on-white standard automated perimetry (SAP), frequency doubling technology perimetry (FDP), short-wavelength automated perimetry (SWAP), and rarebit perimetry (RBP) [83, 84]. Bengtsson et al. suggested that SAP and SWAP are more sensitive to neuroretinal impairment than ETDRS-VA chart [85]. Safi et al. reported that by using microperimetry, it might detect a reduction of foveal sensitivity in diabetic patients with preclinical stage of DR [82].

4.1.4. Color vision test

Many color vision tests have been assessed in diabetic patients with and without retinopathy diabetes, including Lanthony desaturated D-15, Farnsworth-Munsell 100-Hue, and chromatography tests. However, studies recommended that Farnsworth-Munsell 100-hue test has higher sensitivity than the other tests. This test has been recommended as a screening test for DR patients [82].

4.1.5. Visual evoked potential

Visual evoked potential (VEP) is a noninvasive test that evaluates the visual pathways by recording the electric signal in response to a bright flash of light [86, 87]. Changes of amplitudes and latencies in VEP reflects impairment in ganglion cells and optic nerve [88]. Clinical conditions that cause a delay in VEP latencies include papillitis, neuritis, toxic optic neuropathies, multiple sclerosis, glaucoma, and conditions affecting conducting media [89].

Khatoon observed that the pattern of VEP responses may provide early diagnosis of optic nerve involvement in DR and define the prognosis [88]. Onset of diabetes blood glucose control might affect the result of VEP [89]. In diabetic patients, VEP amplitude was reduced progressively with an increase of latency as the years pass [87]. Farisa et al. showed that P100 latency was prolonged among diabetic patients compared to nondiabetic subjects [88].

Progressive delay in VEP latency reflects damage of ganglion cell, even before the first ophthalmoscopically noticeable signs arise. VEP should be done as a screening tool for detecting optic nerve involvement in DR. Thus, early and proper management can be done to prevent further ocular damage [88].

4.2. Structural test

4.2.1. Fundus photography

Fundus photography is a noninvasive examination for documenting clinical signs and monitoring the progression or improvement of retinal diseases over time. One of the purposes of fundus photography is screening DR in diabetic patients. This method is useful for illustrating normal and abnormal morphology of the retina [90, 91]. Some signs of neurodegeneration in DR patients could be screened by fundus photography, including papilledema and macular edema. However, the result of fundus photography is a two-dimensional image; thus, it is difficult to accurately assess the detailed morphology of the retina leading to a high false-positive rate. In addition, in the condition of vitreous hemorrhage or low-quality image, some part of the retina could not be evaluated [10, 48].

4.2.2. Fundus fluorescein angiography

Fundus fluorescein angiography (FFA) is an invaluable imaging method demonstrating an interaction of fluorescent within the anatomic structure of ocular fundus. FFA is the gold standard in evaluating retinal vascularization. FFA has early and late phase. Early phase demonstrates following the injection until complete filling of retinal arteries, arterioles, and capillaries, while the late phase demonstrates filling of veins until gradual elimination of the fluorescent from the retinal vasculature. Hypofluorescence occurs due to a vascular filling defect or a secondary condition of a blocking effect, while hyperfluorescence may occur due to fluorescein leakage, staining, or pooling [10, 24, 36].

4.2.3. Optical coherence tomography

Optical coherence tomography (OCT) is a high-resolution imaging modality to measure retinal morphology, including vitreoretinal interface, neurosensory retina, and subretinal space [48]. We can measure the retinal layer thickness and segmentation [92, 93]. OCT provides an accurate assessment with low specificity value [48]. OCT is divided into two types: spectral domain (SD) and time domain (TD) [2]. TD-OCT is mostly used in neuro-ophthalmology to measure peripapillary retinal nerve fiber layer (RNFL) thickness. Peripapillary RNFL thickness increases in disc edema and decreases in optic nerve atrophy [94]. The results of OCT can be used as a guide for making therapeutic decision.

4.2.4. Optical coherence tomography angiography

Optical coherence tomography angiography (OCT-A) is a three-dimensional noninvasive chorioretinal vascular imaging to observe the microvascular structures of new vessels, including

NVD and NVE [95]. OCT-A can analyze blood flow in the vessels without dye injections. In FFA, it sometimes showed artifacts due to dye leakage effect. OCT-A is superior to FFA in determining the number, course, size, and extension of NVD [96].

5. Conclusion

Changes in the optic nervous system may start prior to classic clinical manifestation of DR. The development of an integrated multimodal approach for detecting optic nerve involvement in DR is important for early diagnosis in preclinical stage DR and reducing diabetic complications.

Conflict of interest

There are no conflicts of interest in this chapter.

Author details

Andi Arus Victor

Address all correspondence to: arvimadao@yahoo.com

Department of Ophthalmology, Faculty of Medicine, Universitas Indonesia, Cipto Mangunkusumo National General Hospital, Jakarta, Indonesia

References

[1] Abcouwer SF, Gardner TW. Diabetic retinopathy: Loss of neuroretinal adaptation to the diabetic metabolic environment. Annals of the New York Academy of Sciences. 2014;**1311**: 174-190. DOI: 10.1111/nyas.12412

[2] Mazumder AG, Chatterjee S, Chatterjee S, Gonzalez JJ, Bag S, Ghosh S, et al. Spectro-pathology-corroborated multimodal quantitative imaging biomarkers for neuroretinal degeneration in diabetic retinopathy. Journal of Clinical Ophthalmology. 2017;**11**:2073-2089. DOI: 10.2147/OPTH.S140110

[3] Nentwich MM, Ulbig MW. Diabetic retinopathy—ocular complications of diabetes mellitus. World Journal of Diabetes. 2015;**6**(3):489-499. DOI: 10.4239/wjd.v6.i3.489

[4] Wild S, Roglic G, Green A, Sicree R, King H. Global prevalence of diabetes. Diabetes Care. 2004;**27**(5):1047-1053. DOI: 10.2337/diacare.27.5.1047

[5] Wu L, Fernandez-Loaiza P, Sauma J, Hernandez-Bogantes E, Masis M. Classification of diabetic retinopathy and diabetic macular edema. World Journal of Diabetes. 2013;**4**(6):290-294. DOI: 10.4239/wjd.v4.i6.290

[6] Barber AJ, Lieth E, Khin SA, Antonetti DA, Buchanan AG, Gardner TW. Neural apoptosis in the retina during experimental and human diabetes. The Journal of Clinical Investigation. 1998;**102**(4):783-791

[7] Barber AJ, Gardner TW, Abcouwer SF. The significance of vascular and neural apoptosis to the pathology of diabetic retinopathy. Investigative Ophthalmology & Visual Science. 2011;**52**:1156-1163

[8] Chen X, Nie C, Gong Y, Zhang Y, Jin X, Wei S, et al. Peripapillary retinal nerve fiber layer changes in preclinical diabetic retinopathy: A meta-analysis. PLoS One. 2015;**10**(5):e0125919. DOI: 10.1371/journal.pone.0125919

[9] Pekel E, Tufaner G, Kaya H, Kasikci A, Deda G, Pekel G. Assessment of optic disc and ganglion cell layer in diabetes mellitus type 2. Medicine. 2017;**96**(29):e7556. DOI: 10.1097/MD.0000000000007556

[10] Gregori B, Galié E, Pro S, Clementi A, Accornero N. Luminance and chromatic visual evoked potentials in type I and II diabetes: Relationships with peripheral neuropathy. Neurological Sciences. 2006;**27**:323-327

[11] Zheng Y, He M, Congdon N. The worldwide epidemic of diabetic retinopathy. Indian Journal of Ophthalmology. 2012;**60**(5):428-431. DOI: 10.4103/0301-4738.100542

[12] Pemp B, Palkovits S, Howorka K, Pumprla J, Sacu S, Garhöfer G, et al. Correlation of retinal neurodegeneration with measures of peripheral autonomic neuropathy in type 1 diabetes. Acta Ophthalmologica. 2018:1-7. DOI: 10.1111/aos.13733. DOI: 10.1111/aos.13733

[13] Joltikov KA, deCastro VM, Davila JR, Anand R, Khan SM, Farbman N, et al. Multidimensional functional and structural evaluation reveals neuroretinal impairment in early diabetic retinopathy. Investigative Ophthalmology & Visual Science. 2017;**58**:BIO277-BIO290. DOI: 10.1167/iovs.17-21863

[14] Neriyanuri S, Pardhan S, Gella L, Pal SS, Ganesan S, Sharma T, et al. Retinal sensitivity changes associated with diabetic neuropathy in the absence of diabetic retinopathy. The British Journal of Ophthalmology. 2017;**101**(9):1174-1178. DOI: 10.1136/bjophthalmol-2016-309641

[15] Adams AJ, Bearse MA. Retinal neuropathy precedes vasculopathy in diabetes: A function-based opportunity for early treatment intervention? Clinical and Experimental Optometry. 2012;**95**(3):256-265

[16] Heng LZ, Comyn O, Peto T, Tadros C, Ng E, Sivaprasad S, et al. Diabetic retinopathy: Pathogenesis, clinical grading, management and future developments. Diabetic Medicine. 2013;**30**:640-650. DOI: 10.1111/dme.12089

[17] Jiao C, Abramoff MD, Lee K. Diabetes induced neurodegeneration in the retina and the brain of mice are associated and independent of microvasculopathy. Investigative Ophthalmology and Visual Science. 2017;**58**:5195

[18] Rajala RVS, Anderson RE. Rhodopsin-regulated insulin receptor signaling pathway in rod photoreceptor neurons. Molecular Neurobiology. 2010;**42**(1):39-47. DOI: 10.1007/s12035-010-8130-8

[19] Rajala RVS. Phosphoinositide 3-kinase signaling in the vertebrate retina. Journal of Lipid Research. 2010;**51**(1):4-22. DOI: 10.1194/jlr.R000232

[20] Stem MS, Gardner TW. Neurodegeneration in the pathogenesis of diabetic retinopathy: Molecular mechanisms and therapeutic implications. Current Medicinal Chemistry. 2014; **20**(26):3241-3250

[21] Kergoat H, Hérard ME, Lemay M. RGC sensitivity to mild systemic hypoxia. Investigative Ophthalmology & Visual Science. 2006;**47**(12):5423-5427. DOI: 10.1167/iovs.06-0602

[22] Abcouwer SF. Angiogenic factors and cytokines in diabetic retinopathy. Journal of Clinical and Cellular Immunology. 2013;**11**:1. DOI: 10.4172/2155-9899

[23] Victor AA, Sitompul R. Proliferative diabetic retinopathy: An overview of vitreous immune and biomarkers. In: Tsin A, editor. Early Events in Diabetic Retinopathy and Intervention Strategies Andrew Tsin. IntechOpen; 2018. pp. 71-91. DOI: 10.5772/intechopen.74366. Available from: https://www.intechopen.com/books/early-events-in-diabetic-retinopathy-and-intervention-strategies/proliferative-diabetic-retinopathy-an-overview-of-vitreous-immune-and-biomarkers

[24] Catanzaro OL, Capponi JA, Di Martino I, Labal ES, Sirois P. Oxidative stress in the optic nerve and visual area of steptozocin-induced diabetic Wistar rats: Blockade with selective bradykinin B1 receptor antagonist. Neuropeptides. 2017;**66**:97-102. DOI: 10.1016/j.npep.2017.10.003

[25] Kadłubowska J, Malaguarnera L, Wąż P, Zorena K. Neurodegeneration and neuroinflammation in diabetic retinopathy: Potential approaches to delay neuronal loss. Current Neuropharmacology. 2015;**14**:831-839. DOI: 10.2174/1570159X14666160614095559

[26] Yu Y, Chen H, Su SB. Neuroinflammatory responses in diabetic retinopathy. Journal of Neuroinflammation. 2015;**12**:141. DOI: 10.1186/s12974-015-0368-7

[27] Amano S, Kaji Y, Oshika T, Oka T, Machinami R, Nagai R, et al. Advanced glycation end products in human optic nerve head. The British Journal of Ophthalmology. 2001; **85**:52-55

[28] Madsen-Bouterse SA, Kowluru RA. Oxidative stress and diabetic retinopathy: Patho physiological mechanisms and treatment perspectives. Reviews in Endocrine & Metabolic Disorders. 2008;**9**(4):315-327. DOI: 10.1007/s11154-008-9090-4

[29] Simó R, Hernández C. Neurodegeneration in the diabetic eye: New insights and therapeutic perspectives. Trends in Endocrinology and Metabolism. 2014;**25**(1):23-33. DOI: 10.1016/j.tem.2013.09.005

[30] Xiao C, He M, Nan Y, Zhang D, Chen B, Guan Y, et al. Physiological effects of superoxide dismutase on altered visual function of retinal ganglion cells in db/db mice. PLoS One. 2012;**7**(1):e30343. DOI: 10.1371/journal.pone.0030343

[31] Fukumoto M, Nakaizumi A, Zhang T, Lentz SI, Shibata M, Puro DG. Vulnerability of the retinal microvasculature to oxidative stress: Ion channel-dependent mechanisms. American Journal of Physiology. Cell Physiology. 2012;**302**(9):C1413-C1420. DOI: 10.1152/ajpcell.00426.2011

[32] Li Q, Puro DG. Diabetes-induced dysfunction of the glutamate transporter in Müller cells. Investigative Ophthalmology & Visual Science. 2002;**43**(9):3109-3116

[33] Ng YK, Zeng XX, Ling EA. Expression of glutamate receptors and calcium-binding proteins in the retina of streptozotocin-induced diabetic rats. Brain Research. 2004;**1018**(1): 66-72. DOI: 10.1016/j.brainres.2004.05.055

[34] Santiago AR, Gaspar JM, Baptista FI, Cristóvão AJ, Santos PF, Kamphuis W, et al. Diabetes changes the level of ionotropic glutamate receptors in the rat retina. Molecular Vision. 2009;**15**:1620-1630

[35] Kaur C, Foulds WS, Ling EA. Hypoxia-ischemia and retinal ganglion cell damage. Clinical Ophthalmology. 2008;**2**(4):879-889

[36] Zhang L et al. Alterations in retrograde axonal transport in optic nerve of type I and type II diabetic rats. The Kobe Journal of Medical Sciences. 1998;**44**:205-215. [PubMed: 10401224]

[37] Fernandez DC et al. Early distal axonopathy of the visual pathway in experimental diabetes. The American Journal of Pathology. 2012;**180**:303-313. DOI: 310.1016/j.ajpath. 2011.1009.1018. Epub 2011 Nov 1010. [PubMed: 22079928]

[38] Sokol S, Moskowitz A, Skarf B. Contrast sensitivity in diabetics with and without background retinopathy. Archives of Ophthalmology. 1985;**103**(1):51-54

[39] Katz G, Levkovitch-Verbin H, Treister G, et al. Mesopic foveal contrast sensitivity is impaired in diabetic patients without retinopathy. Graefe's Archive for Clinical and Experimental Ophthalmology. 2010;**248**(12):1699-1703

[40] Racette L, Sample PA. Short-wavelength automated perimetry. Ophthalmology Clinics of North America. 2003;**16**:227-236. vi-vii

[41] Lynch SK, Abràmoff MD. Diabetic retinopathy is a neurodegenerative disorder. Vision Research. 2017;**139**(2017):101-107. DOI: 10.1016/j.visres.2017.03.003

[42] Peduzzi M, Melli M, Fonda S, Codeluppi L, Guerrieri F. Comparative evaluation of blood viscosity in diabetic retinopathy. International Ophthalmology. 1984;**7**(1):15-19

[43] Rimmer T, Fleming J, Kohner EM. Hypoxic viscosity and diabetic retinopathy. British Journal of Ophthalmology. 1990;**74**:400-404

[44] Victor AA, Gondhowiardjo TD, Waspadji S, Wanandi SI, Bachtiar A, Suyatna FD, et al. Effect of laser photocoagulation and bevacizumab intravitreal in proliferative diabetic retinopathy: Review on biomarkers of oxidative stress. Medical Journal of Indonesia. 2014;**23**(2):79-86

[45] Bandello F, Rosangela L, Zucchiatti I, Del Turco C. Pathophysiology and treatment of diabetic retinopathy. Acta Diabetologica. 2013;**50**(1):1-20

[46] Antonetti DA, Klein R, Gardner TW. Mechanisms of disease diabetic retinopathy. The New England Journal of Medicine. 2012;**366**:1227-1239

[47] Tarr JM, Kaul K, Chopra M, Kohner EM, Chibber R. Pathophysiology of diabetic retino pathy. ISRN Ophthalmology. 2013;**2012**:1-13

[48] Ghanchi F, Bailey C, Chakravarthy U, Cohen S, Dodson P, Gibson J, et al. Diabetic Retino pathy Guidelines. London: The Royal College of Ophthalmologists; 2012. pp. 9-64

[49] Sayin N, Kara N, Pekel G. Ocular complications of diabetes mellitus. World Journal of Diabetes. 2015;**6**(1):92-108. DOI: 10.4239/wjd.v6.i1.92

[50] Slagle WS, Musick AN, Eckermann DR. Diabetic papillopathy and its relation to optic nerve ischemia. Optometry and Vision Science. 2009;**86**:E395-E403. DOI: 1040-5488/09/8604-0395/0

[51] Giuliari GP, Sadaka A, Chang PY, Cortez RT. Diabetic papillopathy: Current and new treatment options. Current Diabetes Reviews. 2011;**7**(3):171-175

[52] Barbera LG, Weiss MJ, Hofeldt AJ. Diabetic retinopathy and diabetic papillopathy. Seminars in Neurology. 1996;**16**(2):179-185

[53] Ciulla TA, Amador AG, Zinman B. Diabetic retinopathy and diabetic macular edema: Pathophysiology, screening, and novel therapies. Diabetes Care. 2003;**26**:2653-2664

[54] Bayraktar Z, Alacali N, Bayraktar S. Diabetic papillopathy in type II diabetic patients. Retina. 2002;**22**:752-758

[55] Hayreh SS, Zimmerman MB. Nonarteritic anterior ischemic optic neuropathy: Clinical characteristics in diabetic patients versus nondiabetic patients. Ophthalmology. 2008;**115**:1818-1825

[56] Brancato R, Menchini U, Bandello FM. Diabetic papillopathy: Fluorangiographic aspects. Metabolic, Pediatric, and Systemic Ophthalmology. 1986;**9**:57-61

[57] Regillo CD, Brown GC, Savino PJ, Byrnes GA, Benson WE, Tasman WS, et al. Diabetic papillopathy: Patient characteristics and fundus findings. Archives of Ophthalmology. 1995;**113**:889-895

[58] Shin SY, Kim DS, Ko MK. Fluorescein angiographic features of choroidal insufficiency in anterior ischemic optic neuropathy. Korean Journal of Ophthalmology. 1999;**13**:100-104

[59] Ostri C, Lund-Andersen H, Sander B, Hvidt-Nielsen D, Larsen M. Bilateral diabetic papillopathy and metabolic control. Ophthalmology. 2010;**117**:2214-2217. DOI: 10.1016/j.ophtha.2010.03.006

[60] Lubow M, Makley T. Pseudopapilledema of juvenile diabetes mellitus. Archives of Ophthalmology. 2007;**85**:417-422

[61] Appen RE, Chandra SR, Klein R, Myers FL. Diabetic papillopathy. American Journal of Ophthalmology. 1980;**90**:203-209

[62] Freund M, Carmon A, Cohen AM. Papilledema and papillitis in diabetes: Report of two cases. American Journal of Ophthalmology. 1965;**60**:18-20

[63] Ciulla TA, Harris A, Latkany P, Piper HC, Arend O, Garzozi H, et al. Ocular perfusion abnormalities in diabetes. Acta Ophthalmologica Scandinavica. 2002;**80**:468-477

[64] Yanko L, Ticho U, Ivry M. Optic nerve involvement in diabetes. Acta Ophthalmologica. 1972;**50**:556-564

[65] Kim M, Lee JH, Lee SJ. Diabetic papillopathy with macular edema treated with intravitreal ranibizumab. Clinical Ophthalmology. 2013;**7**:2257-2260

[66] Al-Hinai AS, Al-Abri MS, Al-Hajri RH. Diabetic papillopathy with macular edema treated with intravitreal bevacizumab. Oman Journal of Ophthalmology. 2011;**4**:135-138

[67] Al-Dhibi H, Khan AO. Response of diabetic papillopathy to intravitreal bevacizumab. Middle East African Journal of Ophthalmology. 2011;**18**:243-245

[68] Willerslev A, Munch IC, Larsen M. Resolution of diabetic papillopathy after a single intravitreal injection of ranibizumab. Acta Ophthalmologica. 2012;**90**:e407-e409

[69] Mansour AM, El-Dairi MA, Shehab MA, Shahin HK, Shaaban JA, Antonios SR. Periocular corticosteroids in diabetic papillopathy. Eye (London, England). 2005;**19**:45-51

[70] Yassur Y, Pickle LW, Fine SL, Singerman L, Orth DH, Patz A. Optic disc neovascularisation in diabetic retinopathy: A system for grading proliferation at the optic nerve head in patients with proliferative diabetic retinopathy. British Journal of Ophthalmology. 1980;**64**:69-76

[71] Jeganathan VSE, Wardrop D. A paradigm shift in the management of neovascular glaucoma. New Frontiers in Ophthalmology. 2016;**2**(3):119-124. DOI: 10.15761/NFO.1000128

[72] Jeganathan VSE, Wang JJ, Wong TY. Ocular associations of diabetes other than diabetic retinopathy. Diabetes Care. 2008;**31**(9):1905-1912. DOI: 10.2337/dc08-0342

[73] Rodrigues GB, Abe RY, Zangalli C, Sodre SL, Donini FA, Costa DC, et al. Neovascular glaucoma: A review. International Journal of Retina and Vitreous. 2016;**2**:26. DOI: 10.1186/s40942-016-0051-x

[74] Hayreh SS. Neovascular glaucoma. Progress in Retinal and Eye Research. 2007;**26**:470-485

[75] Akiyama H, Li D, Shimoda Y, Matsumoto H, Kishi S. Observation of neovascularization of the disc associated with proliferative diabetic retinopathy using OCT angiography. Japanese Journal of Ophthalmology. 2018;**62**(3):286-291. DOI: 10.1007/s10384-018-0571-z

[76] Dubey S, Pegu J. Management of neovascular glaucoma. Journal of Current Glaucoma Practice. 2009;**3**(3):27-34

[77] Venkatramani DV, Amula GM, Gandhi RA. Optic Atrophy. Kerala Journal of Ophthalmology. 2010;**22**(1):7-12

[78] Gandhi R, Amula GA. Optic Atrophy. Medscape. 2016. Available from: https://emedicine.medscape.com/article/1217760-overview#a4

[79] Adachi M, Takahashi K, Nishikawa M, Miki H, Uyama M. High intraocular pressure-induced ischemia and reperfusion injury in the optic nerve and retina in rats. Graefe's

Archive for Clinical and Experimental Ophthalmology. 1996;**234**:445-451. DOI: 10.1007/bf02539411

[80] Joachim SC, Wax MB, Boehm N, Dirk DR, Pfeiffer N, Grus FH. Upregulation of antibody response to heat shock proteins and tissue antigens in an ocular ischemia model. Investigative Ophthalmology & Visual Science. 2011;**52**:3468-3474. DOI: 10.1167/iovs.10-5763

[81] Renner M, Stute G, Alzureiqi M, Reinhard J, Wiemann S, Schmid H, et al. Optic nerve degeneration after retinal ischemia/reperfusion in a rodent model. Frontiers in Cellular Neuroscience. 2017;**11**:254. DOI: 10.3389/fncel.2017.00254

[82] Safi H, Safi S, Hafezi-Moghadam A, Ahmadieh H. Early Detection of Diabetic Retinopathy. Survey of Ophthalmology. 2018;**63**(5):601-608. DOI: 10.1016/j.survophthal.2018.04.003

[83] Anderson AJ, Johnson CA. Mechanisms isolated by frequencydoubling technology perimetry. Investigative Ophthalmology & Visual Science. 2002;**43**:398-401

[84] Frisen L. New, sensitive window on abnormal spatial vision: Rarebit probing. Vision Research. 2002;**42**:1931-1939

[85] Bengtsson B, Heijl A, Agardh E. Visual fields correlate better than visual acuity to severity of diabetic retinopathy. Diabetologia. 2005;**48**:2494-2500

[86] Kumar KVSH, Ahmad FMH, Sood S, Mansingh S. Visual evoked potential to assess retinopathy in gestational diabetes mellitus. Canadian Journal of Diabetes. 2015:1-4

[87] Nasralah Z, Robinson W, Jackson GR, Barber AJ. Measuring visual function in diabetic retinopathy: Progress in basic and clinical research. Journal of Clinical and Experimental Ophthalmology. 2013;**4**:306. DOI: 10.4172/2155-9570.1000306

[88] Shankar U, Gunasundari R. A review on electrophysiology based detection of diabetic retinopathy. Procedia Computer Science. 2015;**48**:630-637

[89] Kumar R, Sundararajan D, Ponraj RS, Srinivasan M. A study on early detection of changes in visual pathway due to diabetes mellitus by visual evoked potential. International Journal of Medical Research and Health Sciences. 2014;**3**(1):161-164

[90] Vujosevic S, Simo R. Local and systemic inflammatory biomarkers of diabetic retinopathy: An integrative approach. Investigative Ophthalmology & Visual Science. 2017;**58**(6): Bio68-bio75

[91] Kaviarasan K, Jithu M, Arif Mulla M, et al. Low blood and vitreal BDNF, LXA4 and altered Th1/Th2 cytokine balance are potential risk factors for diabetic retinopathy. Metabolism. 2015;**64**(9):958-966

[92] Demirkaya N, van-Dijk HW, van-Schuppen SM, Abràmoff MD, Garvin MK, Sonka M, et al. Effect of age on individual retinal layer thickness in normal eyes as measured with spectral-domain optical coherence tomography. Investigative Ophthalmology and Visual Science. 2013;**54**(7):4934-4940

[93] Tawse KL, Hedges TR, Gobuty M, Mendoza-Santiesteban C. Optical coherence tomography shows retinal abnormalities associated with optic nerve disease. Brazilian Journal of Ophthalmology. 2014;**98**(Suppl 2):ii30-ii33. DOI: 10.1136/bjophthalmol-2013-304301

[94] Lamirel C, Newman NJ, Biousse V. Optical coherence tomography (OCT) in optic neuritis and multiple sclerosis. Revista de Neurologia. 2010;**166**(12):978-986. DOI: 10.1016/j.neurol.2010.03.024

[95] Ishibazawa A, Nagaoka T, Yokota H, Takahashi A, Omae T, Song Y, et al. Characteristics of retinal neovascularization in proliferative diabetic retinopathy imaged by optical coherence tomography angiography. Investigative Ophthalmology & Visual Science. 2016;**57**:6247-6255. DOI: 10.1167/iovs.16-20210

[96] Savastano MC, Federici M, Falsini B, Caporossi A, Minnella AM. Detecting papillary neovascularization inproliferative diabetic retinopathy using opticalcoherence tomography angiography. Acta Ophthalmologica. 2018;**96**(3):321-323. DOI: 10.1111/aos.13166

8

Novel Insight into Morphological Features and Vascular Profile of Selected Macular Dystrophies Using Swept-Source Optical Coherence Tomography and Optical Coherence Tomography Angiography

Magdy Moussa and Mahmoud Leila

Abstract

Our perception of macular dystrophies has evolved overtime from collective grouping into hereditary disorders of unclear etiology and no effective treatment to avid search for the underlying pathogenic mechanism that would provide base for future therapy. A causal conjunction between abnormalities in the photoreceptors layer and the RPE—Bruch's membrane complex and abnormal profile of the retinal vascular plexuses and the choriocapillaris—stands out as a plausible theory of pathogenesis. The recently introduced swept-source optical coherence tomography (SS-OCT) technology incorporates long-wavelength (1050-nm) scanning light, less susceptibility to sensitivity roll-off, and ultrahigh-speed image acquisition. These features enabled in vivo noninvasive visualization of different strata of the outer retina and the choriocapillaris with unprecedented finesse. Furthermore, the SS-OCT technology incorporated a blood flow detection algorithm; OCTARA that in tandem with the deeper penetration and superior axial resolution of SS-OCT enabled detailed assessment of the retinal capillary plexuses and the choriocapillaris in terms of structure and density. This novel technology could help explore yet undiscovered frontiers in the pathophysiology of macular dystrophies and guide future therapeutic approaches. This chapter includes a review of literature along with the authors' experience in imaging selected macular dystrophies using SS-OCT and SS-OCT angiography (SS-OCTA).

Keywords: imaging macular dystrophies, SS-OCTA in Stargardt's, SS-OCTA in Best's disease, OCTARA algorithm, swept-source OCT

1. Introduction

Macular dystrophy is a unifying term used to describe a group of hereditary fundus disorders that exhibits Mendelian inheritance pattern and has varying degrees of expressivity and penetrance. These disorders share common criteria in that they are isolated, that is, confined to the eye with no systemic association, limited to the anatomic macula, exhibit bilateral involvement with striking symmetry, and have characteristic biomicroscopic features that manifest universally along with visual symptoms or often discovered on routine examination before symptoms develop. The classic tools for the diagnosis and follow-up of macular dystrophies were largely based on clinical appearance, electrophysiologic findings, and fundus fluorescein angiography (FFA). More recently, fundus autofluorescence (FAF) increasingly became an invaluable noninvasive tool in the follow-up scheme of these patients [1–7]. FAF captures the stimulated emission of light from lipofuscin molecules that accumulate excessively in cases of retinal pigment epithelium (RPE) dysfunction and depicts specific autofluorescence patterns that are characteristic for each disease [8–11]. To date, there is no known effective treatment for macular dystrophies other than the management of complications, for example, choroidal neovascularization (CNV) secondary to Best's disease and visual rehabilitation using low-vision aids [1, 2].

2. Theories of pathogenesis of vascular changes in macular dystrophies

Histopathological studies in humans affected with macular dystrophies and in animal models of retinal degeneration demonstrated a wide-spread loss of the photoreceptors and the RPE, in addition to extensive vascular remodeling of the retinal vascular plexuses and the choriocapillaris [1, 2, 12]. These findings purported a cause–effect relationship between the morphological changes seen in retinal microstructure and the status of vascular nourishment, in the sense that one pathology is a consequence of the other, though the exact mechanism remains debatable [13–15]. One theory proposes that the progressive demise of photoreceptors and RPE causes a thinning out of the retina with subsequent progressive atrophy of retinal vasculature and choriocapillaris as part of a downregulation process due to a reduced vascular demand [16]. Another proposed mechanism is that retinal thinning due to the loss of photoreceptors and RPE allows more oxygen influx into the inner retinal layers from the choroidal circulation. The ensuing retinal hyperoxic state induces vasoconstriction and vascular rarefaction [12]. Another plausible theory is that progressive RPE loss results in a decreased release of vascular endothelial growth factor (VEGF) and other signaling factors that are essential for the viability of the choriocapillaris, hence precipitating choriocapillaris atrophy [17–19]. Finally, some researches propose that mechanical compression by the lipofuscin-laden RPE and accumulation of hyaline deposits between the RPE and Bruch's membrane exerts mechanical compression on the choriocapillaris with subsequent atrophy and loss [16].

3. Optical coherence tomography angiography (OCTA): a new imaging frontier

The prospect of an abnormal vascular profile going on in tandem with the morphological changes in retinal microstructure in macular dystrophies turned our attention to the diagnostic and therapeutic potentials of the early detection of abnormal changes in the retinal vascular plexuses and the choriocapillaris. Currently, the available diagnostic modalities rely on inference extrapolated from indirect evidence to determine disease stage and progression. For instance, FFA depicts disease patterns based on varying degrees of fluorescence; FAF identifies diseased or dead RPE cells based on varying intensities of lipofuscin autofluorescence, whereas electrophysiology records the amplitude and latency of electric transduction in retinal layers to identify different dystrophies [1–3, 8–11]. The common factor among these diagnostic tools is that they reveal useful information only when retinal function due to a given dystrophy has already been compromised. In comparison, OCTA offers direct noninvasive visualization of the vascular profile in macular dystrophies and thus has the clear advantages of screening vulnerable population and detecting the disease process in its nascence. Though no therapeutic line is currently available for macular dystrophies, the identification of early disease phases based on the integrity of the vascular profile helps selecting patients who would be best candidates for on-going research trials on gene therapy and pluripotent stem cell transplantation. On the other hand, identifying patients with severely compromised vascular profile, and in whom favorable outcome of these therapies is unlikely, will help avoid biased results and reduce the economic burden on health-care institutions.

4. Swept-source optical coherence tomography (SS-OCT), SS-OCT angiography (SS-OCTA), and OCTARA algorithm

SS-OCTA incorporates a blood flow detection algorithm; OCTARA (Optical Coherence Tomography Angiography Ratio Analysis); Topcon Corporation, Tokyo, Japan. OCTARA uses decorrelation motion contrast between rapidly repeated SS-OCT B-scans to detect moving erythrocytes in relation to static tissue [20]. SS-OCTA is integrated in the SS-OCT technology which incorporates a long-wavelength (1050-nm) scanning light, reduced sensitivity roll-off feature, and ultrahigh-speed image acquisition. These implements enable deeper penetration with minimal light scattering, hence superior axial resolution and segmentation of different retinal layers. The result is the generation of ultrahigh-definition images of the retinal microstructure, retinal vascular plexuses, and the choriocapillaris, while obviating the need for dye injection. It is worth noting that OCTARA algorithm generates SS-OCTA images by registering B-scan repetition at each scan location, thereby computing a ratio-based result between corresponding image pixels. This method preserves the integrity of the OCT spectrum and does not result in compromised axial resolution, an inherent disadvantage of other OCTA technologies [20–25]. In addition, SS-OCTA software generates color-coded flow density maps of the retinal vascular plexuses and the choriocapillaris, each layer separately.

In this map, vessel density in a given area is inferred from the decorrelation motion contrast signal provided by SS-OCTA, where high flow is represented by an increased vessel density and vice versa. Different vessel densities are then given color codes and numeric percentage values that reflect the percentage area occupied by blood vessels, where bright red color represents areas of highest density and hence a high numeric percentage, whereas dark blue represents areas of no detectable vessels and hence low or zero numeric percentage. Intermediate color shades represent variable grades of vessel density [26, 27].

5. SS-OCTA depiction of retinal vascular plexuses and the choriocapillaris in normal individuals

Normally, the retinal superficial capillary plexus (SCP) appears on SS-OCTA as an interlacing network of horizontal arterioles and venules connected by transverse capillaries and anastomosing together to form the peri-foveal capillary circle. Arterioles are surrounded by a wider capillary-free zone compared to venules. The retinal deep capillary plexus (DCP) appears as polygonal lobules or vortices composed of capillaries converging radially on an epicenter. The choriocapillaris appears as a homogeneous hyperintense layer composed of densely packed capillaries with no intervening dark spaces [21, 27, 28].

6. Spectral domain OCT (SD-OCT) and OCTA features of selected macular dystrophies

6.1. Stargardt's disease

Stargardt's disease is considered the most common inherited childhood dystrophy. The pattern of inheritance is an autosomal-recessive one and represents the mildest form of ABCA4 gene mutation. The mutated gene causes malfunction of the ATP-binding cassette proteins that have key role in cell transport processes within the photoreceptors layer. The resultant disruption of photoreceptors visual cycle leads to over-accumulation of a metabolic byproduct, namely lipofuscin in the RPE cell layer. Clinically, patients present with bilateral and symmetrical involvement of the posterior pole by characteristic yellowish flecks at the level of the RPE resembling fish scales. Occasionally, two adjacent flecks join in an obtuse angle reminiscent of a fish tail, hence the term pisciform. The end stage is characterized by resorption of flecks and ensuing atrophic maculopathy with a substantial visual loss. To date, no known treatment exists for Stargardt's disease [1, 2].

SD-OCT in Stargardt's disease demonstrates thinning of the outer retina including the photoreceptor layer and the RPE, and altered choroidal morphology in which the normal bowl-shaped contour of the choroidoscleral interface, with maximum thickness at the sub-foveal area, is replaced by an abnormal S-shaped contour due to a marked reduction of sub-foveal choroidal thickness and displacement of the thickest point of the choroid away from the fovea [13]. On the other hand, OCTA imaging reveals generalized attenuation of the vascular layers of the ocular fundus, though the most significant vascular changes are located in the choriocapillaris, which exhibit generalized loss of the normal homogeneous hyperintense texture with the development of vascular rarefaction and flow-void areas. These morphological changes are attributed to the patchy loss of choriocapillaris or to the masking effect of the pisciform flecks [15, 29]. In some cases, there is enhanced visualization of the underlying Sattler's layer [16]. In terms of retinal capillary plexuses, vascular alterations of the SCP layer include rarefaction of the peri-foveal arcade with the enlargement of the foveal avascular zone (FAZ), and generalized reduction of vessel density in the SCP and the DCP layers, though these changes are most pronounced in the DCP layer [15, 28, 29].

6.2. Best's disease (vitelliform macular dystrophy)

Best's disease is an autosomal-dominant disorder whose primary target tissue is the RPE cell layer. The condition is caused by mutation in the BEST1 gene which causes the production of abnormal bestrophin protein. Normally located in the RPE plasma membrane, bestrophin acts as a calcium-dependent chloride channel and is responsible for normal ionic conduction across the RPE cell. Abnormal bestrophin formation causes the disruption of the ionic conduction within the RPE and interferes with the normal calcium metabolism that is essential for adhesiveness between interphotoreceptor matrix and the RPE layer. The end result is the deposition of abnormal amorphous vitelliform or egg yolk-like material in the photoreceptors' outer segments, within the RPE and sub-RPE. Though considered the hallmark of Best's disease, the origin of the vitelliform material remains uncertain. One plausible theory is that it is derived from the accumulation of lipofuscin material within over-shed photoreceptors' outer segments due to abnormal phagocytosis by RPE cell layer. Clinically, the disease is characterized by a solitary sub-retinal vitelliform lesion occupying the macular area. Less commonly, lesions may be multiple or eccentric in location. With time, the vitelliform lesion undergoes degeneration and may even get resorbed completely, with ensuing atrophic changes and scarring. Vision remains unaffected in early stages with most individuals maintaining reading and driving vision well into adult life until the atrophic or cicatricial stages develop. The abnormal ionic conduction in Best's disease is responsible for the characteristic loss of light response and abnormal Arden ratio on electro-oculogram (EOG) examination [1, 2].

SD-OCT in early stages of the disease shows a sub-retinal smooth dome-shaped amorphous optically opaque material. As the disease progresses, degenerative changes ensue on the vitelliform structure causing it to break down. The corresponding SD-OCT features consist of irregular optically—opaque amorphous deposits alternating with optically—translucent areas that correspond to the resorbed vitelliform material. In addition, RPE irregularities could be detected including irregular thickened RPE layer, and solitary or multiple RPE detachment(s) (PED). The atrophic stage of the disease is marked by diffuse disruption of the outer retinal layers including the external limiting membrane (ELM), inner segment/outer segment (IS/OS) photoreceptor junction, and marked atrophy or even disappearance of RPE cell layer [30, 31].

OCTA in Best's disease demonstrates generalized rarefaction of the SCP and the DCP layers along with a reduced vessel density. The mechanism of vascular rarefaction in Best's disease is controversial. One explanation is that the vitelliform material causes centrifugal displacement of blood vessels in the macular area with resultant progressive atrophy due to mechanical compression. Occasionally, the DCP layer shows a central area of hypointense signal caused by vascular rarefaction and a reduced vessel density surrounded by an annulus of hyperintense signal. This peculiar configuration could be due to overcrowding of vessels being displaced by the vitelliform lesion, or due to compensatory dilatation of the para-macular vascular bed secondary to vessel rarefaction in the macula, with consequent increased blood flow. Likewise, the choriocapillaris shows vascular rarefaction with multiple hypointense flow-void areas, which could be explained by vascular impairment due to degenerative changes induced by mechanical compression or due to masking effect by the accumulating vitelliform material [30–35].

6.3. Choroidal neovascularization secondary to Best's disease: a diagnostic predicament

The most dreadful complication of Best's disease is CNV formation, which could develop in some cases secondary to compromised RPE/Bruch's complex [30, 32–34]. The advent of CNV on top of Best's disease could pose a diagnostic challenge due to overlapping fluorescein patterns of the vitelliform material and PEDs in Best's disease and the fibrovascular and neovascular components of CNV. Likewise, SD-OCT could yield inconclusive results, even when deploying the ultrahigh-definition versions, due to similar backscattering light intensity properties between the amorphous vitelliform and the CNV. OCTA helps disentangle this overlap by its ability to separate erythrocytes from the surrounding static tissue, hence displaying flow in a vascular network that is pathognomonic of CVN formation. In addition, OCTA integrates light-scattering reduction technology (reduced sensitivity roll-off) that preserves the integrity of the incident infra-red laser beam, hence allowing deeper penetration, layer segmentation, and delineation of the neovascular network of CNV from the surrounding vitelliform material [20, 27, 36–40].

7. Authors' case reports

Over the past year, the authors studied 40 patients with macular dystrophies (27 patients with Best's disease and adult-onset vitelliform foveomacular dystrophy, and 13 patients with Stargardt's disease). SS-OCT and SS-OCTA images were acquired using the DRI OCT Triton machine version 10.11 (Topcon Corporation, Tokyo, Japan). Herein, we present representative cases to demonstrate our findings regarding the morphological alteration in retinal microstructure, retinal vascular plexuses, and choriocapillaris in different stages of both diseases.

7.1. SS-OCT and SS-OCTA findings in Stargardt's disease

Case 1. Early stage of Stargardt's disease. A 26-year-old male presented with defective vision in both eyes of approximately 1-year duration. His best-corrected visual acuity (BCVA) was 20/63 and 20/50 in the right eye (RE) and the left eye (LE), respectively. Fundus examination revealed bilateral numerous yellowish discrete flecks in the macular area at the level of the RPE. The lesions were identical in appearance though more numerous in the RE. SS-OCT examination revealed bilateral foveal thinning, disrupted ELM and IS/OS photoreceptor junction, and thinning of the choriocapillaris with enhanced visualization of the larger choroidal vessels. SS-OCTA revealed bilateral rarefaction of the SCP and the DCP layers. Affection was more pronounced in the DCP layer. The choriocapillaris showed a moth-eaten appearance instead of the normal hyperintense homogeneous texture, due to the presence of multiple black areas that could correspond to areas of flow void or masking effect by the pisciform lesions. The corresponding flow density maps showed a reduced vessel density that corresponded to vascular rarefaction in the SCP, the DCP, and the choriocapillaris (**Figures 1** and **2**).

Case 2. Late stage of Stargardt's disease. A 58-year-old female who was a known case of Stargardt's disease presented for follow-up with complaints of defective vision in both eyes of approximately 2-year duration. Her BCVA was 20/400 and 20/200 in the RE and the LE, respectively. Fundus examination of the RE revealed a sharply circumscribed area of geographic atrophy occupying the macula, approximately of 4 disc diameters (DD) in size. On

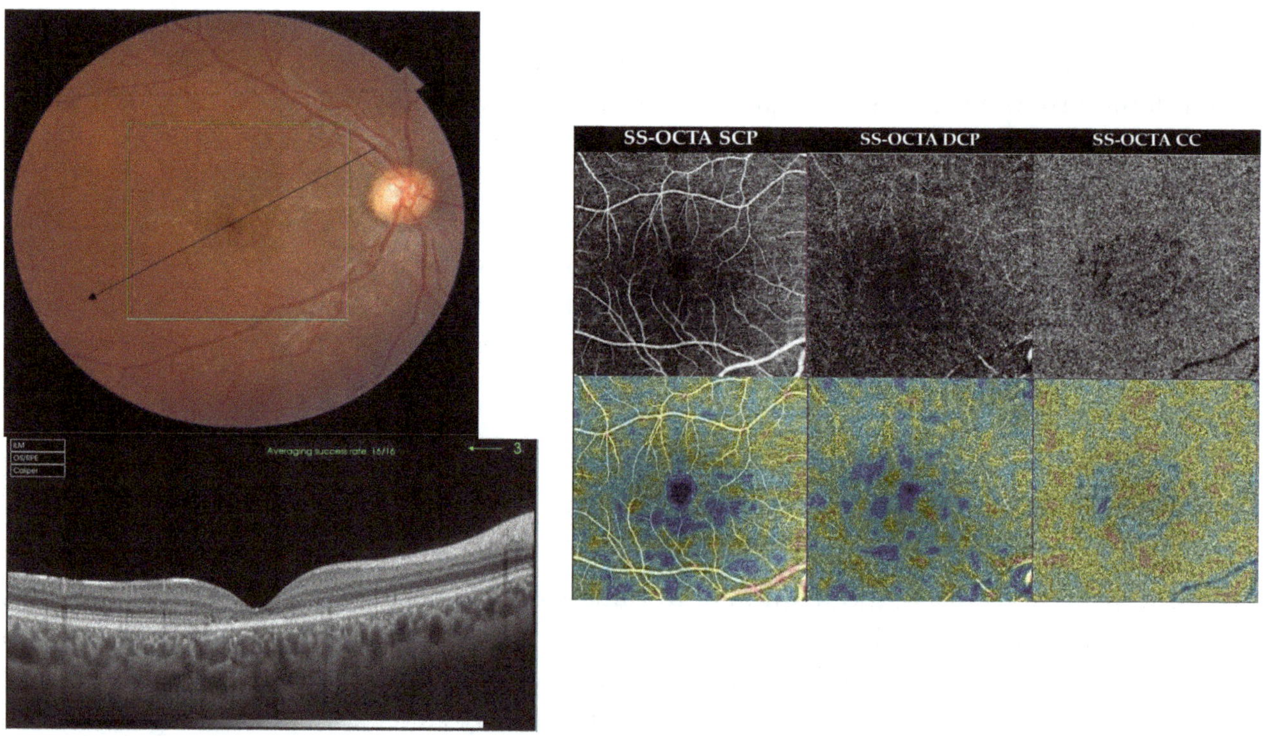

Figure 1. Case 1. Top left, color photograph of the RE of a 26-year-old male in early stage of Stargardt's disease. Note the numerous subretinal pisciform yellowish flecks occupying the macular area. Bottom left, radial scan SS-OCT shows foveal thinning (168 μ), disrupted ELM and IS/OS photoreceptor junction, and thinning of the choriocapillaris with enhanced visualization of the larger choroidal vessels. Right, en face SS-OCTA projection of the SCP, the DCP, and the choriocapillaris in a 6 × 6 mm field (upper row), and the corresponding flow density maps (lower row). The SCP and the DCP layers show vascular rarefaction. Affection is more pronounced in the DCP layer. The choriocapillaris shows a moth-eaten appearance instead of the normal homogeneous hyperintense texture, due to the presence of multiple black areas of flow voids. The corresponding flow density maps show a reduced vessel density that corresponds to vascular rarefaction in the SCP, the DCP, and the choriocapillaris.

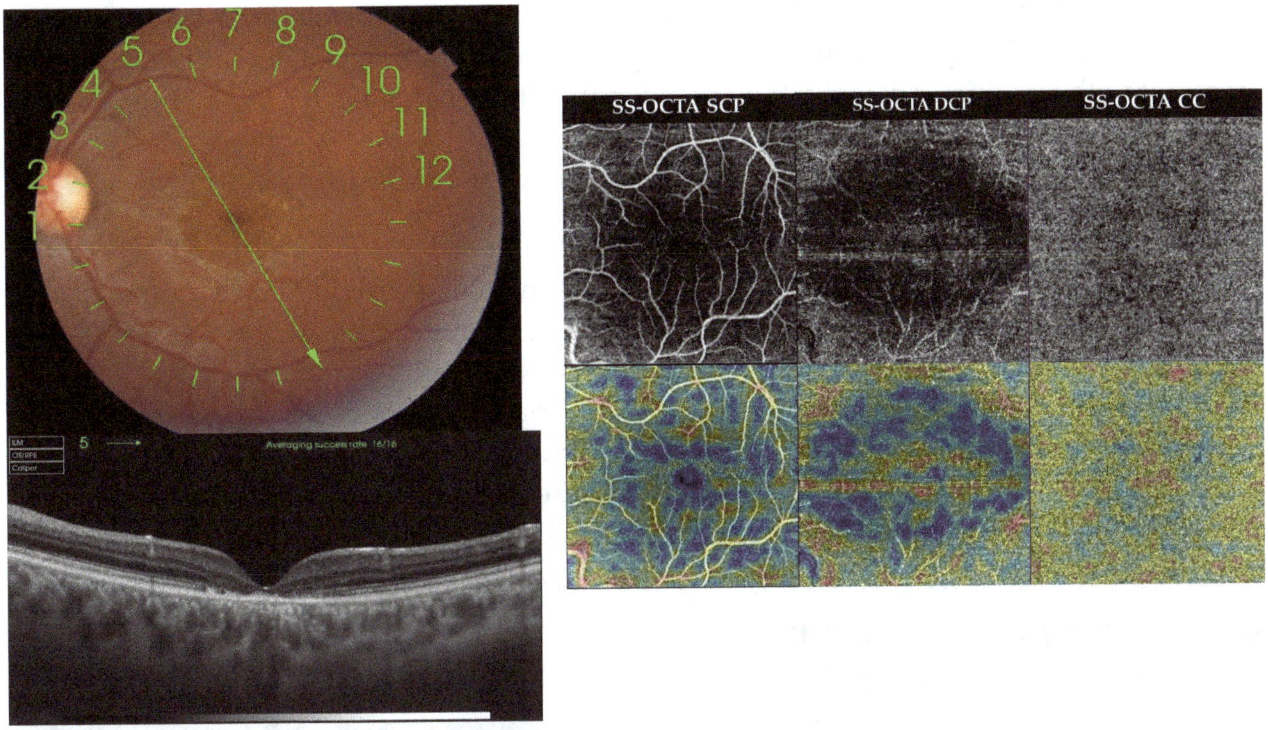

Figure 2. Case 1. Top left, color photograph of the LE of the same patient as in **Figure 1**. The fundus shows identical lesions to those seen in the RE though less numerous. Bottom left, radial scan SS-OCT reveals foveal thinning (144 μ), disrupted ELM and IS/OS photoreceptors junction, and thinning of the choriocapillaris with enhanced visualization of the larger choroidal vessels. Right, en face SS-OCTA projection of the SCP, the DCP, and the choriocapillaris in a 6 × 6 mm field (upper row), and the corresponding flow density maps (lower row). The SCP and the DCP layers demonstrate vascular rarefaction. Affection is more pronounced in the DCP layer. The choriocapillaris shows multiple black areas of flow voids. The corresponding flow density maps show a reduced vessel density that corresponds to vascular rarefaction in the SCP, the DCP, and the choriocapillaris.

FFA, the lesion seen in the color photograph demonstrated that the RPE in the center of the lesion has virtually disappeared with unveiling of the underlying large choroidal vessels. More peripheral areas of the lesion demonstrated transmission fluorescence. SS-OCT of the same eye showed foveal thinning, wiping-out of the ELM, and the IS/OS layer in the subfoveal area. The RPE layer was extremely rarified with extensive loss of the choriocapillaris and enhanced visualization of the underlying choroidal vessels. SS-OCTA of the SCP and the DCP layers of the same eye showed vascular rarefaction and reduced vessel density. These changes were most pronounced in the DCP layer. SS-OCTA at the level of the choriocapillaris showed complete loss of the vessels in the central portion of the lesion with clear view of the larger choroidal vessels. This peculiar configuration could be explained by severe atrophy of the choriocapillaris and Sattler's layer, and visualization of an anteriorly displaced Haller's layer to the level of the choriocapillaris. The central region was surrounded by an annulus of hypointense flow-void areas and vessel rarefaction (arrows). The LE had a similar lesion though slightly smaller in size (3DD) and less advanced in terms of the extent of geographic atrophy. SS-OCT of the same eye showed fairly preserved ELM though disrupted IS/OS layer and marked RPE thinning. The diffuse atrophy of the choriocapillaris resulted in irregular thickening of the choroid with loss of the normal bowl-shaped configuration of the choroidoscleral junction. SS-OCTA of the LE reflected the relatively less advance disease compared to the RE, especially in the choriocapillaris layer which showed multiple flow-void areas but with less diffuse atrophy than noted in the RE (**Figures 3** and **4**).

7.2. SS-OCT and SS-OCTA findings in Best's disease and adult-onset vitelliform foveomacular dystrophy

Case 3. Adult-onset vitelliform foveomacular dystrophy. A 61-year-old female presented with defective vision in the RE of approximately 6-month duration. Her BCVA was 20/100 and 20/400 in the RE and the LE, respectively. Fundus examination of the RE revealed a sub-foveal plaque of amorphous yellowish-white material surrounded by numerous satellite lesions varying in size and in shape, and scattered in the anatomic macula region. On the corresponding FFA, the sub-foveal lesion showed blocked hypofluorescence with multiple pinpoint hyperfluorescent spots due to leakage within PED. The satellite lesions seen in the color

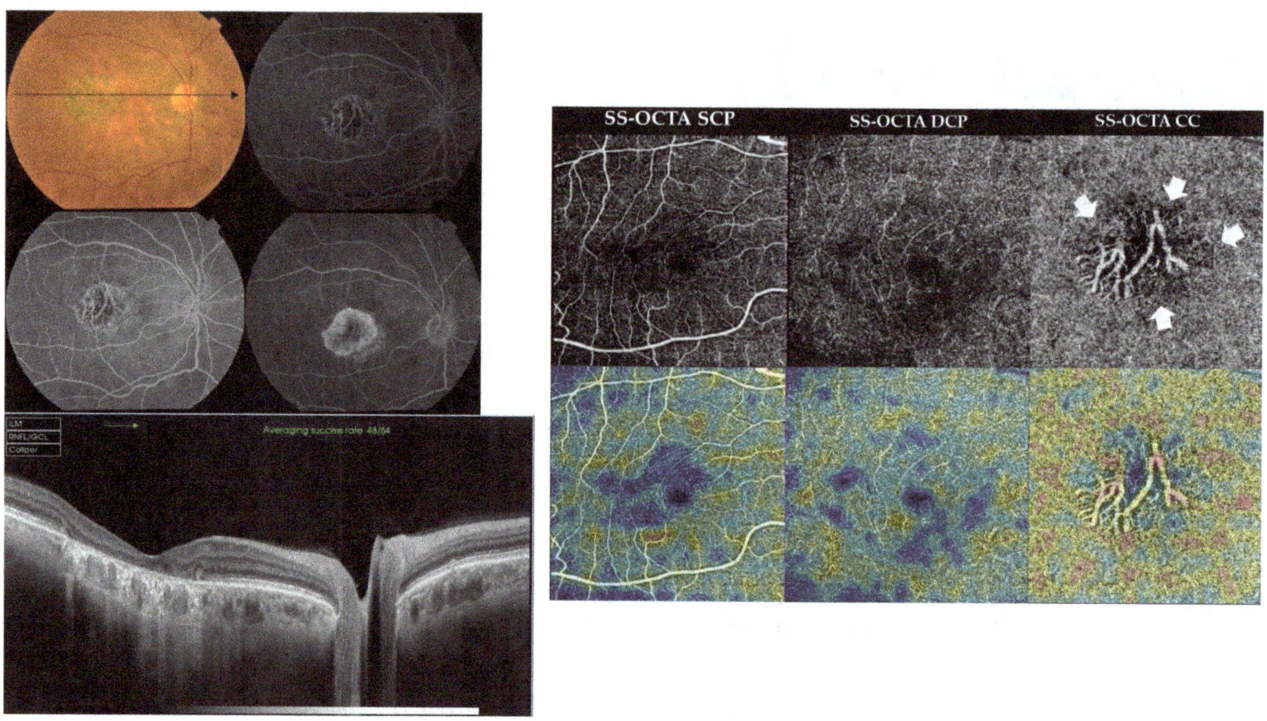

Figure 3. Case 2. Top left, color photograph and FFA of the RE of a 58-year-old female in late stage of Stargardt's disease. The fundus shows a sharply circumscribed area of geographic atrophy occupying the macula, approximately 4 DD in size. On FFA, the RPE in the center of the lesion has virtually disappeared with unveiling of the large choroidal vessels. More peripheral areas of the lesion demonstrated transmission fluorescence. Bottom left, high-definition line scan (12.0 mm) SS-OCT of the same eye shows marked foveal thinning (84 μ), wiping out of the ELM and the IS/OS layer in the sub-foveal area. The RPE layer is extremely rarified with extensive loss of the choriocapillaris and enhanced visualization of the underlying choroidal vessels. Right, en face SS-OCTA projection of the SCP, the DCP, and the choriocapillaris in a 6 × 6 mm field (upper row), and the corresponding flow density maps (lower row). The SCP and the DCP layers show vascular rarefaction and reduced vessel density. These changes are most pronounced in the DCP layer. The choriocapillaris shows complete loss of vessels in the central portion of the lesion with clear view of the larger choroidal vessels. The central region is surrounded by an annulus of hypointense flow-void areas and vessel rarefaction (arrows).

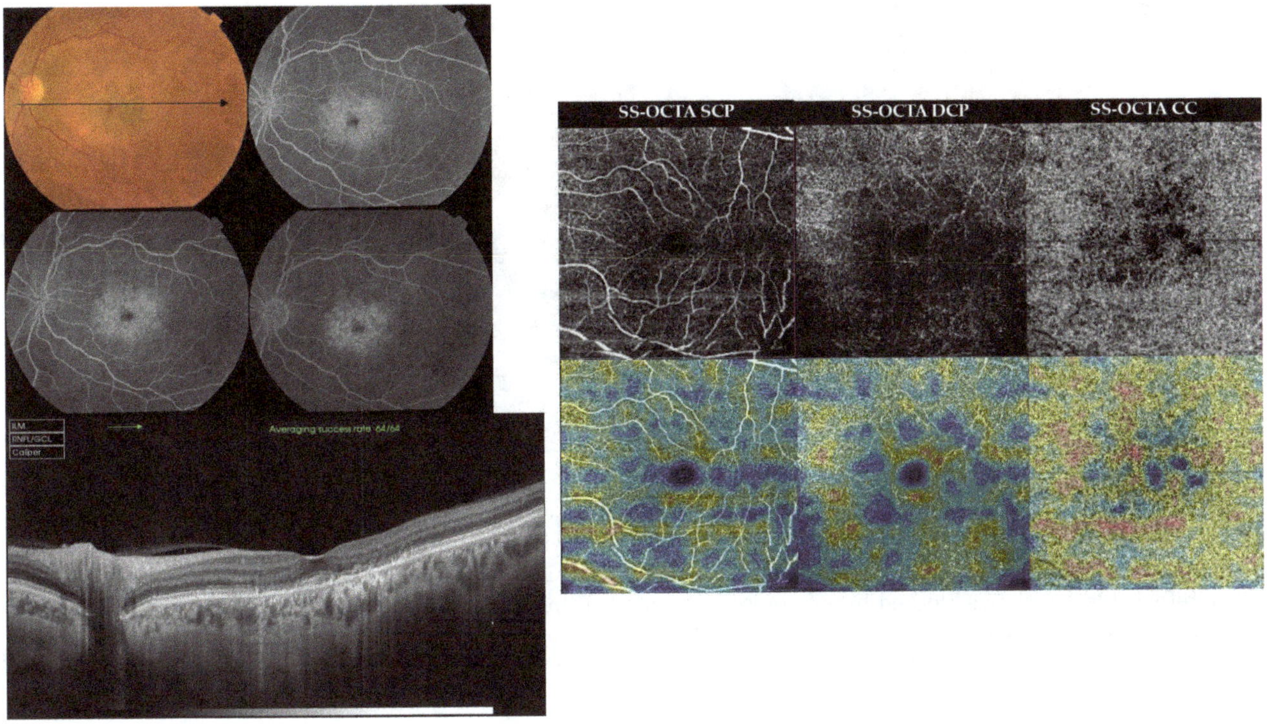

Figure 4. Case 2. Top left, color photograph and FFA of the LE of the same patient as in **Figure 3**. The fundus shows a sharply circumscribed area of geographic atrophy occupying the macula, approximately 3 DD in size. FFA in the macular area demonstrated transmission fluorescence due to marked RPE attenuation. Bottom left, high-definition line scan (12.0 mm) SS-OCT of the same eye shows foveal thinning (177 μ), wiping out of the IS/OS layer in the sub foveal area. The RPE layer was extremely rarified with extensive loss of the choriocapillaris and enhanced visualization of the underlying choroidal vessels. The diffuse atrophy of the choriocapillaris resulted in irregular thickening of the choroid with loss of the normal bowl-shaped configuration of the choroidoscleral junction. Sub-foveal choroidal thickness is 257 μ. Right, en face SS-OCTA projection of the SCP, the DCP, and the choriocapillaris in a 6 × 6 mm field (upper row), and the corresponding flow density maps (lower row). The SCP and the DCP layers show vascular rarefaction and reduced vessel density. These changes are most pronounced in the DCP layer. The choriocapillaris shows vascular rarefaction with development of multiple hypointense flow-void areas.

photograph demonstrated hyperfluorescence caused by a combination of staining, pooling in PED, and transmission fluorescence due to RPE atrophy. SS-OCT of the same eye showed a dome-shaped hyper-reflective sub-foveal lesion corresponding to the yellowish vitelliform deposits seen in the color fundus photograph. The entire lesion was optically opaque except for a small optically lucent area caused by breakdown of the vitelliform material. The underlying RPE was thickened and irregular with multiple PED formation and marked thinning of the underlying choriocapillaris. SS-OCTA of the SCP layer was essentially normal in appearance apart from irregularity of the FAZ (arrow) and scattered flow-void areas (circles). The DCP layer showed centrifugal displacement of the peri-foveal vessels with extensive vascular rarefaction and enlargement of the FAZ (arrows). The para-foveal area showed hyperintense signal derived from abnormally high flow within the overcrowded vessels due to lateral displacement by the vitelliform material (asterisk). The choriocapillaris showed patchy hypointense areas that corresponded to the abovementioned vitelliform lesions. The hypointense signal might represent flow-void areas due to choriocapillaris atrophy or due to masking by the vitelliform material. The LE had rather similar fundus changes though FFA revealed more extensive RPE atrophy (**Figures 5** and **6**).

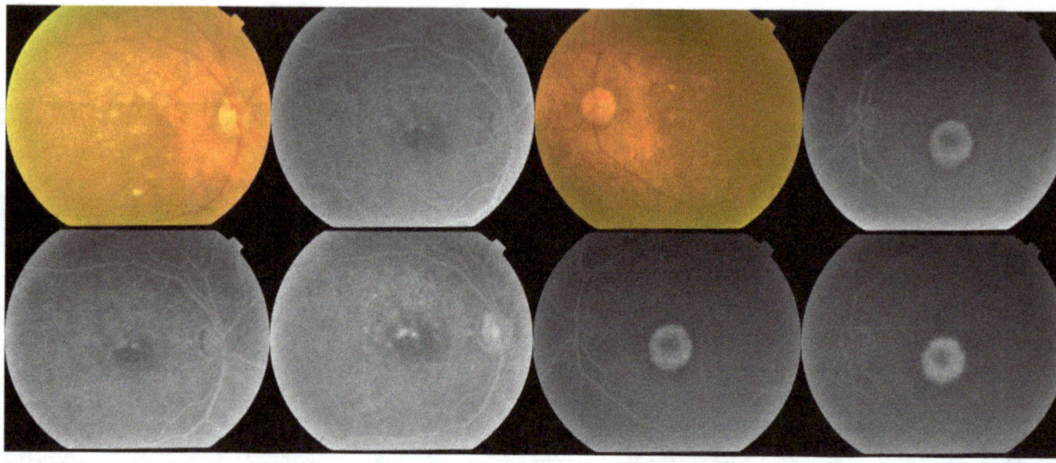

Figure 5. Case 3. Color photograph and FFA of the RE and the LE of a 61-year-old female in the vitelliruptive stage of Best's disease. The fundus of the RE shows a sub-foveal plaque of amorphous yellowish-white material surrounded by numerous satellite lesions varying in size and shape, and scattered in the anatomic macula. On the corresponding FFA, the sub-foveal lesion shows blocked hypofluorescence with multiple pin-point hyperfluorescent spots due to leakage within PED. The satellite lesions seen in the color photograph demonstrate hyperfluorescence caused by a combination of staining, pooling in PED, and transmission fluorescence due to RPE atrophy. The LE had rather similar fundus changes though FFA revealed more extensive RPE atrophy.

Case 4. Cicatricial stage of Best's disease. A 30-year-old female presented with defective vision in both eyes of 3–6 months duration. Her BCVA was 20/80 and 20/100 in the RE and the LE, respectively. Fundus examination of the LE revealed a sub-foveal sharply circumscribed ovoid area of RPE changes with central scarring. The lesion measured approximately 1 DD. On the corresponding FFA, the lesion seen in the color photograph demonstrated transmitted fluorescence due to RPE attenuation with late staining of scar tissue. The RPE in the center of the lesion has virtually disappeared with unveiling of the large choroidal vessels in earlier phases of the angiogram. SS-OCT of the same eye showed marked thinning of the fovea with a hyper-reflective scar tissue replacing the sub-foveal outer retinal layers, the choriocapillaris, and extending well into the underlying choroid. The immediate para-foveal area showed a sub-retinal pouch of optically lucent space with optically opaque sub-retinal clumps representative of degenerative changes peculiar of an earlier vitelliruptive stage. SS-OCTA of the DCP layer showed extensive vascular rarefaction in the area previously occupied by the vitelliform material. The choriocapillaris shows a central hypointense flow-void area surrounded by an outer zone of vascular rarefaction. The RE had rather similar fundus changes. The corresponding FFA revealed foveal RPE atrophy with on outer rim of blocked fluorescence due to RPE hyperplasia (**Figures 7** and **8**).

Case 5. CNV complicating cicatricial stage of Best's disease. A 28-year-old female complaining of recent diminution of vision in the RE 10 days ago. Her BCVA was 20/80 and 20/400 in the RE and the LE, respectively. Fundus examination of the RE showed an area of shallow neurosensory detachment in the foveal region, approximately 1.5 DD. The lesion showed yellowish-white precipitates gravitating in its inferior portion. On FFA, the lesion seen in the color photograph demonstrated early well-defined disc-shaped hyperfluorescence inferiorly with progressively increasing fluorescence intensity suggestive of classic CNV formation. The lesion was surrounded by diffuse and fuzzy hyperfluorescence due to pooling in

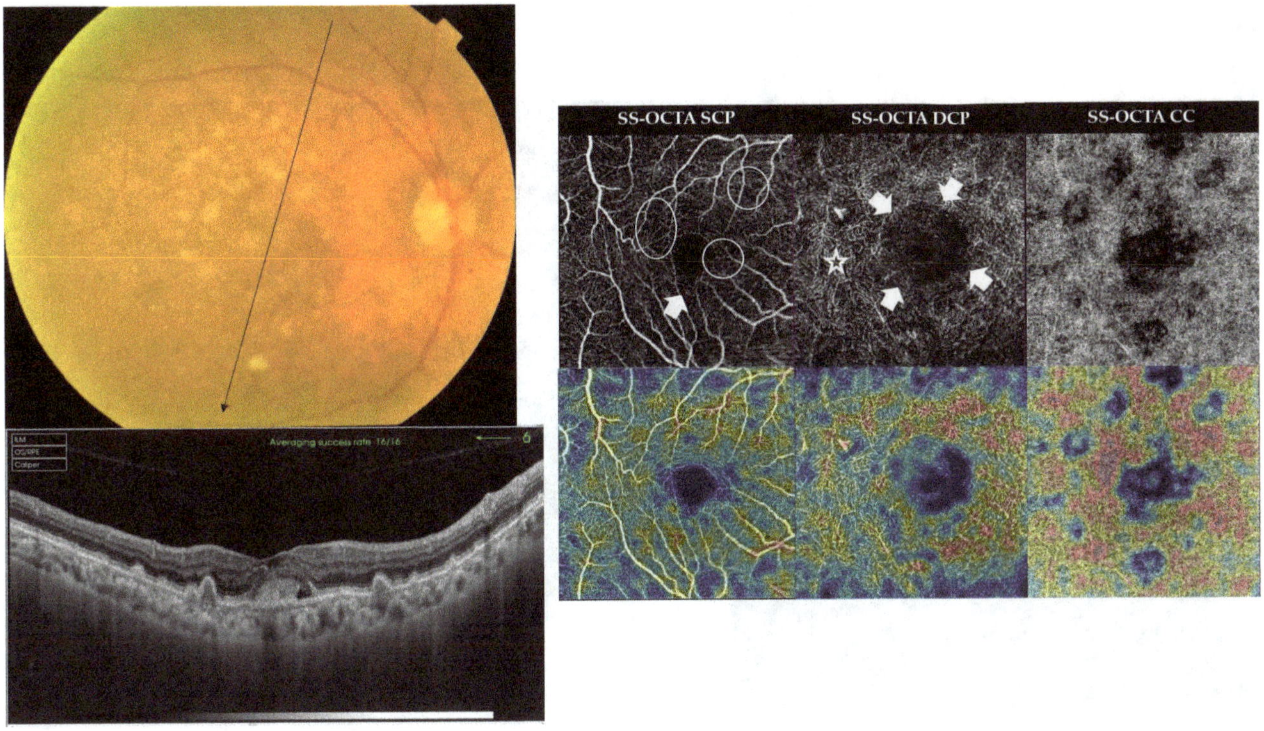

Figure 6. Case 3. Left, radial scan SS-OCT of the RE of the same patient as in **Figure 5**. Note the dome-shaped hyper-reflective sub-foveal lesion. The entire lesion is optically opaque except for a small optically lucent area caused by breakdown of the vitelliform material. The underlying RPE is thickened and irregular with multiple PED formation and marked thinning of the underlying choriocapillaris. Sub-foveal choroidal thickness measured 159 μ. Right, en face SS-OCTA projection of the SCP, the DCP, and the choriocapillaris in a 4.5 × 4.5 mm field (upper row), and the corresponding flow density maps (lower row). The SCP layer is essentially normal in appearance apart from irregularity of the FAZ (arrow) and scattered flow-void areas (circles). The DCP layer shows centrifugal displacement of the peri-foveal vessels with extensive vascular rarefaction and enlargement of the FAZ (arrows). Note the hyperintense signal derived from abnormally high flow within overcrowded vessels in the para-foveal area (asterisk). The choriocapillaris shows patchy hypointense flow-void areas that corresponded to the location of the abovementioned vitelliform lesions.

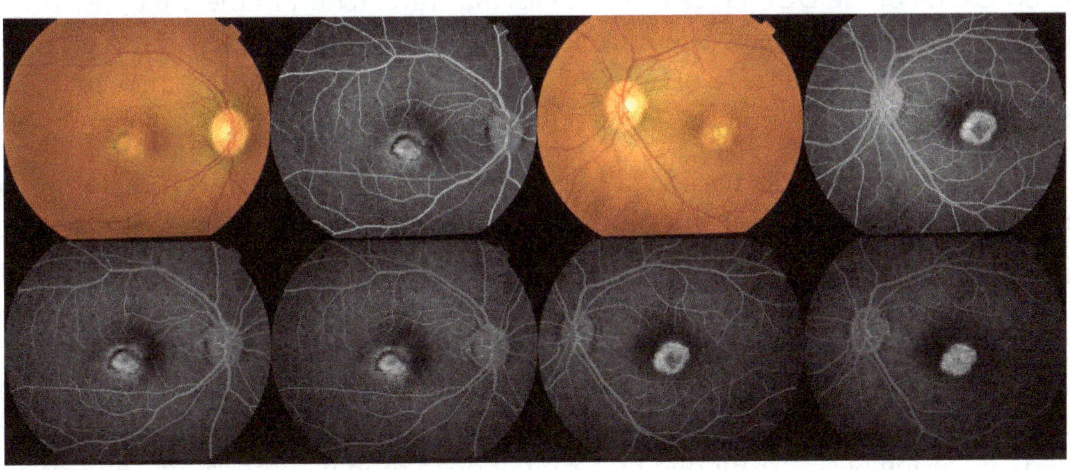

Figure 7. Case 4. Color photograph and FFA of the RE and the LE of a 30-year-old female in the cicatricial stage of Best's disease. The fundus of the LE reveals a sub-foveal sharply circumscribed ovoid area of RPE changes with central scarring. The lesion measures approximately 1 DD. On the corresponding FFA, the lesion demonstrates transmitted fluorescence due to RPE attenuation with late staining of scar tissue. The RPE in the center of the lesion has virtually disappeared with unveiling of the large choroidal vessels in earlier phases of the angiogram. The RE shows rather similar fundus changes. The corresponding FFA reveals foveal RPE atrophy with an outer rim of blocked fluorescence due to RPE hyperplasia.

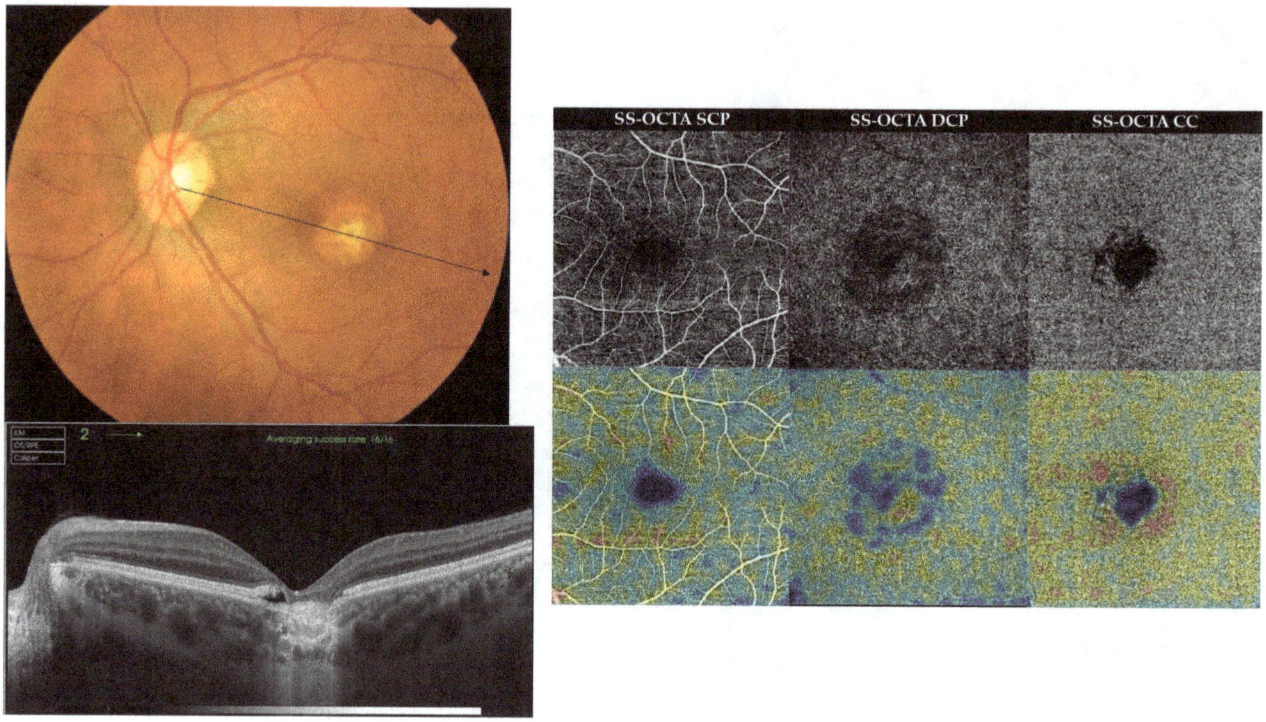

Figure 8. Case 4. Left, radial scan SS-OCT of the LE of the same patient as in **Figure 7**. Note marked thinning of the fovea with a hyper-reflective scar tissue replacing the sub-foveal outer retinal layers, the choriocapillaris, and extending well into the underlying choroid. Right, en face SS-OCTA projection of the SCP, the DCP, and the choriocapillaris in a 6 × 6 mm field (upper row), and the corresponding flow density maps (lower row). The DCP layer shows extensive vascular rarefaction in the area previously occupied by the vitelliform material. The choriocapillaris shows a central hypointense flow-void area surrounded by an outer zone of vascular rarefaction.

the neurosensory detachment cavity. An inferior rim of transmission fluorescence is noted. SS-OCT of the same eye showed sub-foveal shallow neurosensory detachment with hyper-reflective amorphous lesion, along with disrupted outer retinal layers and marked atrophy of the RPE. SS-OCTA of the DCP layer showed vascular rarefaction in the area previously occupied by the vitelliform material. The normally avascular outer retina showed a para-central hyperintense signal characteristic of active CNV formation. The LE had a macular scar with corresponding transmission fluorescence on FFA (**Figures 9** and **10**).

Case 6. CNV complicating cicatricial stage of Best's disease. A 9-year-old male presented to our clinic complaining of recent diminution of vision in the RE of few days duration. The patient was a known case of Best's disease. His BCVA was 20/200 and 20/400 in the RE and the LE, respectively. Fundus biomicroscopy examination of both eyes showed the typical scrambled-egg lesion occupying the macular area. The lesion was surrounded by residual neurosensory detachment and showed inferior migration of yellowish material and RPE alteration. The entire lesion measured approximately 2 DD in size. In the RE, the inferior portion of the scrambled-egg lesion was surrounded by a ring of deep retinal hemorrhage. FFA of both eyes demonstrated stippled fluorescence pattern due to RPE alteration, late staining of the yellowish material, and pooling of the dye in the neurosensory detachment but without conclusive evidence of CNV formation. SS-OCT of both eyes showed the typical dome-shaped hyper-reflective lesion at the level of RPE extending into—and surrounded by—empty sub-retinal space. On the other hand, SS-OCTA of the RE at the plane of the outer retina demonstrated

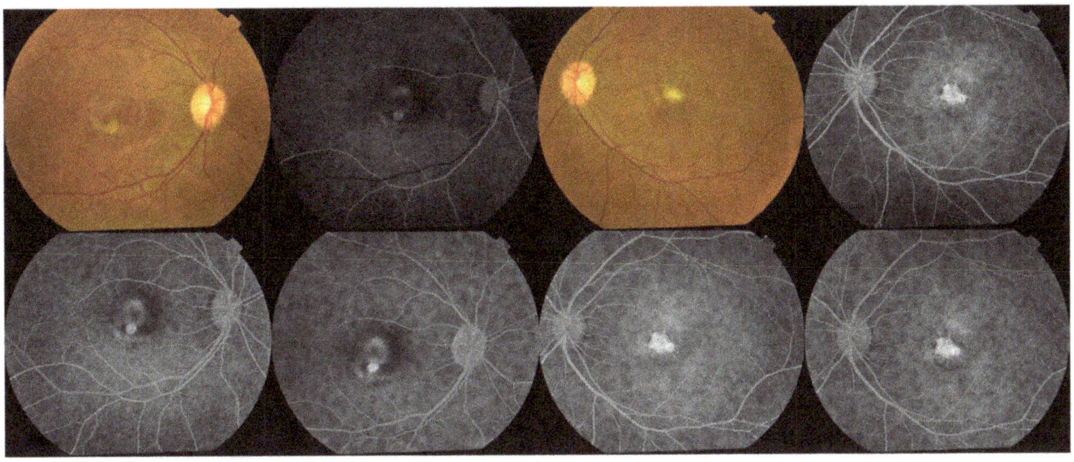

Figure 9. Case 5. Color photograph and FFA of the RE and the LE of a 28-year-old female with CNV secondary to cicatricial stage of Best's disease. The fundus of the RE shows an area of shallow neurosensory detachment in the foveal region, approximately 1.5 DD. The lesion shows yellowish-white precipitates gravitating in its inferior portion. The corresponding FFA demonstrates early well-defined disc-shaped hyperfluorescence inferiorly with progressively increasing fluorescence intensity suggestive of classic CNV. The LE had a macular scar with corresponding transmission fluorescence on FFA.

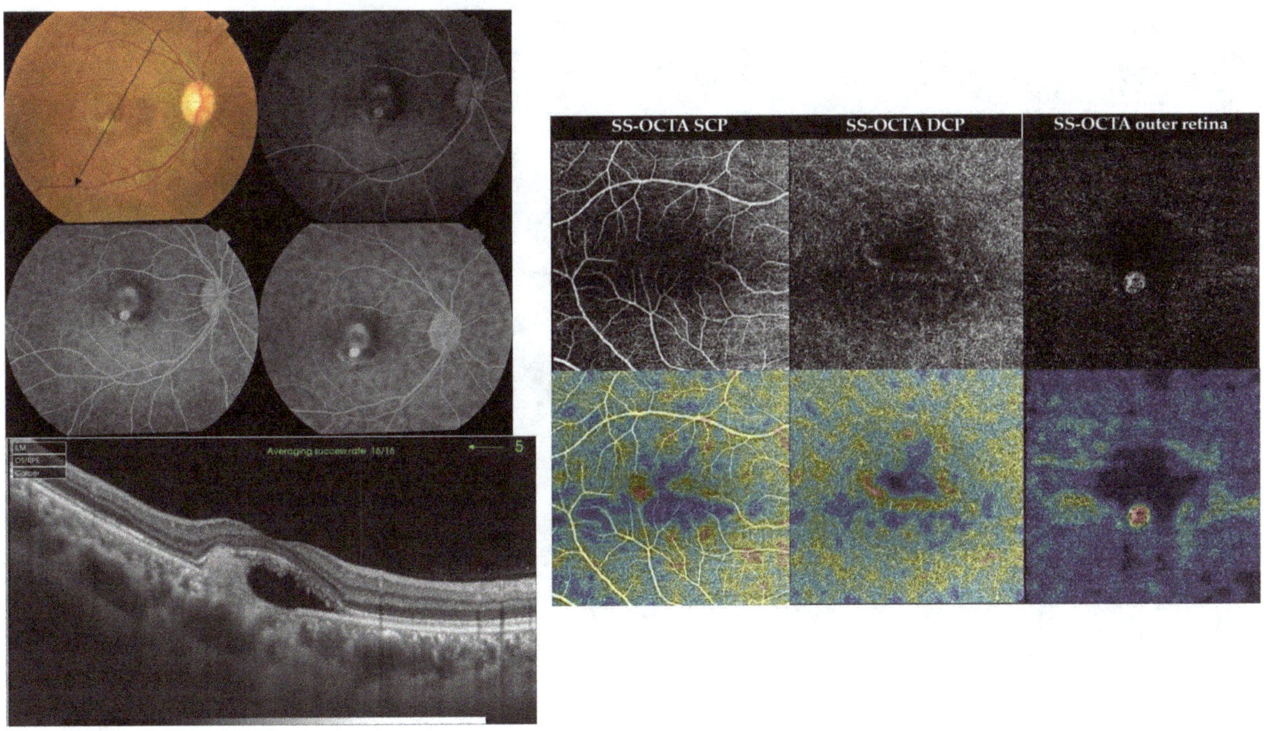

Figure 10. Case 5. Left, radial scan SS-OCT of the RE of the same patient as in **Figure 9**. Note the sub-foveal shallow neurosensory detachment with hyper-reflective amorphous lesion, along with disrupted outer retinal layers and marked atrophy of the RPE. Right, en face SS-OCTA projection of the SCP, the DCP, and the outer retina in a 6 × 6 mm field (upper row), and the corresponding flow density maps (lower row). The DCP layer shows vascular rarefaction in the area previously occupied by the vitelliform material. The outer retina shows a Para-central hyperintense signal characteristic of active CNV formation.

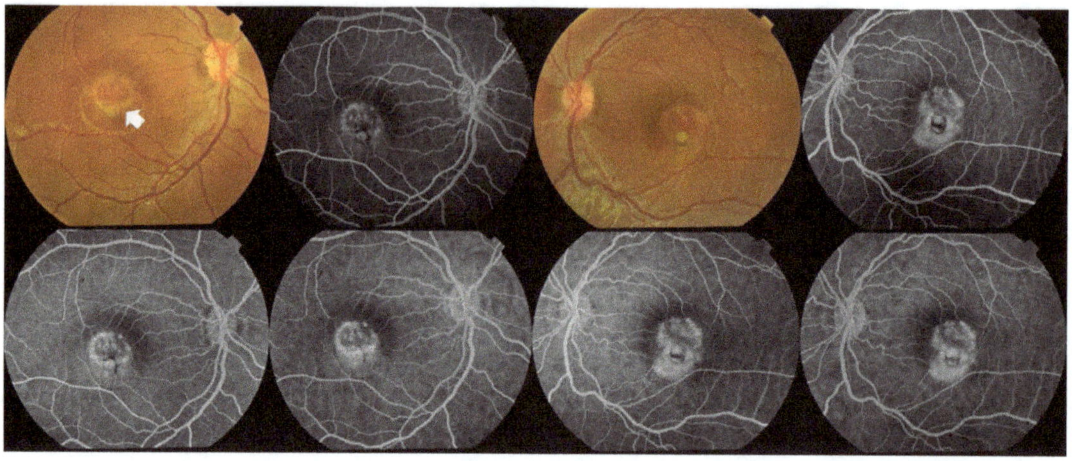

Figure 11. Case 6. Left, color fundus photograph and FFA of the RE shows a scrambled-egg lesion of vitelliform macular dystrophy surrounded by residual neurosensory detachment. The entire lesion measures approximately 2 DD in size. Note the inferior migration of the yellowish material with a ring of deep retinal hemorrhage (arrow). The corresponding FFA in arteriovenous phase of the same eye shows early transmitted fluorescence corresponding to RPE mottling seen in color photograph. Late phases of FFA show staining of the scrambled-egg lesion and residual sub-retinal yellowish deposits. Note the late pooling of the dye into the neurosensory detachment seen at the inferior edge of the vitelliform lesion. Right, color fundus photograph and FFA of the LE show essentially similar features to the RE.

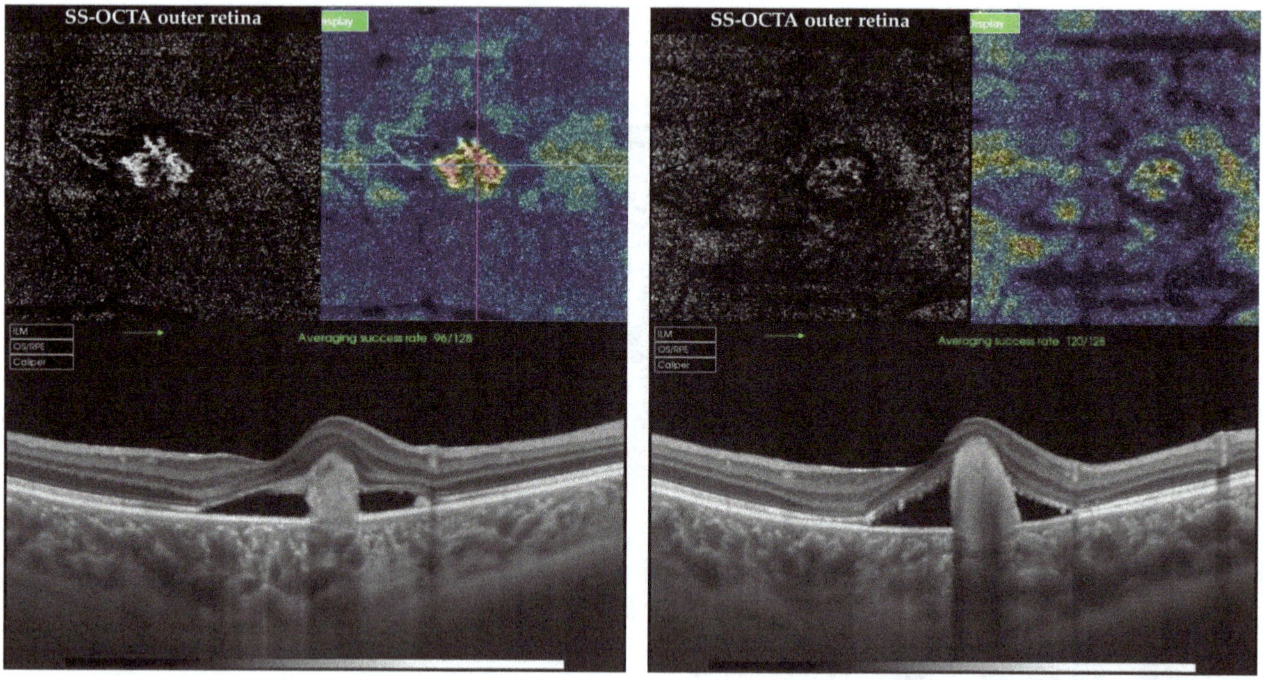

Figure 12. Case 6. Left, en face SS-OCTA projection of the outer retina and the corresponding flow density map in a 3 × 3 mm field of the RE of the same patient as in **Figure 11**. Note the hyperintense signal due to high flow within an interlacing curvilinear neovascular tuft characteristic of active CNV. Note the bright red color code denoting high vessel density. Corresponding SS-OCT shows the hyper-reflective lesion in the sub-retinal space. Right, en face SS-OCTA projection of the outer retina and the corresponding flow density map in a 3 × 3 mm field of the LE demonstrating hyperintense signal due to flow within an inactive lesion (vascularized disciform scar). Note the much less vessel density represented by a faint yellow color code compared to the RE signal intensity. The quality of SS-OCTA image of the LE is degraded by motion artifacts due to poor fixation. Corresponding SS-OCT shows the hyper-reflective lesion in the sub-retinal space.

a distinct active neovascular complex which appeared as a small tuft of bright high-flow (hyperintense signal) curvilinear vessels, whereas SS-OCTA of the LE at the plane of the outer retina demonstrated flow within inactive lesion (vascularized disciform scar). It is worth noting that in this case, both FFA and SS-OCT were inconclusive in confirming the diagnosis and the state of activity of CNV; meanwhile, SS-OCTA unequivocally displayed active CNV in the RE and vascularized disciform scar in the LE (**Figures 11** and **12**).

8. Limitations of SS-OCTA in imaging macular dystrophies

Despite the obvious advantages of OCTA as a noninvasive risk-free technology, an important consideration is that a sizeable portion of the population, targeted by OCTA imaging in macular dystrophies, is in the pediatric age group. Often, children are unable to maintain steady fixation during OCTA examination; hence, the quality of the image could be degraded by motion artifacts and segmentation errors. Future advances in eye tracking and segmentation algorithms, and introduction of portable machines for examination under anesthesia could improve the versatility of OCTA technology in imaging macular dystrophies.

9. Conclusion

The appearance of clinical changes on fundus examination of patients with macular dystrophies is synonymous with the already established damage of a certain level with consequent visual morbidity. Until the present date, OCTA has proven its efficacy in imaging macular dystrophies and identifying the morphological alteration in the vascular layers of the ocular fundus associated with different disease stages. Moreover, SS-OCTA is an essential imaging tool whenever FFA and SS-OCT reveal inconclusive results in the advent of CNV development secondary to vitelliform macular dystrophy. The future of OCTA in imaging macular dystrophies lies in its potential for screening target population and identifying patients at incipient disease stages well in advance of visible clinical changes by depicting specific OCTA pattern or OCTA *signature* that is diagnostic for a particular macular dystrophy. The objective is to identify patients who would be best candidates for the ongoing trials on gene therapy and stem cell transplantation before irreversible visual dysfunction sets in.

Author details

Magdy Moussa[1,2*] and Mahmoud Leila[3]

*Address all correspondence to: magdymoussa60@gmail.com

1 Ophthalmology Department, Faculty of Medicine, Tanta University, Tanta, Egypt

2 MEDIC Eye Center, Tanta, Egypt

3 Retina Department, Research Institute of Ophthalmology, Giza, Egypt

References

[1] Sohn EH, Mullins RF, Stone EM. Macular dystrophies. In: Ryan SJ, editor. Retina. 5th ed. Philadelphia: Saunders; 2013. pp. 852-886

[2] Agarwal A, JDM G. Heredodystrophic disorders affecting the pigment epithelium and retina. In: Gass' Atlas of Macular Diseases. 5th ed. Philadelphia: Saunders; 2012. pp. 239-436

[3] Richard G, Soubrane G, Yannuzzi LA. Hereditary disorders. In: Fluorescein and ICG Angiography. Textbook and Atlas. 2nd ed. New York: Thieme; 1998. pp. 200-225

[4] von Rückman A, Fitzke FW, Bird AC. Distribution of fundus autofluorescence with a scanning laser ophthalmoscope. The British Journal of Ophthalmology. 1995;**79**(5):407-412

[5] Delori FC, Dorey CK, Staurenghi G, Arend O, Goger DG, Weiter JJ. In vivo fluorescence of the ocular fundus exhibits retinal pigment epithelium lipofuscin characteristics. Investigative Ophthalmology & Visual Science. 1995;**36**(3):718-729

[6] Delori F, Greenberg JP, Woods RL, Fischer J, Duncker T, Sparrow J, Smith RT. Quantitative measurements of autofluorescence with the scanning laser ophthalmoscope. Investigative Ophthalmology & Visual Science. 2011;**52**:9379-9390

[7] Greenberg JP, Duncker T, Woods RL, Smith RT, Sparrow JR, Delori FC. Quantitative fundus autofluorescence in healthy eyes. Investigative Ophthalmology & Visual Science. 2013;**54**:5684-5693

[8] Burke TR, Duncker T, Woods RL, et al. Quantitative fundus autofluorescence in recessive Stargardt disease. Investigative Ophthalmology & Visual Science. 2014;**55**:2841-2852

[9] Duncker T, Lee W, Tsang SH, et al. Distinct characteristics of inferonasal fundus autofluorescence patterns in stargardt disease and retinitis pigmentosa. Investigative Ophthalmology & Visual Science. 2013;**54**:6820-6826

[10] Smith RT, Gomes NL, Barile G, et al. Lipofuscin and autofluorescence metrics in progressive STGD. Investigative Ophthalmology & Visual Science. 2009;**50**:3907-3914

[11] Khan KN, Kasilian M, Mahroo OAR, Tanna P, Kalitzeos A, Robson AG, Tsunoda K, Iwata T, Moore AT, Fujinami K, Michaelides M. Early patterns of macular degeneration in ABCA4–Associated retinopathy. Ophthalmology. 2018;**125**(5):735-746

[12] Rezaei KA, Zhang Q, Chen CL, Chao J, Wang RK. Retinal and choroidal vascular features in patients with retinitis pigmentosa imaged by OCT based microangiography. Graefe's Archive for Clinical and Experimental Ophthalmology. 2017;**255**:1287-1295

[13] Adhi M, Read SP, Ferrara D, Weber M, Duker JS, Waheed NK. Morphology and vascular layers of the choroid in Stargardt disease analyzed using spectral-domain optical coherence tomography. American Journal of Ophthalmology. 2015;**160**(6):1276-1284

[14] Giani A, Pellegrini M, Carini E, Peroglio Deiro A, Bottoni F, Staurenghi G. The dark atrophy with indocyanine green angiography in Stargardt disease. Investigative Ophthalmology & Visual Science. 2012;**53**(7):3999-4004

[15] Mastropasqua R, Toto L, Borrelli E, Di Antonio L, Mattei PA, Senatore A, Di Nicola M, Mariotti C. Optical coherence tomography angiography findings in Stargardt disease. PLoS One. 2017;**12**(2):e0170343. DOI: 10.1371/journal.pone.0170343

[16] Guduru A, Lupidi M, Gupta A, Jalali S, Chhablani J. Comparative analysis of autofluorescence and OCT angiography in Stargardt disease. The British Journal of Ophthalmology. 2017;**0**:1-4. DOI: 10.1136/bjophthalmol-2017-311000

[17] Korte GE, Reppucci V, Henkind P. RPE destruction causes choriocapillary atrophy. Investigative Ophthalmology & Visual Science. 1984;**25**(10):1135-1145

[18] Neuhardt T, May CA, Wilsch C, Eichhorn M, Lutjen-Drecoll E. Morphological changes of retinal pigment epithelium and choroid in rd-mice. Experimental Eye Research. 1999; **68**(1):75-83

[19] Blaauwgeers HG, Holtkamp GM, Rutten H, et al. Polarized vascular endothelial growth factor secretion by human retinal pigment epithelium and localization of vascular endothelial growth factor receptors on the inner choriocapillaris. Evidence for a trophic paracrine relation. The American Journal of Pathology. 1999;**155**:421-428

[20] Stanga PE, Tsamis E, Papayannis A, Stringa F, Cole T, Jalil A. Swept-source optical coherence tomography angiography™ (Topcon Corp, Japan): Technology review. Developments in Ophthalmology. 2016;**56**:13-17

[21] Bonnin S, Mané V, Couturier A, Julien M, Paques M, Tadayoni R, Gaudric A. New insight into the macular deep vascular plexus imaged by optical coherence tomography angiography. Retina. 2015;**35**:2347-2352

[22] Grulkowski I, Liu JJ, Potsaid B, Jayaraman V, Lu CD, Jiang J, Cable AE, Duker JS, Fujimoto JG. Retinal, anterior segment and full eye imaging using ultrahigh speed swept source OCT with vertical-cavity surface emitting lasers. Biomedical Optics Express. 2012;**3**:2733-2751

[23] Gao SS, Liu G, Huang D, Jia Y. Optimization of the split-spectrum amplitude-decorrelation angiography algorithm on a spectral optical coherence tomography system. Optics Letters. 2015;**40**:2305-2308

[24] Kuehlewein L, Tepelus TC, An L, Durbin MK, Srinivas S, Sadda SR. Noninvasive visualization and analysis of the human parafoveal capillary network using swept source OCT optical microangiography. Investigative Ophthalmology & Visual Science. 2015;**56**: 3984-3988

[25] Savastano MC, Lumbroso B, Rispoli M. In vivo characterization of retinal vascularization morphology using optical coherence tomography angiography. Retina. 2015;**35**: 2196-2203

[26] Pechauer AD, Jia Y, Liu L, Gao SS, Jiang C, Huang D. Optical coherence tomography angiography of peripapillary retinal blood flow response to hyperoxia. Investigative Ophthalmology & Visual Science. 2015;**56**:3287-3291

[27] Sambhav K, Grover S, Chalam KV. The application of optical coherence tomography angiography in retinal diseases. Survey of Ophthalmology. 2017;**62**:838-866

[28] De Carlo TE, Adhi M, Salz DA, Joseph T, Waheed NK, Seddon JM, Duker JS, Reichel E. Analysis of choroidal and retinal vasculature in inherited retinal degenerations using optical coherence tomography angiography. Ophthalmic Surgery, Lasers & Imaging Retina. 2016;**47**:120-127

[29] Parodi MB, Cicinelli MV, Rabiolo A, Pierro L, Bolognesi G, Bandello F. Vascular abnormalities in patients with Stargardt disease assessed with optical coherence tomography angiography. The British Journal of Ophthalmology. 2017;**101**:780-785

[30] Querques G, Zambrowski O, Corvi F, Miere A, Semoun O, Srour M, Souied EH. Optical coherence tomography angiography in adult-onset foveomacular vitelliform dystrophy. The British Journal of Ophthalmology. 2016;**100**:1724-1730

[31] Parodi MB, Rabiolo A, Cicinelli MV, Iacono P, Romano F, Bandello F. Quantitative analysis of optical coherence tomography angiography in adult-onset foveomacular vitelliform dystrophy. Retina. 2018;**38**:237-244

[32] Parodi MB, Romano F, Cicinelli MV, Rabiolo A, Arrigo A, Pierro L, Iacono P, Bandello F. Retinal vascular impairment in best vitelliform macular dystrophy assessed by means of optical coherence tomography angiography. American Journal of Ophthalmology. 2018;**187**:61-70

[33] Lupidi M, Coscas G, Cagini C, Coscas F. Optical coherence tomography angiography of a choroidal neovascularization in adult onset foveomacular vitelliform dystrophy: Pearls and pitfalls. Investigative Ophthalmology & Visual Science. 2015;**56**:7638-7645

[34] Guduru A, Gupta A, Tyagi M, Jalali S, Chhablani J. Optical coherence tomography angiography characterization of best disease and associated choroidal neovascularization. The British Journal of Ophthalmology. 2018;**102**:444-447

[35] Treder M, Lauermann JL, Alnawaiseh M, Heiduschka P, Eter N. Quantitative changes in flow density in patients with adult-onset foveomacular vitelliform dystrophy: An OCT angiography study. Graefe's Archive for Clinical and Experimental Ophthalmology. 2018;**256**:23-28

[36] Demirel S, Yanık Ö, Nalcı H, Batıoğlu F, Özmert E. The use of optical coherence tomography angiography in pachychoroid spectrum diseases: A concurrent comparison with dye angiography. Graefe's Archive for Clinical and Experimental Ophthalmology. 2017;**255**:2317-2324

[37] Tan ACS, Tan GS, Dennsiton AK, Keane PA, Ang M, Milea D, Chakravarthy U, Cheung CMG. An overview of the clinical applications of optical coherence tomography angiography. Eye. 2018;**32**:262-286

[38] El-Maftouhi MQ, El Maftouhi A, Eandi CM. Chronic central serous chorioretinopathy imaged by optical coherence tomographic angiography. American Journal of Ophthalmology. 2015;**160**(3):581-587.e1

[39] Moussa M, Leila M, Khalid H, Lolah M. Detection of silent type I choroidal neovascular membrane in chronic central serous chorioretinopathy using en face swept-source optical coherence tomography angiography. Journal of Ophthalmology. 2017; Article ID 6913980:1-10. doi.org/10.1155/2017/6913980

[40] Moussa M, Leila M. Swept-source optical coherence tomography angiography in pediatric patients. European Ophthalmology News. 09.2016.XXXIV congress of the ESCRS report

9

Intraoperative OCT in Lamellar Corneal Transplants (DALK, DSAEK, DMEK)

Jorge Luis Domene Hinojosa,
Jorge L. Domene-Hickman and
Nuria Judith Alemán Hurtado

Abstract

An explanation of this new technology, consisting of optical coherence tomography integrated to the microscope in both anterior and posterior lamellar corneal transplants (DALK, DSAEK, DMEK). The advantages of visualizing the different layers of the host and donor cornea, with specific emphasis in the Descemet-stroma interphase, are explained in the written work and captured in the intraoperative images. This technology makes the procedure safer, increases the surgery success rate and consequently improves the postoperative results in the patient. The surgical technique of the lamellar transplants and its benefits are explained. The advantages of this new technology are analyzed, including visualizing the corneal planes, checking the tissue orientation and ensuring the correct execution of critical surgical steps; all of these help in reducing the technical difficulty of the procedure. Likewise, it is explained that by providing direct transurgical visualization in a screen, there is a potential teaching and academic advantage.

Keywords: deep anterior lamellar keratoplasty (DALK), Descemet stripping automated endothelial keratoplasty (DSAEK), Descemet membrane endothelial keratoplasty (DMEK), optical coherence tomography (OCT), lamellar transplant, Descemet-stroma interphase

1. Introduction

We are familiarized with the term *penetrating keratoplasty* (PK), which is a transplant of the full thickness of the cornea. Nowadays, lamellar transplants are widely accepted because of its many advantages like a decreased probability for immunologic rejection, higher resistance to trauma, anatomic integrity maintenance, better refractive stability, a quicker rehabilitation and a surgery with fewer risks. Anterior lamellar transplants have evolved into the deep anterior lamellar keratoplasty (DALK), which is the substitution of the entire stroma while maintaining the recipient's Descemet membrane and endothelium. Endothelial transplants have also seen a wide range of changes throughout the years. In the present day, the most widely performed techniques are Descemet stripping automated endothelial keratoplasty (DSAEK), in which the recipient's endothelium and a thin layer of posterior stroma are replaced, and Descemet membrane endothelial keratoplasty (DMEK), in which only the Descemet and endothelium are replaced. Even though lamellar transplants have a wide array of advantages, these techniques are not always offered by the ophthalmologist due to the complexity and the difficult learning curve of the surgical technique, which requires a precise dissection of the corneal anatomic layers. The use of a transurgical optical coherence tomography (OCT) may help the surgeon to visualize the corneal layers and hence increase the rate of success in lamellar transplants.

2. Historical background

2.1. DALK

The firts anterior lamellar keratoplasty was performed in 1905 [1]. In the second half of the twentieth century [1], PK became the surgical gold standard to treat the majority of the axial diseases in the cornea. Meanwhile in Colombia at the start of the 1950s, José Barraquer et al. began dissecting two-thirds of the stroma in both the donor and the recipient's cornea [2], but the technique did not gain popularity due to the poor final visual acuity in patients due to irregularities of the interphase.

Beginning in 1984, Eduardo Arenas Archila created the term *deep anterior lamellar keratoplasty* (DALK) by using intrastromal air to dissect the corneal tissue [3]. This technique has evolved over time, and currently surgical techniques achieve the complete separation of the stroma-Descemet interphase with few risks, maintaining the integrity of the Descemet with no stromal residue, which is extremely important to reach a high-quality visual acuity.

In 2002, Anwar developed the *Big Bubble* technique, which is the most widely used one nowadays [2]. This technique allows the separation of the corneal stroma and Descemet with an injection of air into the deep stroma with a #30 cannula after a partial trepanation (80% deep), in this way modifying Archila's technique [4]. The key step in this procedure is the correct injection of air into the recipient's pre-Descemet space to facilitate the removal of the stromal tissue. This technique has been widely accepted worldwide due to its easy reproducibility and high success rate. Nevertheless, it has a steep learning curve that has slowed its adoption [5]. In 2012, Ghanem describes the *pachy-bubble* technique, in which he used transurgical pachymetry to penetrate 90% of the corneal thickness with a diamond scalpel to reach with the air the pre-Descemet space with a higher success rate [6].

2.2. DSAEK

In 1956, Tillen introduced the concept of replacing the corneal endothelium by describing the first case of a posterior lamellar keratoplasty [7]. He described how he performed a lamellar dissection of the recipient's cornea and afterward inserted the donor's endothelium to the anterior chamber, suturing it to the recipient's cornea and finally injecting air to apply pressure on the donor endothelium. In 1980, Barraquer modified this technique and trepanated the posterior stroma and sutured to it a posterior lenticule from the donor [8].

Melles is credited with the current success of the endothelial transplant and with the concept of posterior lamellar keratoplasties through a posterior approach [8]. He was the first surgeon to successfully place an endothelial graft to the recipient's stroma without the use of sutures, which allowed better visual results. The procedure was adapted, modified and popularized by Price, which named it *Descemet stripping endothelial keratoplasty* (DSEK). Gorovoy modified this technique by dissecting the donor cornea with a microkeratome, hence the name *descemet stripping automated endothelial keratoplasty* (DSAEK) and is nowadays the most popular technique for endothelial transplants. With the wide acceptance of these techniques, eye banks have begun offering precut donor tissue, facilitating the procedure for surgeons into a one-step procedure.

2.3. DMEK

In 2002, Melles introduced the concept of DMEK [9]. He reported a simpler method for dissecting the stroma of the recipient, by just removing the Descemet and endothelium and placing the endothelium graft behind the recipient's stroma and injecting air into the anterior chamber to hold the graft in place.

3. Indications

3.1. DALK

The DALK procedure is the technique of choice for many diseases in the anterior stroma of the cornea such as [8]:

- keratoconus and other ectasias
- postsurgical corneal ectasia
- partial thickness leukoma
- anterior corneal dystrophies

3.2. DSAEK/DMEK

The indications to perform an endothelial transplant are those that implicate an endothelial dysfunction such as [8]:

- postsurgical bullous keratopathy
- Fuchs dystrophy
- posterior polymorphous corneal dystrophy
- corneal transplant rejection
- traumatic endothelial dysfunction
- iridocorneal endothelial syndrome

4. Advantages

4.1. DALK

The advantages of performing DALK corneal transplants are [1] as follows:

- no immunologic endothelial rejection
- extra-ocular procedure
- higher transurgical safety
- higher resistance to traumatic injuries (**Figure 1**)
- endothelium preservation
- less postsurgical use of steroids
- better refractive stability

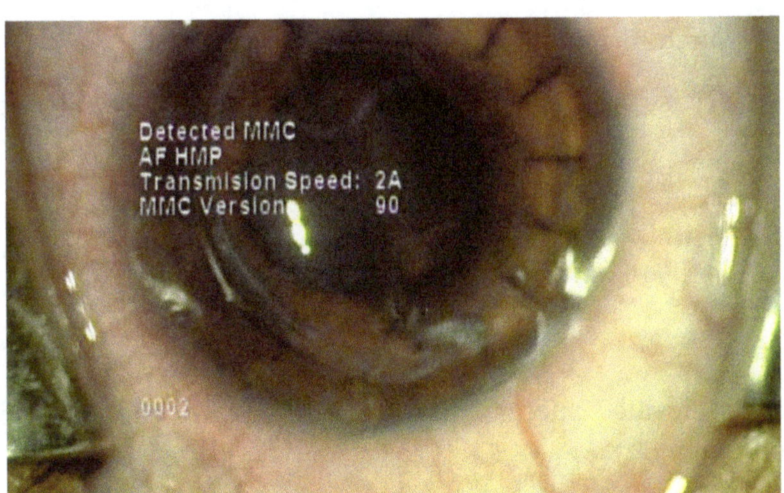

Figure 1. Wound dehiscence in a patient with DALK surgery. The patient received an ocular trauma 1 month postsurgery and eight stitches broke, yet the Descemet remained intact without aqueous humor leakage.

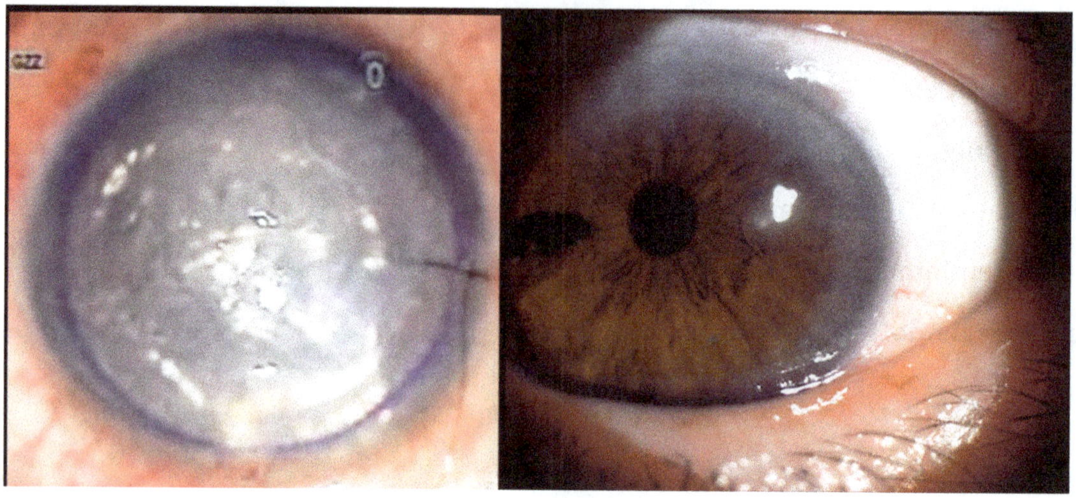

Figure 2. Clinical photographs of an endothelial transplant. On the left a photograph taken at the end of the surgery and on the right the same eye 12 months later.

4.2. DSAEK/DMEK

The advantages of performing endothelial transplants are [8] as follows:

- lower immunologic rejection rate
- less transurgical risks
- small incision
- less sutures or absence of them
- less complications related to ocular surface
- preservation of the corneal innervation
- preservation of the anatomic integrity of the cornea
- visual acuity recovery is faster, more stable and more predictable (**Figure 2**)

5. Surgical technique

5.1. DALK

Nowadays, due to its elevated success rate, the authors use the pachy-bubble technique, which will be described here.

The technique begins with a partial trepanation of 80% of the corneal thickness and an average diameter of 8 mm. Afterward, an ultrasound pachymeter is utilized to measure the corneal thickness in MXII, at a distance of 3 mm from the visual axis. The diamond scalpel is calibrated for 90% of the pachymetric measurement and a 4-mm incision is performed in this area. Air is injected into the anterior chamber, which will help verify the formation of the big bubble. A specially designed cannula is inserted and moved through the pre-Descemet plane until the visual axis is reached. It is in this zone were air will be injected. Afterward, the stroma is perforated to reach the stroma-Descemet interphase, which is now full of air (**Figure 3**). The stroma is removed and the donor cornea (with no endothelium) is sutured with nylon 10–0.

It is important to mention that to achieve an adequate Descemet detachment, the air injection should be very deep, unfortunately leading to an increased perforation risk [2]. This step continues to be the most challenging part of the surgery.

If the injection of air is too superficial or if it remains in the medium stroma, it will usually disseminate laterally without detaching the Descemet and will give the cornea a diffuse-white appearance. When this happens, the surgeon must try to inject the air deeper or change to a manual dissection (layer by layer) technique, which frequently leads to perforation. This technique is a challenge in advanced keratoconus with a severe corneal thinning or scarring and has a reserved success rate when there are dense corneal opacities due to the bad depth visibility [6].

Some of the disadvantages of this type of transplant are its steep learning curve and its longer surgical time compared to a PK [1]. In many countries, including Mexico, this technique does not have a widespread use secondary to its difficulty and longer time requirements. Nowadays, even a skilled surgeon performs with a risk of perforation between 10 and 30% [10].

The DALK procedure has some complications including [1]:

- Descemet membrane rupture
- double anterior chamber
- loss of endothelial cells secondary to air/gas
- interphase opacities or irregularities

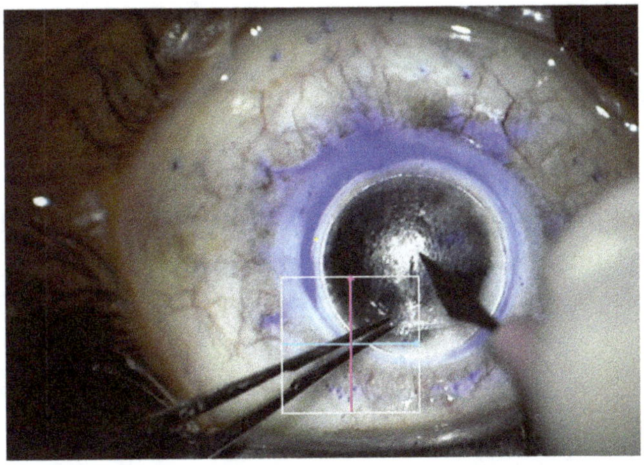

Figure 3. Perforation of the corneal stroma in a DALK corneal transplant.

- detritus, hemorrhage, vascularization, microbial infections and epithelial growth in the interphase
- pupillary block glaucoma secondary to injected air in anterior chamber
- recurrence of the stromal corneal dystrophy
- Difficulty in re-epithelization

5.2. DSAEK

There are many variations to the original endothelial transplant DSAEK technique. The one used by the authors is described here.

The donor cornea is prepared using a Moria microkeratome adapted to an artificial anterior chamber. The ideal thickness is between 90 and 120 μm. Afterward, the donor cornea is trepanated with an average diameter of 8.25 mm.

Once the donor tissue is obtained, surgery begins by inserting an anterior chamber maintainer. Trypan blue solution is inserted to the anterior chamber for better visualization of the Descemet membrane. A circular descemetorhexis is performed with a diameter of 8.25 mm. A 2-mm incision is done on the temporal limbus and a 4-mm incision on the nasal limbus. An iridotomy is performed on the meridian at six o´clock and the donor tissue is inserted through the nasal incision using a Busin glide or any other type of injector designed for this purpose. The temporal incision is used for the instrument used to help during the insertion of the donor tissue. Finally, the anterior chamber is filled with air for adequate fixation of the graft.

The DSAEK procedure has some complications including:

- lack of adherence of the donor tissue
- foldings or tears in the donated tissue
- inverted positioning of the tissue
- endothelial dysfunction secondary to surgical trauma
- pneumatic pupillary block

The most reported complication in endothelial transplants is the lack of adherence of the donor tissue to the recipient's stroma. The key to reducing the dislocation is a meticulous reconstruction of the wound (so that there is no leakage of aqueous humor) and complete removal of fluid from the interphase. Whenever a graft is dislocated, it can be accommodated once again with air injections; nevertheless, this may cause damage to the endothelial cells.

5.3. DMEK

The DMEK technique used by the authors is described below.

To obtain the donor tissue, the Blister technique is used, a technique developed by Eric Abdullayev (Manager of Clinical Development and Innovations at Lions Eye Institute for

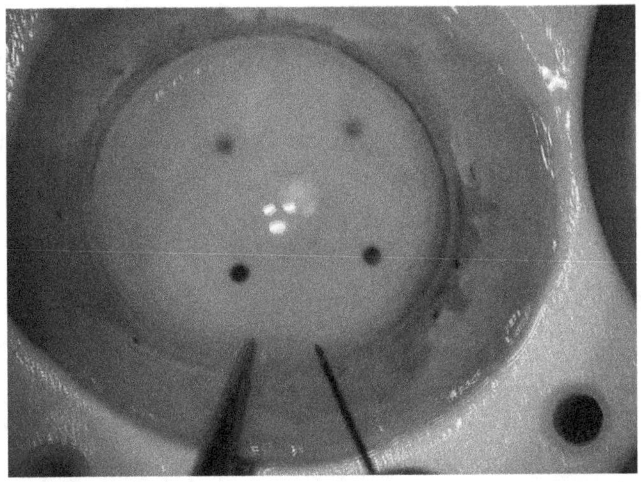

Figure 4. Blister technique for the isolation of corneal Descemet-endothelium prior to a DMEK surgery.

Transplant and Research, Tampa, Florida, USA). In this technique, balanced saline solution is injected to achieve separation of the Descemet membrane (**Figure 4**). Currently, it is possible to get the tissue prepared and preloaded by the staff of some eye banks, which facilitates the procedure and eliminates the risks of tissue preparation in the operating room.

Once the donor tissue is obtained, surgery is performed on the recipient, initiating with the introduction of trypan blue to improve Descemet visualization, then the circular descemetorhexis of an average of 8.25 mm is performed. The Descemet can be extracted using the irrigation-aspiration piece of the phacoemulsification equipment, through a previously performed 3 mm incision. An iridectomy is performed in MVI, and the donor tissue is introduced and unfolded with delicate hydraulic and pressure-counter-pressure maneuvers, finally introducing the air/gas in the anterior chamber once the correct unfolding of the graft has been ensured. The eye must be completely sealed with or without sutures.

The DMEK procedure has some complications including:

- lack of adherence of the donor tissue
- foldings or tears in the donated tissue
- inverted positioning of the tissue
- endothelial dysfunction secondary to surgical trauma
- pneumatic pupillary block

Currently, the number of surgeons performing DMEK is on the rise because of its better visual acuity results when compared to DSAEK.

6. Overview of optical coherence tomography (OCT)

The OCT is based on the principle of low coherence interferometry to measure distances. A light source is used, typically a superluminescent infrared diode with a wavelength between

830 and 1325 nm. OCT has revolutionized clinical ophthalmology, and its development continues providing opportunities for a better diagnosis and even management of eye diseases. Originally introduced in the 1990´s at the Massachusetts Institute of Technology in 1991 as a technique for noninvasive transverse imaging of biological systems, the image of the retina was the first application of this technology [11]. OCT devices have undergone modifications in their original technique to see and measure anterior segment structures such as the cornea, iris, and the lens [12]. In 1994, Izatt described the use of OCT for the anterior segment with a resolution close to histological level [13]. Since then, it has been used for the diagnosis and

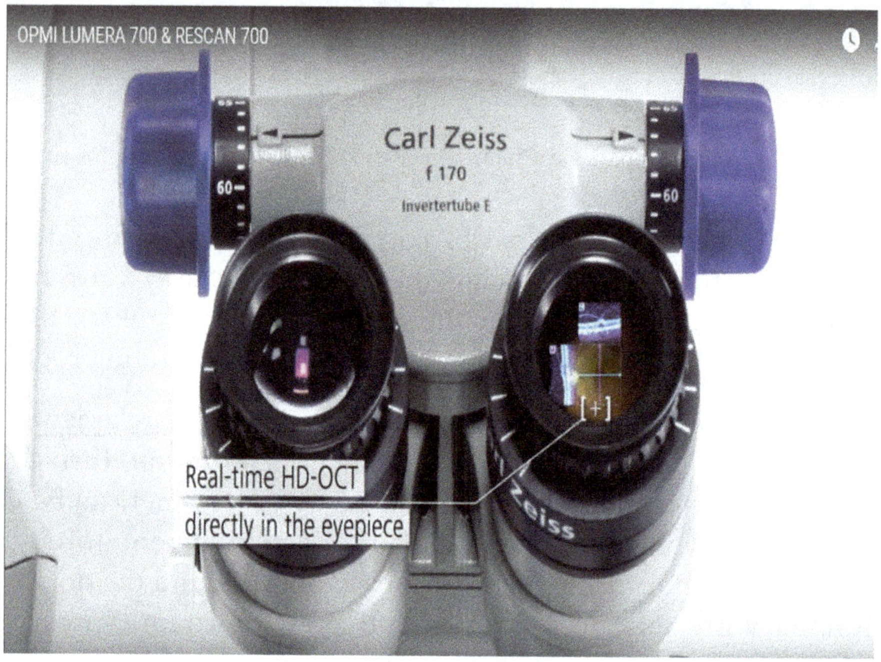

Figure 5. OPMI LUMERA & RESCAN 700 microscope, where OCT images can be observed in real time.

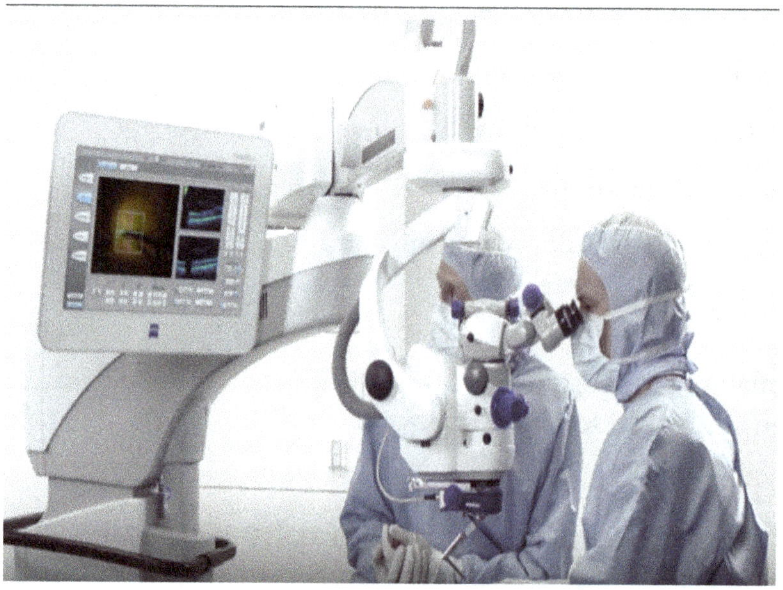

Figure 6. OPMI LUMERA & RESCAN 700 microscope, OCT images can be appreciated for all members of the surgical team.

management of various corneal conditions. Now that it is one of the most important diagnostic tests in ophthalmology, it is natural to use this technology in the operating room, as it provides a unique feedback mechanism in real time and helps facilitate the achievement of surgical objectives.

The authors use the OPMI Lumera® 700 and RESCAN™ microscope from Zeiss (**Figures 5** and **6**), and this microscope includes an integrated OCT system, which optimizes the procedure of deep anterior lamellar keratoplasty and endothelial keratoplasty.

7. Use of transurgical OCT for lamellar transplants (DALK, DSAEK, DMEK)

The application of OCT to lamellar transplant surgery is a useful tool to visualize the tissue planes and depth in the different steps of the surgery. This system optimizes the surgical procedure by letting the surgeon observe high-resolution images both at the eyepiece level of the microscope and at an external screen. By objectively visualizing depth in the different steps of surgery, greater safety is achieved by decreasing the risk of complications and facilitating surgical maneuvers, thereby increasing the success rate.

7.1. DALK

With this new technology, the depth of trepanation can be assessed, avoiding corneal perforations, especially in patients with thickness irregularities, such as keratoconus [14] (**Figure 7**). It is also possible to verify the depth of the cut with the diamond scalpel in the pachy-bubble technique, which is of vital importance to achieve the air injection close to Descemet, avoiding perforation and superficial air injection. Sorcia observed a higher success rate in reaching the pre-Descemet planes when performing DALK pachy-bubble [15]. The measurement of

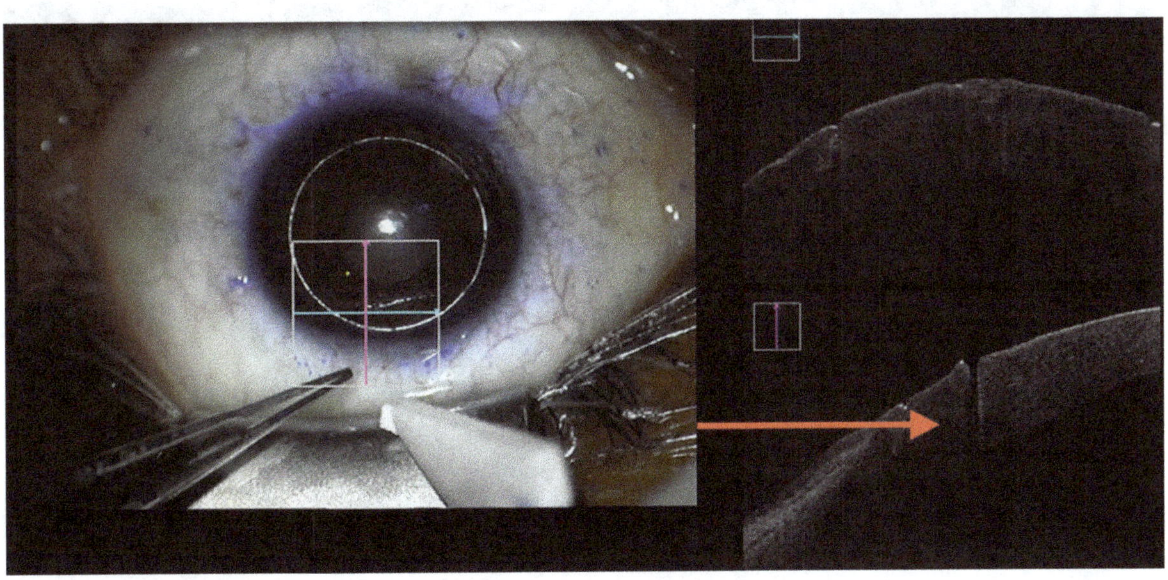

Figure 7. Trepanation depth check (red arrow) by intraoperative OCT.

trepanation seems to be useful to determine if the depth is adequate or there is a need for further dissection to reach the ideal depth for an air injection.

Once air is injected to create the bubble that will separate the Descemet membrane and stroma, OCT images are captured to verify the extent of the dissection, and to check whether it reached the trepanation mark limit. These images will help the surgeon assess if there is risk of perforation or if there exists an inadequate separation of the stroma and the Descemet membrane (**Figures 8–10**).

In cases of poor visibility secondary to injected intrastromal air, the OCT helps to see the extension of the big bubble in the anterior chamber to ensure it is complete and to prevent perforation when removing the stroma (**Figure 11**).

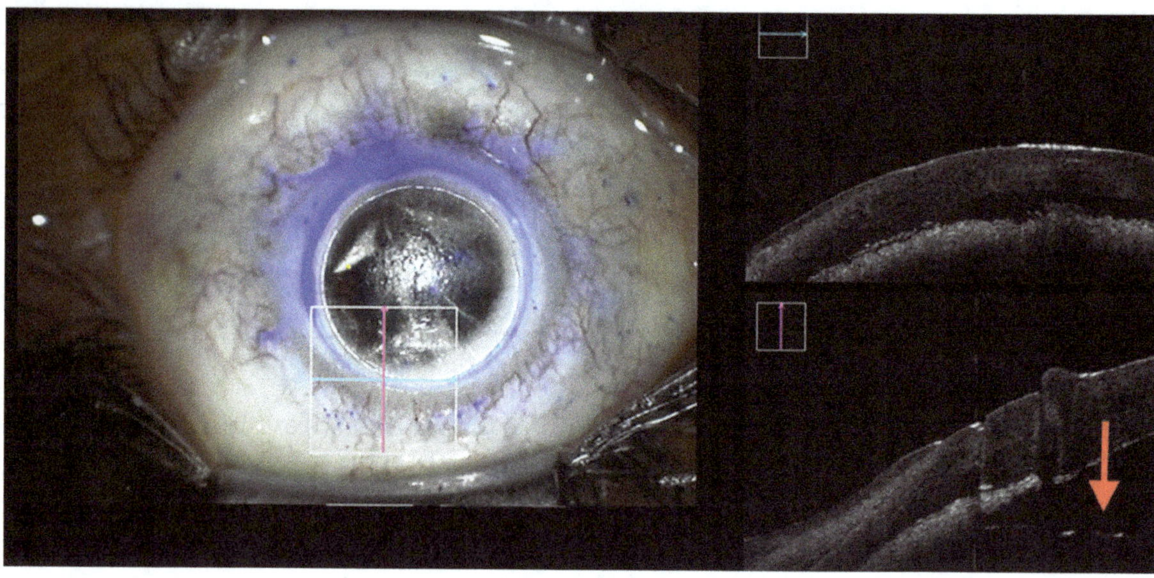

Figure 8. The red arrow points to the Descemet membrane separated from the stroma by air forming the big bubble.

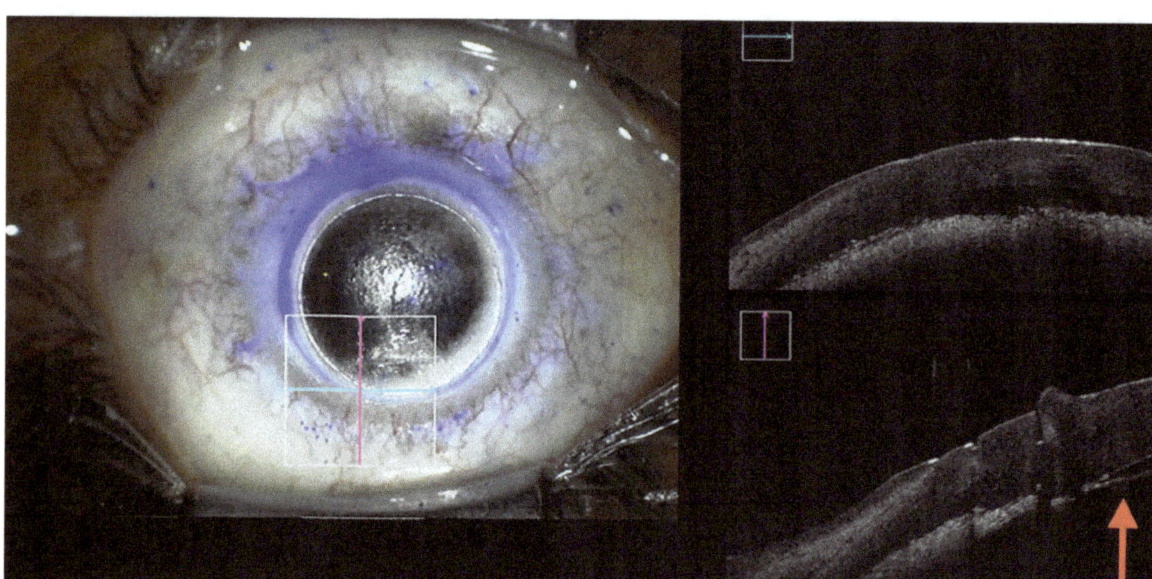

Figure 9. Descemet membrane (red arrow) returning to its original location. This is after the perforation of the stroma.

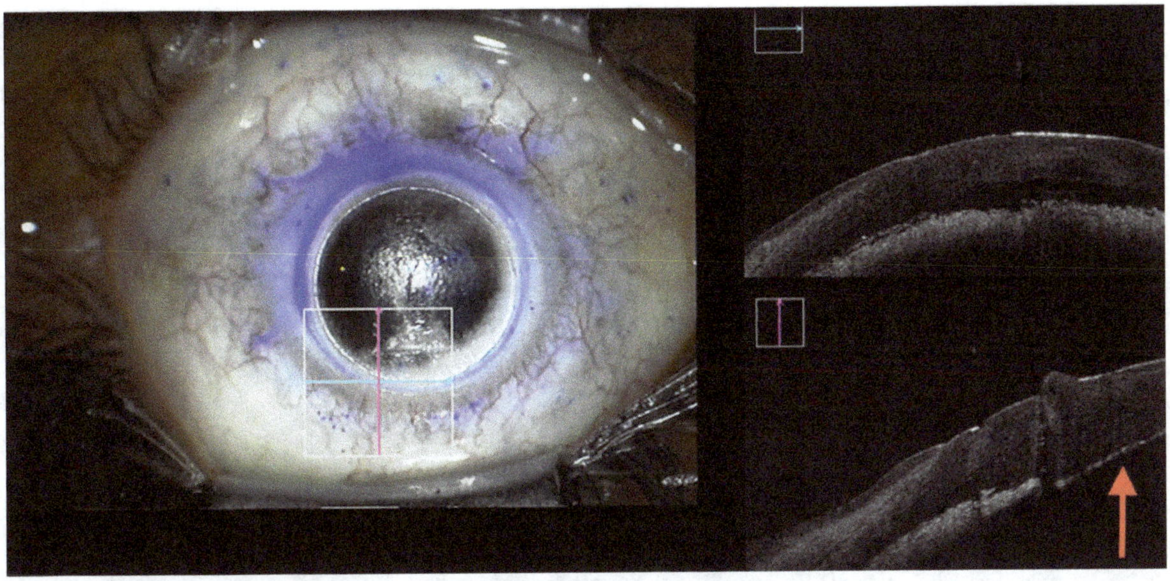

Figure 10. Descemet membrane (red arrow) is completely adhered to the stroma.

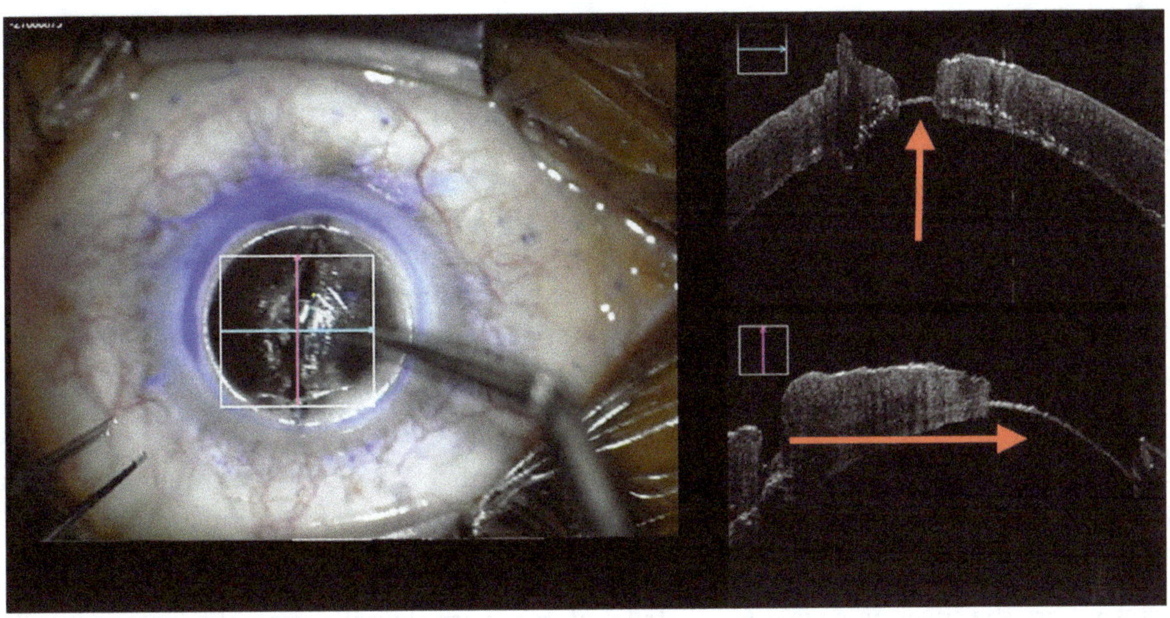

Figure 11. Stromal dissection. The OCT images guide the surgeon to avoid perforation of the Descemet membrane (red arrow).

After the dissection is completed, the surgeon can evaluate if the stroma was completely removed (**Figure 12**). The donor button is allocated and sutured, and the position of both tissues is evaluated. The surgeon should look for irregularities, liquid or air that separates both tissues anywhere. With the OCT system, it is possible to optimize the approximation of graft and host.

7.2. DSAEK/DMEK

When preparing the donor button in the DSAEK transplant, after passing the microkeratome, the residual thickness of the donor can be evaluated with the help of transoperative OCT to guide the surgeon in selecting the ideal blade size for a second cut with the microkeratome [16],

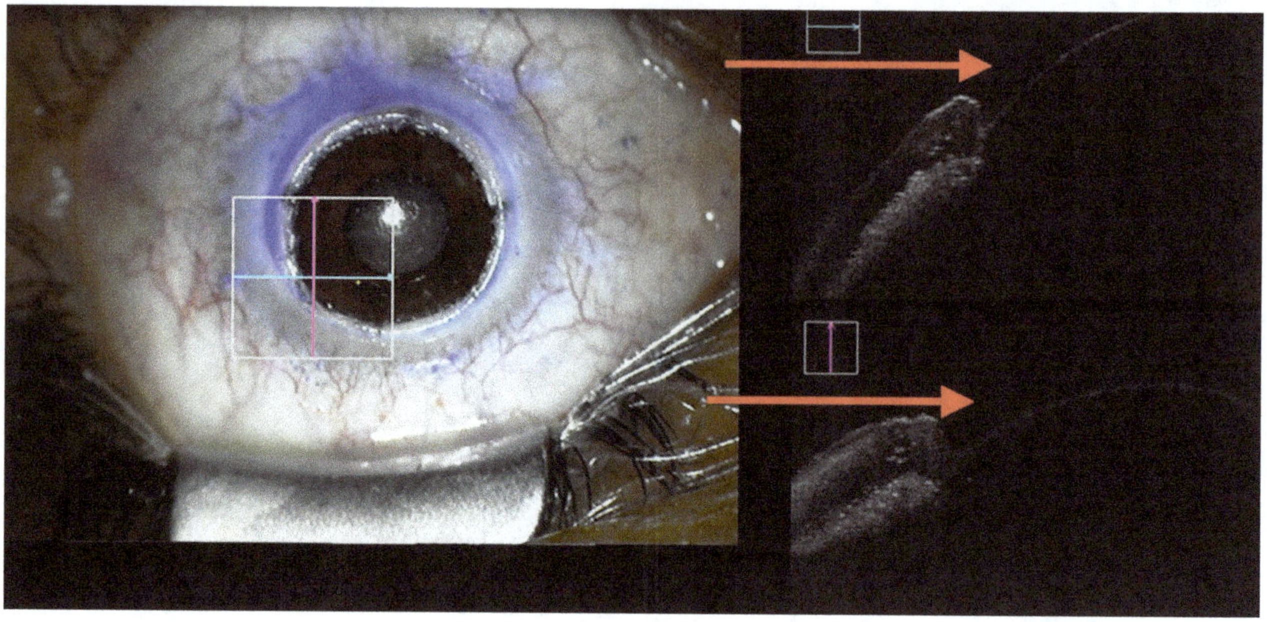

Figure 12. Descemet membrane without any stromal tissue.

in case a thinner donor button is required. Even in cases where the microkeratome is passed once, transoperative OCT evaluates the thickness of the donor cornea and helps to select the ideal size of the blade.

With the transurgical OCT, the state of the donor graft can be observed. In the case of precut grafts for DSAEK, the precut lines are visualized in the corneal images, as well as defects or detritus on the endothelial surface, although these changes have no clinical importance [17]. In the case of DMEK, in addition to showing the space between the endothelium-stroma interphase, another use of transurgical OCT is to prevent cases where the donor button is inverted in the anterior chamber [17].

In donor grafts for DMEK surgery, partial detachments of the Descemet membrane can be observed. Other defects and detritus can also be observed. Therefore, transoperative OCT is an excellent alternative to observe the state of the donor tissue.

In cases where the surgeon's vision is obstructed, for example with corneal edema in a bullous keratopathy, the use of transurgical OCT can help with decision-making inside the operating room [13]. In cases with opaque or edematous corneas, the visualization of the Descemet is difficult, and transurgical OCT can help with its visualization and descemetorhexis. The remaining Descemet membrane can be identified in the case of fibrous or scarred corneas [16]. In this case, transurgical OCT also helps to monitor the insertion and unfolding of the graft, since it can inadvertently have an inverse configuration and result in a failed surgery. With this, the surgeon may ensure an adequate deployment and orientation of the graft, especially in the case of the DMEK surgery in which the graft is much thinner than that of DSAEK (**Figure 13**).

Traditionally, the graft-recipient interphase is reviewed in the slit lamp or in the microscope, but with transoperative OCT, additional information is provided to the surgeon regarding the manipulation of the graft and the final interphase between the graft recipient (**Figure 14**), which can influence the postoperative results.

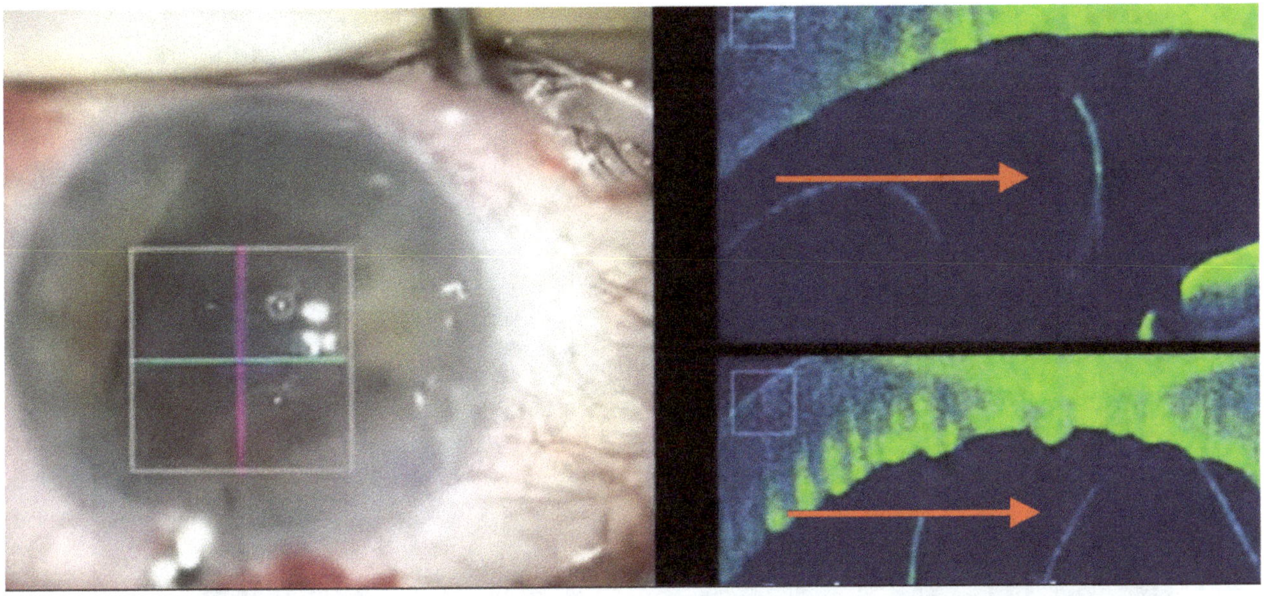

Figure 13. Unfolding of endothelial tissue (red arrow) in DMEK, verifying the tissue orientation. Courtesy of Zeiss.

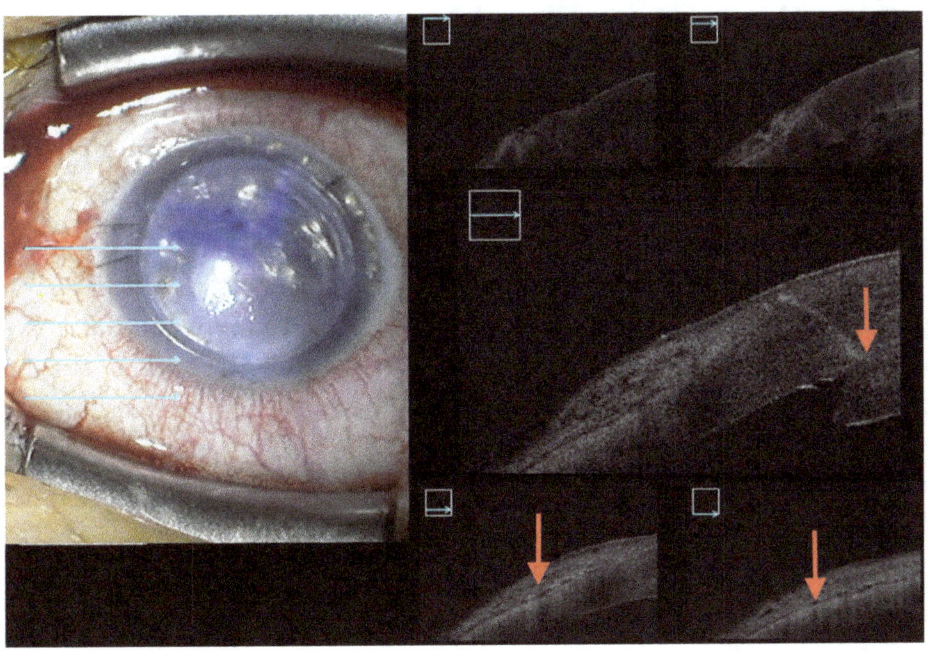

Figure 14. Verification of complete apposition of the donor tissue to the recipient bed, without any space between.

The use of OCT has proved to be useful in detecting any residual space in the interphase at the end of DSAEK surgery. In 2010, Knecht published the first use of transurgical OCT in DSAEK and demonstrated serially the decrease of fluid in the interphase [16], doing manual measurements of the interphase's area of greatest amplitude (between the graft and the recipient). Hallahan correlated the transurgical interphase with the fluid measurements between the graft and the receiver and found that the greater the fluid measurements, the greater the risk for disinsertion and lack of graft adherence in the postoperative period [18].

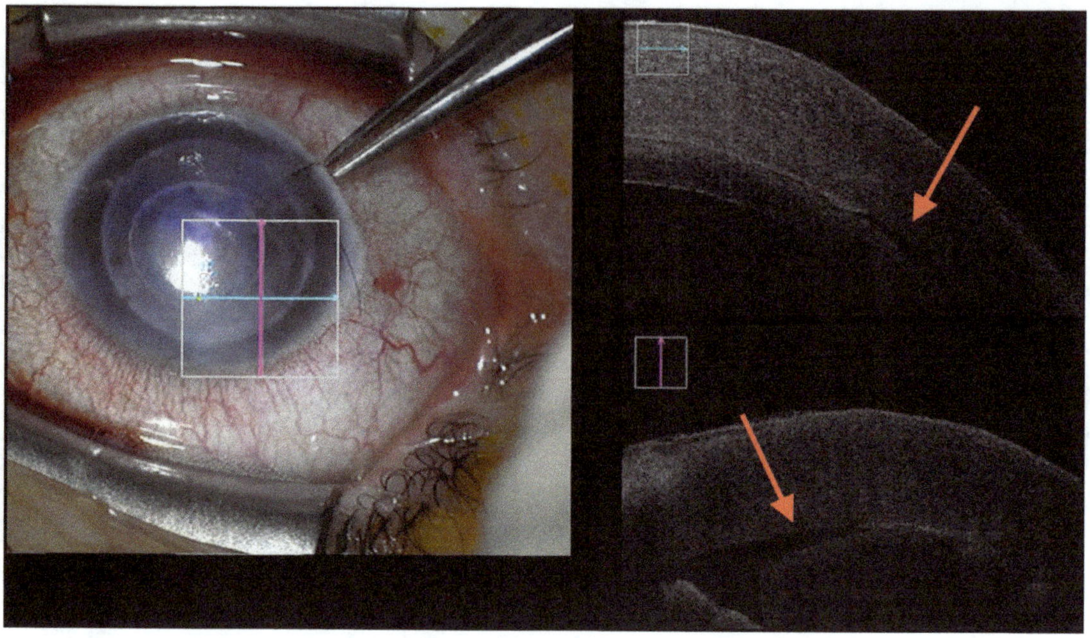

Figure 15. Lack of apposition between donor and recipient tissues, which indicates that additional maneuvers must be performed to achieve correct placement.

If there is an incomplete apposition of the donor lenticule, various maneuvers can be performed such as corneal massage or air tamponade in the anterior chamber to ensure the complete elimination of the fluid between the stroma-Descemet interphase (**Figure 15**). Transoperative OCT helps in determining the efficacy of these maneuvers [16].

A study to determine the feasibility and usefulness of transoperative OCT reported that it indeed helped in decision-making and demonstrated that additional maneuvers were required; this was based on images obtained by OCT in 41% of DSAEK cases. Transoperative OCT revealed persistent fluid in 19% of the cases where the surgeon believed the graft was completely adhered to the stroma. Another finding was that it was indeed adhered in 47% of the cases where the surgeon believed the graft was not completely adhered, therefore reducing the need for further unnecessary surgical manipulation. Transoperative OCT has the potential advantage of decreasing the duration of the surgical event, as well as minimizing graft dislocations [19].

8. Conclusion

The use of this new transoperative OCT technology optimizes the identification of the corneal layer planes by providing a cross section with high-resolution images. These can be observed in real time both in the surgeon's microscope and in an external screen that can be observed by all the staff in the operating room, providing a valuable academic tool. By providing a direct visualization of the critical steps in lamellar transplants (DALK, DSAEK, DMEK), there is an increase in the procedure's safety, it decreases the learning curve of the surgeon in training and facilitates the work of the experienced surgeon by providing detailed visual information in each surgical step, optimizing the decision-making and reducing the surgical event time.

Author details

Jorge Luis Domene Hinojosa[1*], Jorge L. Domene-Hickman[2] and Nuria Judith Alemán Hurtado[1]

*Address all correspondence to: drjldomene@gmail.com

1 Centro Medico Nacional Noreste, Monterrey, Nuevo León, Mexico

2 Tecnologico de Monterrey, Escuela de Medicina y Ciencias de la Salud, Monterrey, Nuevo León, Mexico

References

[1] Reinhart WJ, Musch DC, Jacobs DS. Deep anterior lamellar keratoplasty alternative to penetrating keratoplasty. Opthalmology. 2011;**118**:209-218. DOI: 10.1016/j.ophtha.2010.11.002

[2] Anwar M, Teichmann KD. Deep lamellar keratoplasty: Surgical techniques for anterior lamellar keratoplasty with and without barign of Descemet's membrane. Cornea. 2002;**21**:374-383

[3] Shimmura S, Tsubota K. Deep anterior lamellar keratoplasty. Current Opinion in Ophthalmology. 2006;**17**(4):349-355. DOI: 10.1097/01.icu.0000233953.09595.91

[4] Archila EA. Deep lamellar keratoplasty dissection of host tissue with intrastromal air injecttion. Cornea. 1984-1985;**3**:217-218

[5] Fontana L, Parente G, Tassinari G. Clinical outcomes after deep lamellar keratoplasty using the big bubble technique in patients with keratoconus. American Journal of Ophthalmology. 2007;**143**:117-124. DOI: 10.1016/j.ajo.2006.09.025

[6] Ghanem RC, Ghanem MA. Pachymetry-guided intrastromal air injection ("pachy-bubble") for deep anterior lamellar keratoplasty. Cornea. 2012;**31**:1087-1091. DOI: 10.1097/CO.0b013e31823f8f2d

[7] Tillet CW. Posterior lamellar keratoplasty. American Journal of Ophthalmology. 1956;**41**:530-533

[8] Anshu A, Price MO, Tan DT, Price FW Jr. Endothelial keratoplasty: A revolution in evolution. Survey of Ophthalmology. 2012;**57**:236-252. DOI: 10.1016/j.survophthal.2011.10.005

[9] Melles GR, Lander F, Rietveld FJ. Transplantation of Descemet's membrane carry viable endothelium trough a small scleral incision. Cornea. 2002;**21**:415-418

[10] Trimarchi F, Poppi E, Klersy C, Piacentini C. Deep lamellar keratoplasty. Ophthalmologica. 2001;**215**:389-393. DOI: 10.1159/000050894

[11] Sayegh R, Roberto P. Practical applications of anterior segment optical coherence tomography imaging following corneal surgery. Seminars in Ophtlamology. 2012;**27**:125-132. DOI: 10.3109/08820538.2012.707274

[12] Geerling G, Müller M, Winter C, Hoerauf H. Intraoperative 2-dimensional optical coherence tomography as a new tool for anterior segment surgery. Archives of Ophthalmology. 2005;**123**:253-257. DOI: 10.1001/archopht.123.2.253

[13] Izatt JA, Hee MR, Lin CP. Micrometer - scale resolution imaging of the anterior eye in vivo with optical coherence tomography. Archives of Ophthalmology. 1994;**112**:1584-1589

[14] Domene JL, Ceja SN, Domene Hickman JL. Queratoplastía Lamelar Anterior Profunda (DALK Pachy bubble) guiada por OCT transoperatorio. Caso clínico. Revista Mexicana de Oftalmolgía. Article in press. 2016. DOI: 10.1016/j.mexoft.2016.07.004

[15] Scorcia V, Busin M, Lucisano A. Anterior segment optical coherence tomography-guided big-bubble technique. Ophthalmology. 2013;**120**:471-476. DOI: 10.1016/j.ophtha 2012.08.041

[16] Titiyal JS, Kaur M, Falera R. Intraoperative optical coherence tomography in anterior segment surgieres. Indian Journal of Ophthalmology. 2017;**65**:116-121

[17] Kobayashi A, Yokogawa H, Mori N. Visualization of precut DSAEK and pre-stripped DMEK donor corneas by intraoperative optical coherence tomography using RESCAN 700. BMC Ophthalmology. 2016;**16**:135. DOI: 10.1186/s12886-016-0308-z

[18] Hallahan KM, Cost B, Goshe JM. Intraoperative interface fluid dynamics and clinical outcomes for intraoperative oct-assisted DSAEK from the PIONERR study. American Journal of Ophthalmology. 2017;**173**:16-22. DOI: 10.1016/j.ajo.2016.09.028

[19] Ehlers JP, Goshe J, Dupps WJ. Determination of feasibility and utility of microscope-integrated optical coherence tomography during ophthalmic surgery: The discover study rescan results. JAMA Ophthalmology. 2015;**133**:1124-1132. DOI: 10.1001/jamaoph thalmol.2015.2376

10

Retinal Vasculature Identification and Characterization Using OCT Imaging

Joaquim de Moura, Jorge Novo, José Rouco,
Noelia Barreira, Manuel Penedo and Marcos Ortega

Abstract

The eye fundus is the part of the human body where the blood vessels can be directly observed and studied. For this reason, the analysis and diagnosis of many relevant diseases that affect the circulatory system, for example, reference, hypertension, diabetes or arteriosclerosis can be supported by the use of this source of information, analyzing their degree of severity and impact by the study of the properties of the retinal microcirculation. The development of computer aided-diagnosis tools became relevant over the recent years as they support and facilitate the work of specialists, helping to accurately identify the target structures in many processes of analysis and diagnosis. In that sense, the automatic identification of the retinal vasculature is crucial as its manual identification is an exhaustive and tedious work when it is manually performed by the experts. This chapter presents an analysis of the characteristics of the optical coherence tomography imaging and its potential for the retinal vascular identification and characterization. In that sense, we also analyze computational approaches to automatically obtain and characterize the retinal vasculature and provide an intuitive visualization that facilitates the posterior clinical analysis of relevant diseases such as hypertension or diabetes.

Keywords: computer-aided diagnosis, retinal image analysis, optical coherence tomography, vasculature, retinal microcirculation

1. Introduction

The analysis of the eye fundus is widely used by clinical specialists to identify, analyze and characterize different morphological relevant structures such as the optic disc, the macula or the arterio-venular vasculature. These clinical evaluations allow the doctors to detect and treat different systemic diseases that affect the circulatory system, for example, hypertension

[1], diabetes [2] or arteriosclerosis [3]. Considering the high prevalence and the possible consequences that are directly associated with these diseases, the analysis and monitoring of the retinal microcirculation represents an important task in the diagnostic process [4]. A precise evaluation of the retinal vasculature permits the early identification of several clinical conditions that facilitate an appropriate diagnosis and treatment as well as their prevention [5].

The retinal vessels not only proved their potential in clinical procedures but also in other purposes. Thus, the structure of the retinal vasculature also demonstrated its potential viability as an alternative model for a biometric authentication system [6]. This is due to the complex structure of the retinal vessels, which is unique for each person. Hence, the patterns that were typically used in the identification process are the landmarks of the vasculature [7]. Typically, bifurcations and crossovers are obtained from the retinal vessel tree and used in the identification process [8].

Nowadays, computer-aided diagnosis (CAD) systems are frequently used to improve the accuracy and consistency of different clinical evaluations, facilitating the work of the experts in many relevant diagnostic processes and replacing manual procedures that are tedious and highly time-consuming [9]. These independent decision systems are significantly helpful in the interpretation of several types of medical images, which simplify the doctor's everyday work and improve the quality of patient diagnosis and treatment [10].

Among the different retinal image modalities, optical coherence tomography (OCT) imaging is increasingly in use in clinical services [11]. This imaging modality increased its popularity over the recent years by offering cross-sectional visualizations of the retinal tissues and other relevant structures with a high-resolution and in a reliable noninvasive manner [12]. This technique provides real-time images that are frequently used in the detection, analysis and evaluation of different retinal diseases as, for example, age-related macular degeneration or diabetic retinopathy, which are among the major causes of blindness in the developed countries [13].

The OCT capture technique is based on the principle of the Michelson interferometer to produce the cross-sectional OCT sections, by sequentially collecting reflections from the lateral and longitudinal scans over the retina [14]. The set of OCT sections is complemented with the corresponding near-infrared reflectance (NIR) retinography. Both images are typically captured simultaneously with the OCT capture device by being directly provided to the user for their posterior inspection and use. **Figure 1** shows a representative example of OCT image composed by the NIR image and a corresponding OCT section.

The OCT imaging technique is widely used in the area of ophthalmology, given the facility with which light penetrates in the main ocular structures in both the anterior and posterior segments of the eye [15]. The complete set of information that is provided by this image modality allows the experts to perform a more reliable analysis of the retinal microcirculation that is needed in many processes of diagnosis, treatment and corresponding clinical monitoring [16]. For that reason, a two-dimensional and three-dimensional analysis of the retinal vessel tree in OCT images offers a more precise and coherent information about possible abnormal changes in the retinal vascular architecture that may be derived by a large variability of pathological conditions.

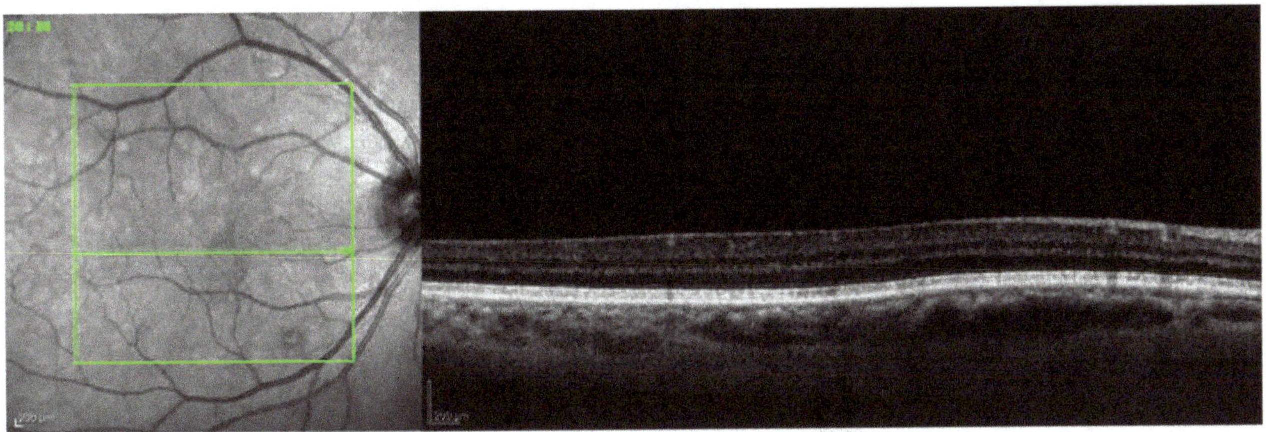

Figure 1. Example of OCT scan. (a) Near-infrared reflectance retinography image and (b) OCT histological section.

In this chapter, we provide an analysis of the characteristics of the OCT image modality and its potential for the retinal vessel tree identification and characterization, which are necessary for many clinical assessments, diagnoses and treatments. In addition, we present a representative computational approach for the automatic detection and characterization of the retinal blood vessels in OCT images, which is combined with an intuitive visualization tool that facilitates the posterior analysis by the clinical specialist in a large variability of diseases. Thus, we motivate the implementation of computational systems and the suitability of the analysis and visualization of their output results.

Section 2 describes the approaches including the extraction of the retinal vasculature and their posterior two-dimensional or three-dimensional reconstruction and visualization. Finally, the conclusion drawn in Section 3 closes this chapter.

2. Automatic extraction and visual reconstruction of the retinal vasculature

The representative system herein described for the vascular extraction and visualization is organized in a set of progressive stages. Firstly, the presence of the retinal vessel tree is automatically identified using the OCT images. In particular, the NIR image and/or the OCT histological sections are analyzed to identify the presence of the vascular structures. Subsequently, the calibers and depth of the vascular profiles are measured. Finally, we use the entire set of extracted information to make a graphical two-/three-dimensional representation, providing an intuitive visualization tool of this complex vascular structure. **Figure 2** illustrates the main parts of the methodology, each stage being detailed in the following subsections.

2.1. Characteristics and variability of the input optical coherence tomography images

Typically, the system receives, as input, a set of OCT images. These images correspond to high-resolution images of the different retinal layers over the macula region approximated by the histological sections. As said, the OCT scan is composed of the NIR image as well as the consecutive OCT histological sections that are often simultaneously obtained by the same capture device, providing sets of images, as illustrated in **Figure 1**. Using these images, we delimited the region where the retinal vessels are located in both modalities.

Recently, several companies have invested in research in the field of ophthalmology especially in the development of OCT capture devices with significant software improvements [17]. Four of the commonly used OCT devices in the daily medical practice are the Cirrus (Carl Zeiss Meditec, Dublin, CA, USA), the Spectralis (Heidelberg Engineering, Heidelberg, Germany), the RTVue (Optovue, Fremont, CA, USA) and the Triton (Topcon, Tokyo, Japan) models. The working principles are similar for all these OCT capture devices; however, they can differ slightly in precision, throughput, depth penetration, acquisition speed, data processing and resolution [18].

In this chapter, we present approaches that were validated mainly with OCT images that are provided by the Spectralis model. Using this OCT capture device, the scan acquisition

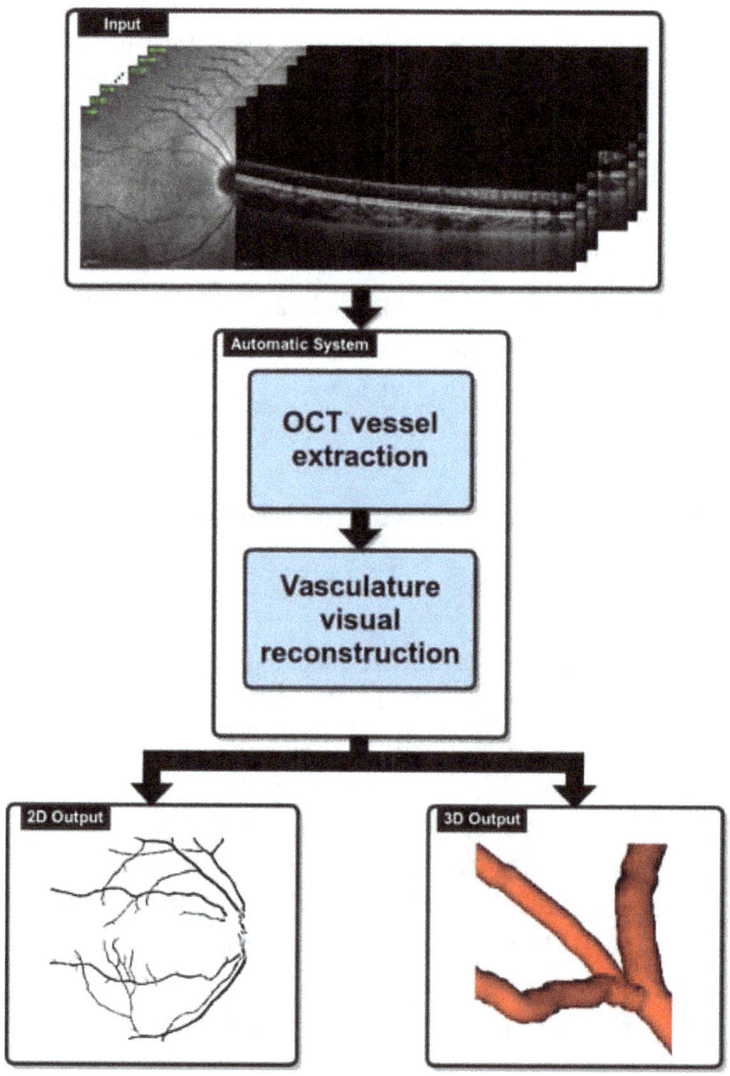

Figure 2. Scheme of the vascular extraction and reconstruction system.

was done by selecting the dense volume scan type over a scan angle of 20°×20°, roughly 6 mm × 6 mm, consisting of 49 B-mode scans acquired utilizing Automatic Real-Time (ART Mean) = 16 (number of scans averaged). B-mode scans are separated by 120 μm from each other and are composed of 1024 A-mode scans, with a separation of 5.5 μm. Each A-mode scan has 496 pixels with 3.8 μm resolution. The system acquires the images at a given frame-rate (8.8 frames/s) and with a given bit depth (32-bits). The approaches herein presented were validated using image datasets including OCT scans with these characteristics. As we can see in the results of the corresponding articles [19, 23], both were satisfactorily tested, demonstrating their suitability for the analyzed issue.

2.2. OCT vessel extraction

Most of the times, the computational systems are provided with both NIR/histological sections. However, there are scenarios where the systems have to perform the analysis with only the availability of the OCT histological sections. For that reason, in this stage, we describe two different and independent approaches for the automatic identification and extraction of the retinal vascular structure, depending on the factor regarding the amount of information of the OCT images provided (see **Figure 3**). The first approach uses the information provided by the NIR image in combination with the histological sections, while the second approach uses only the OCT histological sections for the identification and characterization of the vessel profiles. The characteristics of each approach is detailed in the following subsections.

2.2.1. Vessel extraction using the combination of the near-infrared reflectance image and the histological sections

First, we present a proposal for the identification and segmentation of the retinal vascular structure using the NIR image combined with the histological section images. Generally, the system performs a 2D identification of the vasculature using the NIR image, where we extract the retinal vessel tree and, after that, we obtain the vessel centerline representation. Next, the corresponding calibers of each centerline coordinate are measured. Finally, these identifications are mapped in the corresponding positions of the histological sections to calculate the vascular depths of each vessel coordinate (see **Figure 4**).

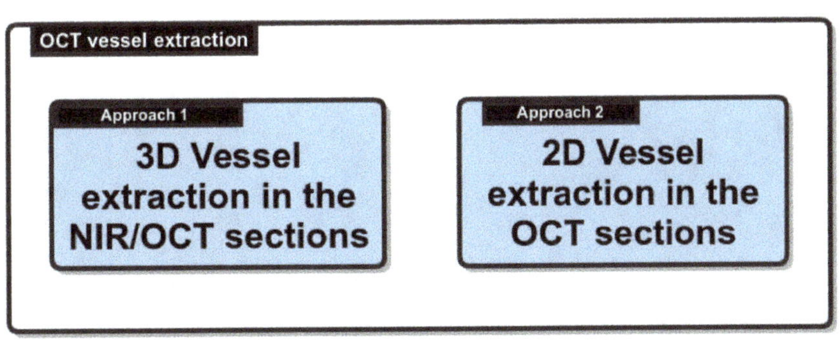

Figure 3. Vessel extraction in OCT images by two different approaches using NIR/OCT sections or only OCT sections.

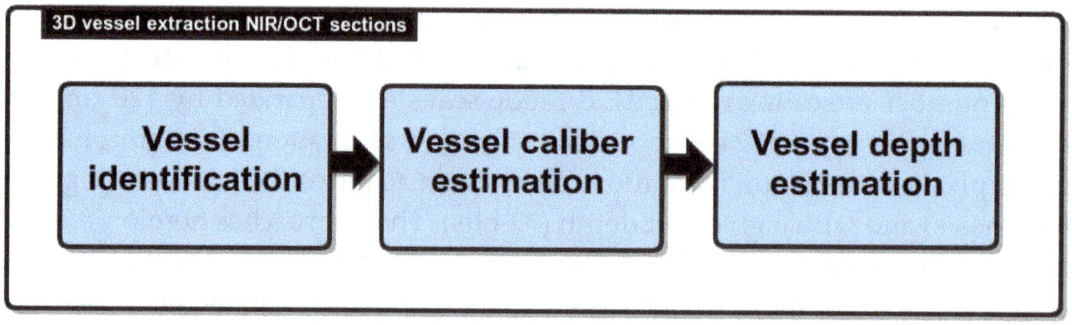

Figure 4. Scheme of 3D vessel extraction using the combination of NIR and the histological sections.

2.2.1.1. *Vessel identification*

Initially, a preprocessing stage is performed to enhance the biggest and darkest structures that characterize the vessels in the NIR images [19]. To achieve this, we use a morphological top-hat transformation (see **Figure 5(b)**). Then, the noise and the vascular reflex are reduced with a median filter (see **Figure 5(c)**). This process facilitates the posterior extraction of the retinal vessels and reinforces the robustness of the method [20].

An initial segmentation was performed by means of a hysteresis-based thresholding technique [21]. A hard threshold (T_h) represents pixels with a high probability of being blood vessel pixels while a weak threshold (T_w) keeps all the pixels of the vascular tree in the surrounding region, even spurious ones. The final segmentation is formed by all the pixels that were included by the T_w threshold connected to, at least, one pixel obtained by the T_h threshold. The values for T_h and T_w are extracted from two characteristics calculated on the NIR images: the percentage of vascular tree and the percentage of background. These thresholds are calculated using percentile values, according to (Eq. (1)).

$$P_k = L_k + \frac{k(n/100) - F_k}{f_k} \times c, \quad k = 1, 2, \ldots, 99 \tag{1}$$

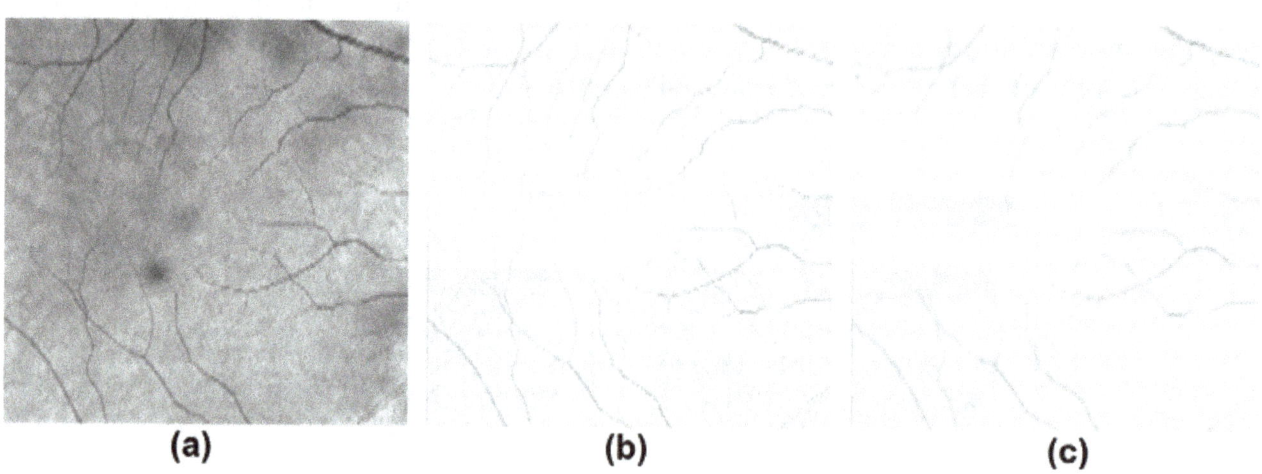

Figure 5. Example of the preprocessing stage in the NIR. (a) Input NIR retinography image; (b) morphological top-hat transformation result and (c) median filter result.

where L_k is the percentile lower limit k, n is the size of the data set, F_k is the accumulated frequency for k - 1 values, f_k depicts the frequency of percentile k and c is the measurement of the size of the percentile interval. In our case, c is equal to 1. A representative example of the vessel segmentation stage using an NIR retinography image is presented in **Figure 6(b)**.

Next, we proceed to identify the centerline of each vessel segment using as baseline the information that was obtained in the previous segmentation. The retinal vessel centerline identification is done using a crease-based strategy. This method follows the idea that vessels can be thought of as creases (ridges or valleys) when images are seen as landscapes [22]. This way, the Multi Local Set of Extrinsic Curvature enhanced by the Structure Tensor (MLSEC-ST) operator is applied with this aim. Then, a skeletonization method is applied to obtain the vessel centerline representation of each vessel by means of one-pixel width segments, as we can see in **Figure 6(c)**.

2.2.1.2. Vessel caliber estimation

In addition to the vessel centerline coordinates, we also need to determine their calibers at each point of the vessel segments, in order to obtain a coherent three-dimensional representation of the retinal vessel tree (see **Figure 7(a)**). The vascular caliber is calculated for each vessel coordinate as the distance between their edges (see **Figure 7(b)**). To this aim, we use the information of the achieved segmentations and the vessel centerlines. These values were previously estimated in the segmentation stage. The vessel orientation θ is calculated as the angle between two consecutive vessel points: $P_1(x_1, y_1)$ and $P_2(x_2, y_2)$. The caliber is then estimated in the perpendicular direction of this angle, see (Eq.(2)).

$$\theta = \arctan\left(\frac{y_2 - y_1}{x_2 - x_1}\right) \tag{2}$$

2.2.1.3. Vessel depth estimation

The depth estimation of the retinal vessels is calculated using the depth information that is provided by OCT histological sections. The shadow projections on the retinal layers indicate

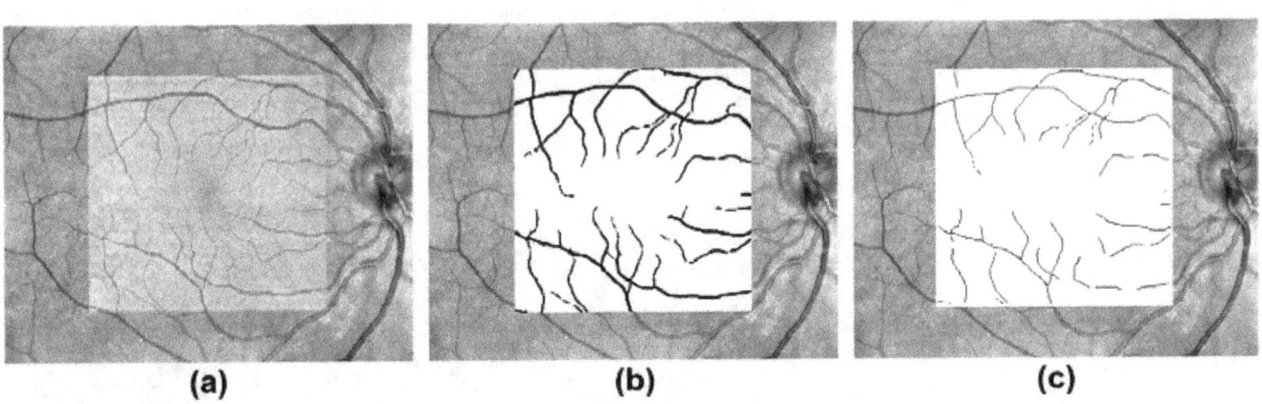

Figure 6. Example of the vessel extraction stage in NIR image. (a) Input NIR retinography image; (b) vessel tree segmentation and (c) vessel tree centerline identification.

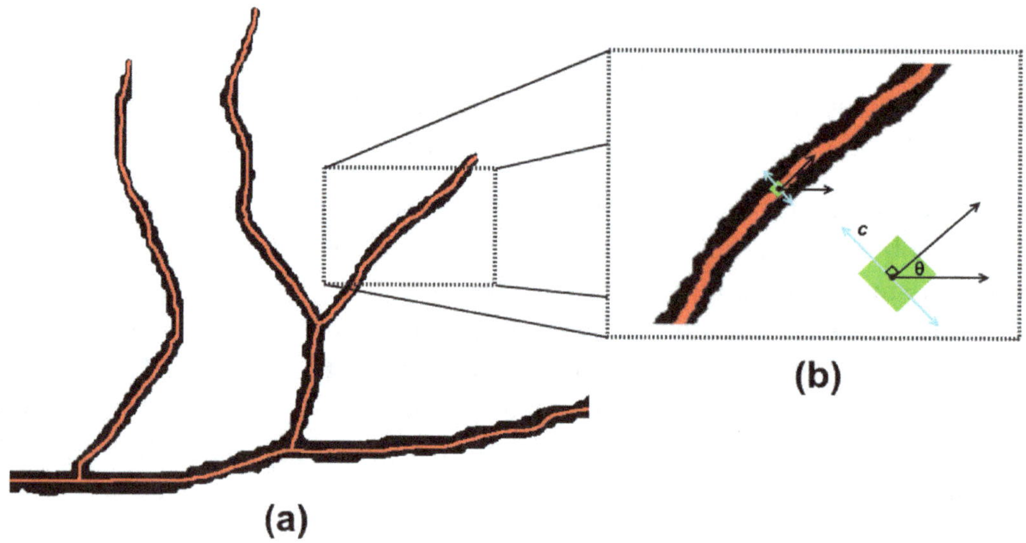

Figure 7. Example of the vessel caliber estimation stage. (a) Vessel centerline overlapping the vessel segments and (b) representation of the analyzed direction at each point of a vessel segment.

the presence of the vessel profiles. In the OCT histological sections, the vessel profiles are the bright spots situated between the retinal layers. To detect these spots, we make a previous mapping process to delimit the vascular region in the OCT section, as is illustrated in **Figure 8**. Then, a search process is performed in this region to determine the precise location of these vessel profiles. The vascular depth Z is estimated by the distance between the vessel profile C_v and the retinal pigment epithelium (RPE) layer P_i, see (Eq.(3)).

$$Z = |C_v - P_i| \tag{3}$$

2.2.2. Vessel extraction using only the OCT histological sections

In many occasions, computational tools are not provided with the entire set of NIR retinography images in combination with their corresponding OCT histological sections. Given this

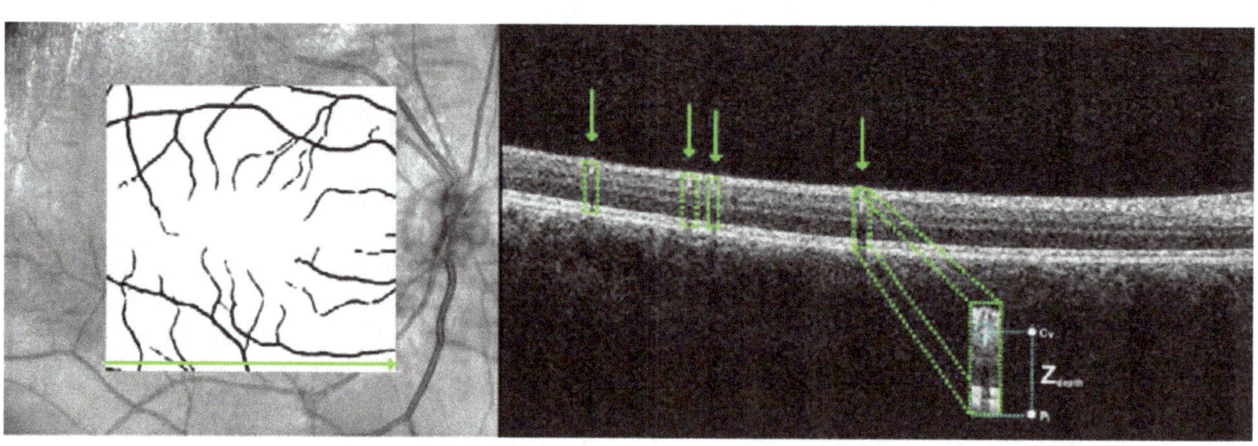

Figure 8. Example of the vessel depth estimation stage with the mapping process and the delimitation of the vascular region.

frequent scenario, that constitutes a limitation, another proposal is also detailed for the automatic detection of retinal vessels using, only, the information that is obtained through the OCT histological sections [23]. To achieve this, the tool bases its performance on the exploitation of the information provided by the shadow projections of the vessels along the retinal layers to identify the presence of vascular structures (see **Figure 9**).

The eye fundus presents a layered structure that contains five main cell types: photoreceptor, horizontal, bipolar, amacrine and ganglion [24]. These cells present different responses to the reflection, transmission and absorption of the light stimuli that are emitted by the OCT capture device. Given this, the presence of the vascular shadows is more prominent in some retinal layers given their brightness, facilitating the detection of the vessel profiles in the OCT sections. In particular, this information is more visible in the region between the Pigment Epithelium Bruch's Complex and the Choroid (RPE/C) layer and the top boundaries of the Ellipsoid (M/E) layer. To achieve the identification of these retinal layers, the method implemented an automated approach using snakes, an active contour-based model [25]. Snake strategies are one of the most common methods that are used in segmentation problems in many issues of medical imaging. This active contour-based model bases its performance on the fact that each vertex of the snake is moved according to inner and outer forces, and the general contour turns stable when the model reaches its local minimum. The mathematical snake model is shown in (Eq.(4)).

$$\xi_{snake}(s) = \int \xi_{\text{internal}}(s)ds + \int \xi_{external}(s)ds \tag{4}$$

The interaction between the snake energies are measured by the energy function ξ_{snake} where $\xi_{internal}$ represents the elasticity energy and $\xi_{external}$ measures the energy of the snake when finding the intensity edges. In **Figure 10**, we can see a representative example with the identification of the RPE/C and M/E retinal layers, delimiting the region of interest where the vascular shadows are identified easily.

Using this identified region of interest, a preprocessing stage is carried out to increase the robustness of the vascular shadow identification process to possible changes in contrast and brightness, a situation that is frequent in OCT images (see **Figure 11**). First, a Gaussian blurring filter is employed to remove the characteristic speckle noise of these images. Next, a

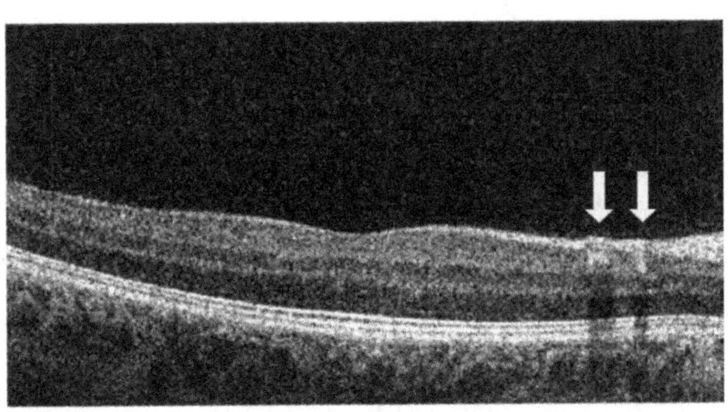

Figure 9. OCT section with the shadow projections of a couple of vessels.

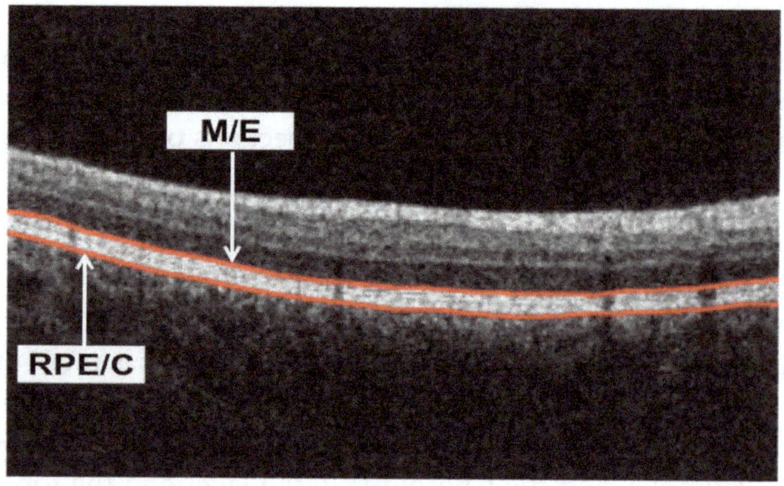

Figure 10. Example of OCT histological section with the identification of the two aimed retinal layers: RPE/C and M/E.

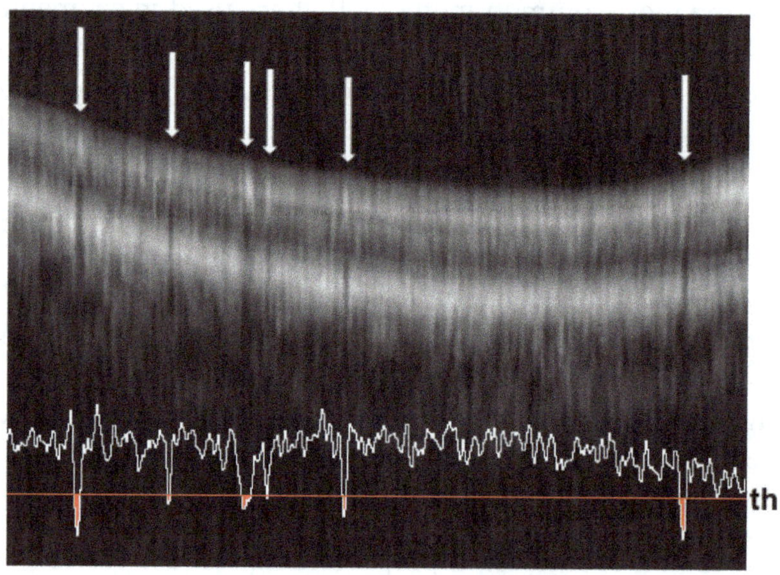

Figure 11. Example of preprocessed OCT section where the vessel profiles are graphically represented as valleys in the mean intensity signal and detected in the region below a fixed threshold.

morphological top-hat transformation is used to enhance the contrast of the vascular shadows. Finally, we calculate the statistical features in the region of interest, features that are used to identify the vascular presence. To achieve this, we analyze the intensity profiles of the vessel shadows in this region. These intensity profiles are calculated using a derived signal, where each point represent the mean of the intensity in each column that is delimited by the mentioned layers RPE/C and M/E. The vessel profiles are identified by means of existing significant local minima along this signal. To achieve this, we use as selection criteria a model that employs a fixed threshold, *th*, as shown in (Eq.(5)).

$$th = \frac{3}{2}(Q_3 - Q_1) + Q_3 \tag{5}$$

where Q_1 represents the first quartile and Q_3 represents the third quartile. As shown in **Figure 11**, the vessel profiles are graphically represented as valleys and detected in the region below a fixed threshold.

2.3. Vasculature visual reconstruction

Nowadays, automatic visualization systems are commonly used by clinical specialists to perform the diagnosis, monitoring and treatment of many diseases. In particular, OCT images provide detailed and relevant information that can be used in the analysis and posterior reconstruction of the retinal vessel tree. Depending on the input image of our system (NIR and/or histological sections), we can obtain more or less information about the characteristics retinal vasculature. Based on the information that is provided by the input scan, we perform the corresponding two-dimensional or three-dimensional visual reconstruction, as we explain in the following sections.

2.3.1. 2D vascular reconstruction

In this stage, we use the information of the vessel profiles that was obtained from a set of OCT histological sections. The information provided by these vascular profiles is used to perform the two-dimensional reconstruction of the entire retinal vessel tree.

First, we make a preliminary binary vessel map with all the vessel profiles that were identified using a set of OCT scans. In this vessel map, each row represents the vascular information obtained for each OCT scan. Then, we scale this binary vessel map to obtain a final representation of the vascular structures with the same dimensions of the original scan (see **Figure 12(a)**). The scaling process is done using the separation value between each OCT scan, if available. This value is a parameter that is selected in the OCT capture device by the clinical expert in the process of obtaining the OCT scans. And finally, we make a two-dimensional reconstruction of the retinal vessel tree using the final binary vessel map obtained, as we can see in **Figure 12(b)**. In this example, we can observe the final two-dimensional identifications over the existing NIR image, for a better illustration of the performance of the approach, despite it not being employed in the identification process.

2.3.2. 3D vascular reconstruction

In this section, we use the information of the vessel profiles provided by the NIR and the histological sections to produce a visual vascular three-dimensional representation. The system represents each vascular structure as a segment S, where each point P of the vascular segment S is represented by the coordinates (x, y, z) and the vessel calibers d, values that were previously calculated [26]. Then, an interpolation by B-splines $S(u)$ is used with the entire set of points P_i connecting them in a curve, see (Eq.(6)).

$$S(u) = \sum_{i=0}^{n} B_{i,m}(u)\, P_i \quad 2 \leqslant m \leqslant n+1 \tag{6}$$

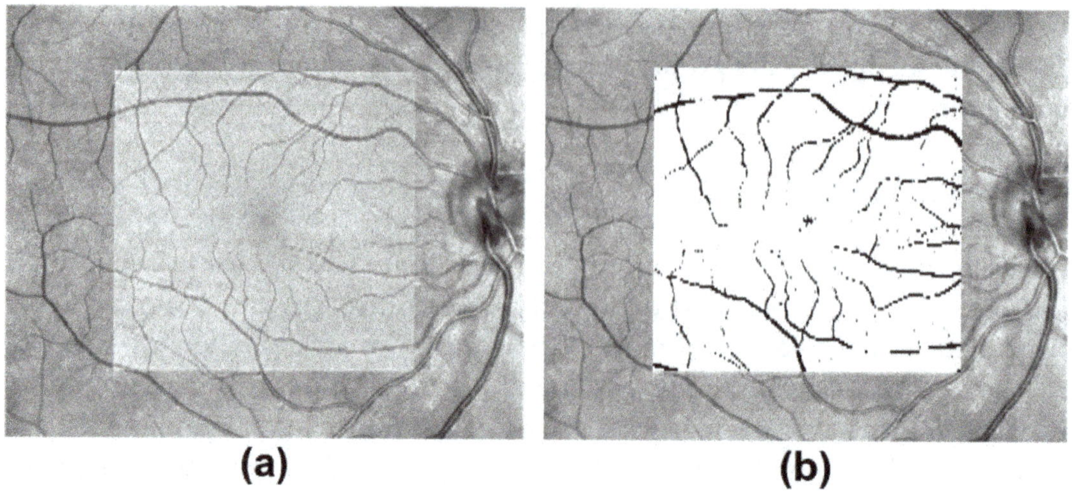

Figure 12. Example of the vessel extraction results in using the approach that uses only the OCT histological sections. (a) NIR retinography image and (b) two-dimensional vascular reconstruction using the vascular identifications.

where P_i is the ith control point of the $(n + 1)$th control point of the curve and $B_{i,m}$ are the B-spline functions, which are polynomials of degree $m - 1$. **Figure 13** shows a representative example of the interpolation process with B-spline curves.

Each vascular segment is represented with a tubular shape centered in the corresponding coordinates (x, y, z) and with a diameter equivalent to its caliber, d. Subsequently, a postprocessing is performed to smooth the transitions between the consecutive vascular coordinates and, therefore, allow a more reliable representation of the vascular structure [27]. **Figure 14** shows this three-dimensional representation process over a given curve.

Finally, this automatic system allows a complete three-dimensional visualization of the complex retinal vessel tree by means of graphical affine transformations including translation,

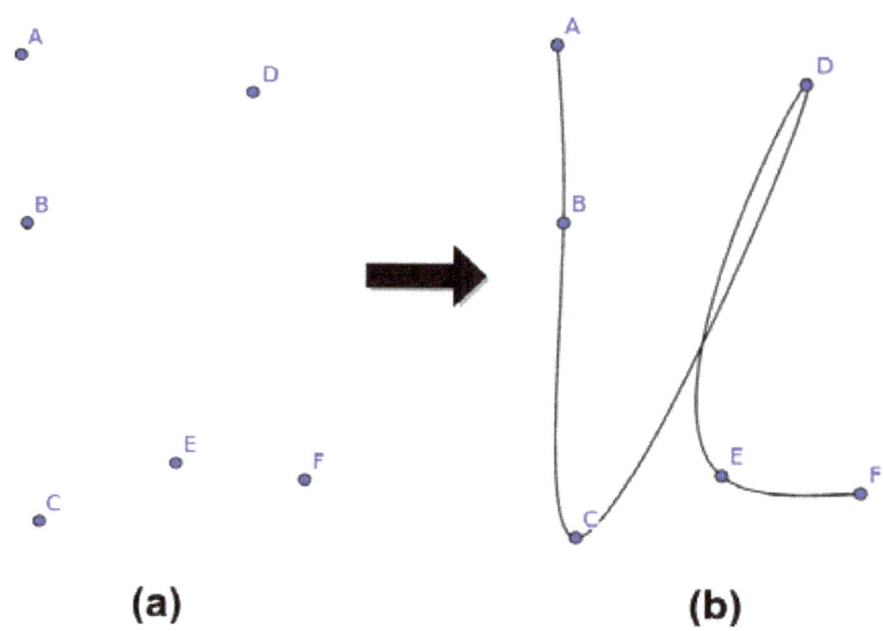

Figure 13. Example of the interpolation process. (a) Set of Cartesian coordinates (x, y, z) and (b) interpolation with B-spline curves between the set of Cartesian coordinates.

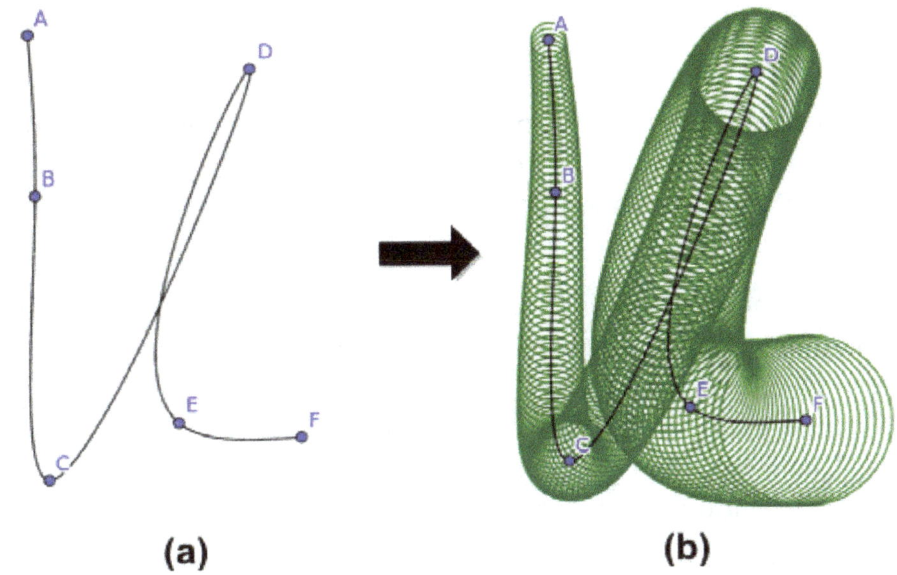

Figure 14. Example of the three-dimensional representation process. (a) Interpolation with B-spline curves between Cartesian coordinates. (b) Representation of a 3D tubular structure associated with the curve.

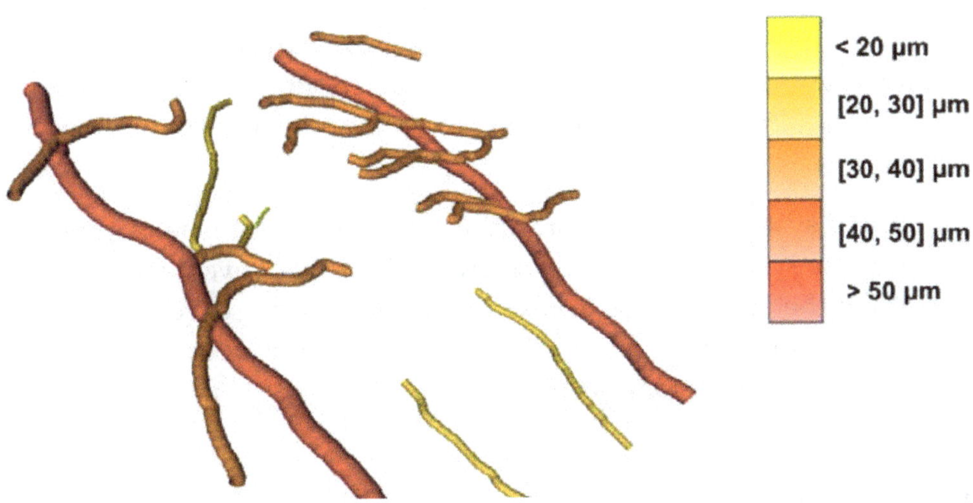

Figure 15. Representative example of the three-dimensional reconstruction of the retinal vessel tree in OCT images.

rotation, scaling and their arbitrary combinations. **Figure 15** shows a representative example of the three-dimensional reconstruction of the retinal vessel tree using the entire set of the OCT scans. The output image also presents the vessels by colors in terms of their calibers. The caliber scales are also presented to facilitate the analysis of the specialists.

3. Conclusions

The retina is a unique region of the human body where the blood vessels can be directly observed and analyzed in vivo and noninvasively. A precise identification and characterization of the retinal vasculature permit an early detection of the presence of several clinical characteristics that facilitate the diagnosis, prevention and treatment of many relevant diseases that affect the retinal microcirculation, such as hypertension, diabetes or arteriosclerosis, among others.

CAD systems have become increasingly important in the assessment of outcomes in the daily clinical practice, mainly in the field of medical imaging-based diagnosis. These systems help the clinical experts in the analysis and interpretation of several modalities of medical images, facilitating and simplifying their work.

OCT is a noninvasive imaging modality capable of producing high-speed three-dimensional cross-sectional imaging of biological tissues with micron-level resolution. This medical image modality enables the precise evaluation of the retinal structure in real time, permitting the detection of alterations in the retinal microcirculation. The OCT devices provide two types of OCT images: the NIR retinography image and the OCT histological sections. These images are frequently acquired simultaneously by the same capture device.

In this chapter, we analyzed the characteristics of the OCT scans and their suitability for the vascular analysis. Additionally, we presented two different and independent approaches for the automatic identification and extraction of the retinal vascular structure to highlight the potential of these computational approaches in the field. The first approach uses the information provided by the NIR retinography image in combination with the histological sections. The second approach uses only the information provided by the OCT histological sections for the characterization of the vessel profiles. Then, both computational approaches perform the corresponding graphical two-dimensional or three-dimensional visual representation of the retinal vessel tree using the extracted information.

These fully automatic systems allow a more accurate and reliable visualization of the complex vascular structure of the retina, and consequently, make an improvement in the visual inspection and analyses of the retinal vessel tree. In addition, the vessel representation permits a more precise analysis of the retinal microcirculation, making the diagnosis of various retinal and systemic pathologies easier for doctors.

Acknowledgements

This work is supported by the Instituto de Salud Carlos III, Government of Spain and FEDER funds of the European Union through the PI14/02161 and the DTS15/00153 research projects and by the Ministerio de Economía y Competitividad, Government of Spain through the DPI2015-69948-R research project. Also, this work has received financial support from the European Union (European Regional Development Fund-ERDF) and the Xunta de Galicia, Centro singular de investigación de Galicia accreditation 2016-2019, Ref. ED431G/01; and Grupos de Referencia Competitiva, Ref. ED431C 2016-047.

Author details

Joaquim de Moura[1,2], Jorge Novo[1,2*], José Rouco[1,2], Noelia Barreira[1,2], Manuel Penedo[1,2] and Marcos Ortega[1,2]

*Address all correspondence to: jnovo@udc.es

1 Department of Computing, University of A Coruña, A Coruña, Spain

2 Research Center of Information and Communication Technologies (CITIC), University of A Coruña, A Coruña, Spain

References

[1] Wong TY, Mitchell P. Hypertensive retinopathy. New England Journal of Medicine. 2004;**351**(22):2310-2317. DOI: 10.1056/NEJMra032865

[2] Nguyen TT, Wong TY. Retinal vascular changes and diabetic retinopathy. Current Diabetes Reports. 2009;**9**(4):277-283. DOI: 10.1007/s11892-009-0043-4

[3] Klein R, Sharrett AR, Klein BE, Chambless LE, Cooper LS, Hubbard LD, Evans G. Are retinal arteriolar abnormalities related to atherosclerosis?: The Atherosclerosis Risk in Communities Study. Arteriosclerosis, Thrombosis, and Vascular Biology. 2000;**20**(6):1644-1650. DOI: 10.1161/01.ATV.20.6.1644

[4] Stevens GA, White RA, Flaxman SR, Price H, Jonas JB, Keeffe J, Leasher J, Naidoo K, Pesudovs K, Resnikoff S, Taylor H. Global prevalence of vision impairment and blindness: Magnitude and temporal trends, 1990-2010. Ophthalmology. 2013;**120**(12):2377-2384. DOI: 10.1016/j.ophtha.2013.05.025

[5] MacGillivray TJ, Trucco E, Cameron JR, Dhillon B, Houston JG, Van Beek EJ. Retinal imaging as a source of biomarkers for diagnosis, characterization and prognosis of chronic illness or long-term conditions. The British Journal of Radiology. 2014;**87**(1040):20130832. DOI: 10.1259/bjr.20130832

[6] Xu Z, Guo X, Hu X, Chen X, Wang Z. The identification and recognition based on point for blood vessel of ocular fundus. In: Proceedings of the International Conference on Biometrics: Advances in Biometrics (ICB 2006); 5-7 January 2006; Hong Kong, China. pp. 770-776

[7] Ortega M, Rouco J, Novo J, Penedo MG. Vascular landmark detection in retinal images. Lecture Notes in Computer Science (EUROCAST 2009); Feb 2009; Canary Islands, Spain. pp. 211-217. DOI: 10.1007/978-3-642-04772-5_28

[8] Ortega M, Penedo MG, Rouco J, Barreira N, Carreira MJ. Personal verification based on extraction and characterisation of retinal feature points. Journal of Visual Languages & Computing. 2009 Apr 1;**20**(2):80-90. DOI: 10.1016/j.jvlc.2009.01.006

[9] Mookiah MR, Acharya UR, Chua CK, Lim CM, Ng EY, Laude A. Computer-aided diagnosis of diabetic retinopathy: A review. Computers in Biology and Medicine. 2013 Dec 1;**43**(12):2136-2155. DOI: 10.1016/j.compbiomed.2013.10.007

[10] Novo J, Hermida A, Ortega M, Barreira N, Penedo MG, López JE, Calvo C. Hydra: A web-based system for cardiovascular analysis, diagnosis and treatment. Computer Methods and Programs in Biomedicine. 2017 Feb 1;**139**:61-81. DOI: 10.1016/j.cmpb.2016.10.019

[11] Adhi M, Duker JS. Optical coherence tomography—Current and future applications. Current Opinion in Ophthalmology. 2013 May;**24**(3):213. DOI: 10.1097/ICU.0b013e32835f8bf8

[12] Huang D, Swanson EA, Lin CP, Schuman JS, Stinson WG, Chang W, Hee MR, Flotte T, Gregory K, Puliafito CA. Optical coherence tomography. Science. 1991 Nov 22;**254**(5035):1178-1181. DOI: 10.1126/science.1957169

[13] Bourne RR, Flaxman SR, Braithwaite T, Cicinelli MV, Das A, Jonas JB, Keeffe J, Kempen JH, Leasher J, Limburg H, Naidoo K. Magnitude, temporal trends, and projections of the global prevalence of blindness and distance and near vision impairment: A systematic review and meta-analysis. The Lancet Global Health. 2017 Sep 1;**5**(9):e888-e897. DOI: 10.1016/S2214-109X(17)30293-0

[14] Michelson AA, Morley EW. On the relative motion of the earth and of the luminiferous ether. Sidereal Messenger. 1887;**6**:306-310. DOI: 10.1366/0003702874447824

[15] Kalev-Landoy M, Day AC, Cordeiro MF, Migdal C. Optical coherence tomography in anterior segment imaging. Acta Ophthalmologica. 2007 Jun 1;**85**(4):427-430. DOI: 10.1111/j.1600-0420.2007.00876.x

[16] Cabrera DeBuc D, Somfai GM, Koller A. Retinal microvascular network alterations: Potential biomarkers of cerebrovascular and neural diseases. American Journal of Physiology-Heart and Circulatory Physiology. 2016 Dec 6;**312**(2):H201-H212. DOI: 10.1152/ajpheart.00201.2016

[17] Fujimoto J, Swanson E. The development, commercialization, and impact of optical coherence tomography. Investigative Ophthalmology & Visual Science. 2016 Jul 1;**57**(9):1-3. DOI: 10.1167/iovs.16-19963

[18] Leite MT, Rao HL, Zangwill LM, Weinreb RN, Medeiros FA. Comparison of the diagnostic accuracies of the Spectralis, Cirrus, and RTVue optical coherence tomography devices in glaucoma. Ophthalmology. 2011 Jul 1;**118**(7):1334-1339. DOI: 10.1016/j.ophtha.2010.11.029

[19] de Moura J, Novo J, Charlón P, Barreira N, Ortega M. Enhanced visualization of the retinal vasculature using depth information in OCT. Medical & Biological Engineering & Computing. 2017;**55**(12):2209-2225. DOI: 10.1007/s11517-017-1660-8

[20] Jackway PT. Improved morphological top-hat. Electronics Letters. 2000;**36**(14):1194-1195. DOI: 10.1049/el:20000873

[21] Jin J, Yang L, Zhang X, Ding M. Vascular tree segmentation in medical images using Hessian-based multiscale filtering and level set method. Computational and Mathematical Methods in Medicine. 2013;**2013**. DOI: 10.1155/2013/502013

[22] Calvo D, Ortega M, Penedo MG, Rouco J. Automatic detection and characterisation of retinal vessel tree bifurcations and crossovers in eye fundus images. Computer Methods and Programs in Biomedicine. 2011 Jul;**103**(1, 1):28-38. DOI: 10.1016/j.cmpb.2010.06.002

[23] de Moura J, Novo J, Rouco J, Penedo MG, Ortega M. Automatic detection of blood vessels in retinal OCT images. In: Proceedings of the International Work-Conference on the Interplay Between Natural and Artificial Computation (IWINAC 2017); 19-23 Jun 2017; A Coruña. 2017. pp. 3-10. DOI: 10.1007/978-3-319-59773-7_1

[24] Masland RH. The fundamental plan of the retina. Nature Neuroscience. 2001;**4**(9):877. DOI: 10.1038/nn0901-877

[25] González-López A, Ortega M, Penedo MG, Charlón P. Automatic robust segmentation of retinal layers in oct images with refinement stages. In: Proceedings of the International Conference Image Analysis and Recognition (ICIAR 2014); 22-24 OCT 2014; Vilamoura, Portugal. 2014. pp. 337-345. DOI: 10.1007/978-3-319-11755-3_38

[26] de Moura J, Novo J, Ortega M, Charlón P. 3D retinal vessel tree segmentation and reconstruction with OCT images. In: Proceedings of the International Conference Image Analysis and Recognition (ICIAR 2016); 13 Jul 2016. pp. 716-726. DOI: 10.1007/978-3-319-41501-7_80

[27] de Moura J, Novo J, Ortega M, Barreira N, Penedo MG. Interactive three-dimensional visualization system of the vascular structure in OCT retinal images. In: Proceedings of the International Conference on Computer Aided Systems Theory (EUROCAST 2017); Feb 2017; Canary Islands, Spain. pp. 306-313. DOI: 10.1007/978-3-319-74727-9_36

11

iOCT in PVR Surgical Management

Salvatore Di Lauro, Salvador Pastor Idoate and
Jose Carlos Pastor

Abstract

Recent advances in optical coherence tomography (OCT) technology have allowed the introduction of OCT into the operating room. Intraoperative OCT (iOCT) has been utilized to visualize the retinal architecture prior, during, and following several retinal surgical technics. The identification of epiretinal, subretinal, and intraretinal changes is one of the crucial points in PVR management. The iOCT can identify intraretinal changes and/or subretinal PVR membranes which cannot be easily peeled as epiretinal membranes. Intraretinal forms are especially difficult to identify preoperatively but their presence may be crucial in surgical management because the attempt to remove the presumed membrane may result in severe retinal tissue damage and iatrogenic tears. Therefore, surgical technique and even tamponade choice may be seriously affected by OCT imaging results.

Keywords: OCT, intraoperative OCT, PVR, retinal detachment, vitreo-retinal surgery

1. Introduction

Optical coherence tomography (OCT) has dramatically changed the diagnosis, classification, and treatment of many vitreo-retinal diseases [1–3]. One of the most recent developments of this technology is the intraoperative OCT (iOCT). The iOCT allows a real-time tomographic visualization of the retina without the need to stop the surgery and without any external machines (microscope-integrated OCT). In this way, the surgeon can see OCT images during the surgery on an external display or directly through the microscope.

iOCT adds microscopic information and visualizes sub-surface structures in a non invasive way. This information can impact surgical decision-making as well as surgical maneuvers in selected cases. In this sense, the intraoperative visualization of the retina opens new surgical and diagnostic possibilities. Vitreo-retinal interphase diseases may especially benefit from iOCT spreading but also retinal detachment (RD) surgery could be positively affected.

Proliferative vitreoretinopathy (PVR) is one of the most severe complications after RD, appearing in 5–10% of them [4]. Despite recent advances in vitreo-retinal surgery, PVR management is still an unsolved issue [4]. The introduction of the iOCT in surgical practice could be useful in improving the management of this important complication.

2. Intraoperative optical coherence tomography (iOCT)

The iOCT is a relatively new technology, and the first relevant study about iOCT applications in ophthalmology was the so named Prospective Intraoperative and Perioperative Ophthalmic Imaging with Optical Coherence Tomography (PIONEER) study [5]. The 2-year results published in 2014 demonstrated the potential advantages and applications of this technology [5]. Nevertheless, in this study, an external OCT system mounted on the operative microscope (Bioptigen SDOIS portable spectral-domain OCT [SD OCT] system; Bioptigen, Research Triangle Park, North Carolina, USA) was used. The most serious inconvenience of this system was the need to pause the surgery to obtain the required images.

Since this study, relevant advances in this technology have been reached to obtain a real microscope-integrated technology. Actually, there are several iOCTs available, including RESCAN 700 (Carl Zeiss Meditec, Inc., Oberkochen, Germany), the EnFocus (Bioptigen/Leica Microsystems, Wetzlar, Germany), and an integrated prototype internally developed at the Cole Eye Institute, Cleveland Clinic Foundation (Cleveland, Ohio) [6]. All these systems allow a real-time OCT imaging during the surgery and provide instantaneous feedback to the surgeon.

The PIONEER and the Determination of Feasibility of Intraoperative Spectral-Domain Microscope Combined/Integrated OCT Visualization during En Face Retinal and Ophthalmic Surgery (DISCOVER) studies have largely demonstrated the iOCT usefulness in the anterior and posterior segment surgery [5, 6]. Surgical procedures and pathologies positively affected by iOCT introduction in surgical practice include Descemet stripping automated endothelial keratoplasty (DSAEK), Descemet membrane endothelial keratoplasty (DMEK), pars plana vitrectomy for epiretinal membrane, proliferative diabetic retinopathy (PDR), rhegmatogenous retinal detachment, macular hole, optic pit maculopathy, chorioretinal biopsy, and Argus (Second Sight Medical Products, Inc., Sylmar, CA) prosthesis implant [5–13]. The DISCOVER study's 3-year results have been recently published [6]. A total of 837 eyes (244 anterior segment/593 posterior segment cases) were included and iOCT successful image acquisition was achieved in 820 eyes (98.0%; 95% confidence interval (CI), 96.8–98.8%). In 43.4% of the anterior segment cases (95% CI, 37.1–49.9%) and 29.2% (95% CI, 25.5–33.0%), the surgeons considered that the iOCT information impacted their surgical decision-making and altered the previous related procedure. Thus, iOCT could be considered a useful technology for ophthalmic surgery. Nevertheless, there are some limitations. The RESCAN 700, the commonest iOCT, is a SD-OCT system with scanning speed of 27,000 A-scans per second, with a wavelength of 840 nm, refresh rate from 5 to 50 Hz, axial resolution of 5.5 μm in tissue, scan depth of 2 mm, and scan length of 6 mm (adjustable from 3 to 16 mm). This means that image quality is still far away from the OCT

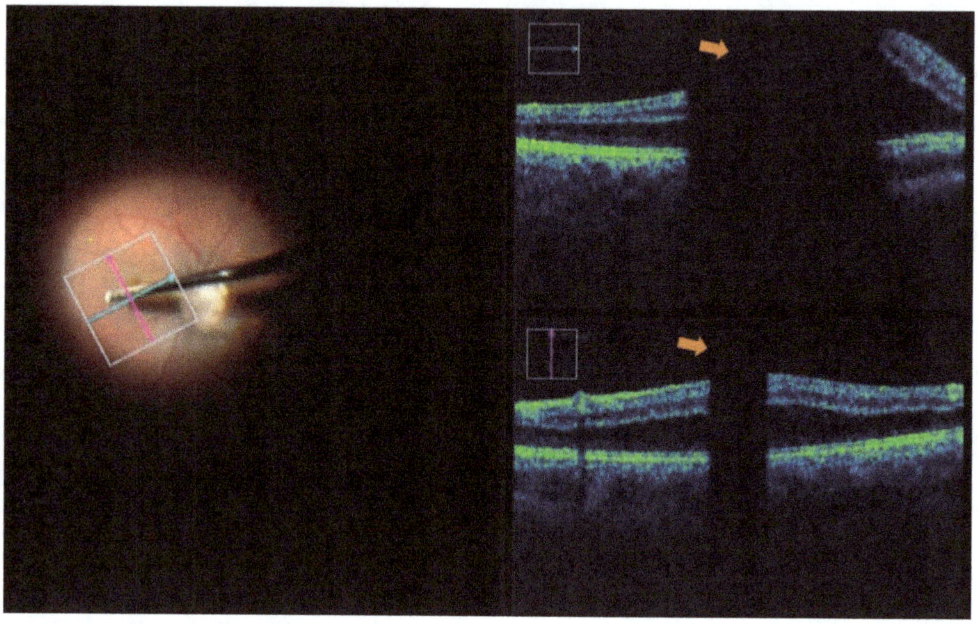

Figure 1. Instrument shadow during intraoperative OCT (iOCT) imaging. Note the shadow (arrow) below the vitreotome probe. Image obtained with the Zeiss Rescan® 700 iOCT (Carl Zeiss Meditec, Oberkochen, Germany).

currently used in clinical practice with axial resolutions of 1 μm and scanning speed of 400,000 A-scans per second. Furthermore, the autofocus and tracking mechanism must be improved to be faster and more accurate. Other limitations include artifacts, instrument shadow during surgery, and function overload with the surgical microscope pedal [6]. Instrument shadow is an important problem limiting the possibility of viewing retinal tissues immediately below the surgical instrument and is related to OCT image caption properties and the materials currently used in vitreo-retinal surgery (**Figure 1**). Nevertheless, new non-metallic instruments made from "OCT-friendly" materials, such as silicone, polycarbonate, and PVC, may allow one to diminish this problem, especially important in vitreo-retinal interface procedures [14, 15]. A valid alternative could be the use of OCT-integrated surgical instruments [14].

3. Proliferative vitreoretinopathy (PVR)

PVR is a complex process involving several risk factors, most of them still unknown. During the last 25 years, and despites the enormous advantages in vitreo-retinal surgery techniques, such as small-gauge instrumentation and new imaging technology, PVR incidence is unchanged and functional and anatomical results are still very poor. PVR is a complex and multifactorial disease, and pharmacological strategies (including anti-inflammatory drugs, antiproliferative agents, antineoplastic, antigrowth factors, and antioxidants) have been considered ineffective and they have been basically abandoned in current practice. Its pathogenesis is divided into several steps: migration of cells, mostly retinal pigment epithelial (RPE) and glial cells; proliferation of these cells; membrane development; contraction of the fibrocellular membrane; extracellular collagen production; and creation of fixed folds in the retina [4]. Several cytokines, growth factors, and single-nucleotide polymorphisms in genes related with inflammation and apoptosis have shown to have a crucial role in PVR development [4, 16–24]. The histopathology of the disease is

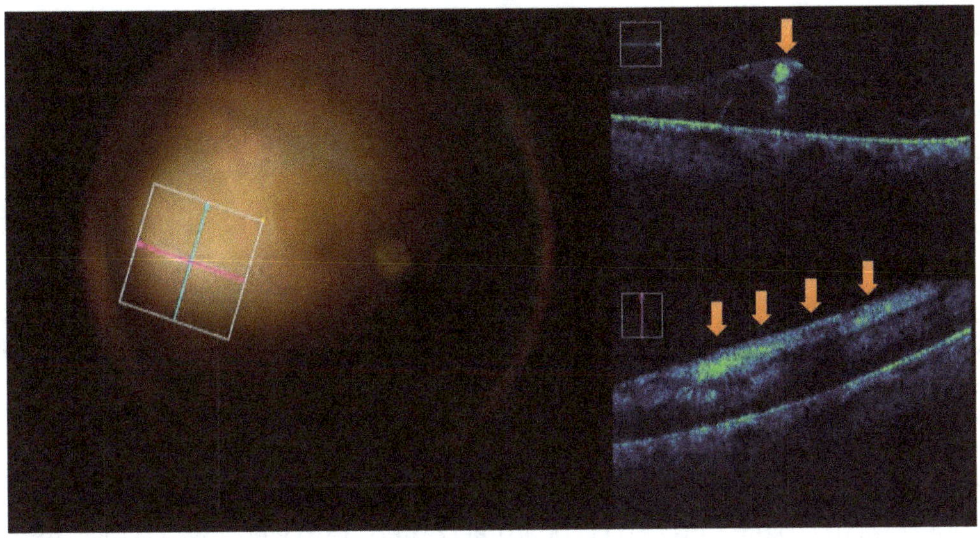

Figure 2. Intraoperative OCT (iOCT) in PVR. iOCT allows intraretinal changes identification (arrows). These membranes cannot be surgically removed. Image obtained with the Zeiss Rescan® 700 iOCT (Carl Zeiss Meditec, Oberkochen, Germany).

characterized by various grades of fibrocellular membrane proliferation with prominent Muller cell activation. These phenomena result in complete retinal architecture alteration with a loss of normal retinal cell organization and function. These membranes may be epi-, intra- or sub-retinal. One of the crucial points is a correct and widely accepted classification which must include intraretinal status [4, 25]. In fact, PVR is characterized by epiretinal, subretinal but also intraretinal proliferation [4, 26, 27]. Intraretinal membranes are especially important because there is no way to remove them during surgery [4], and this increases the risk of surgical failure due to the retinal shortening. Intraretinal PVR must be considered the most severe form in which changes affecting retinal architecture lead to significant dysfunction. Epiretinal or subretinal membranes can be quite easily removed during surgery but intraretinal forms are an unsolved problem. In this sense, iOCT may be awfully valuable in surgical practice allowing the intraoperative assessment of retinal status. The iOCT may be useful to identify intraretinal changes and/or subretinal PVR membranes which cannot be removed with standard techniques (**Figure 2**). This means that it allows a better PVR classification and this can change our surgical attitude intraoperatively for better decision-making about a surgical technique. In fact, trying to remove the presumed membrane can have as consequences severe retinal injury and iatrogenic tears. Thus, surgical technique and even tamponade choice may be seriously affected by iOCT imaging.

Author details

Salvatore Di Lauro[1,2*], Salvador Pastor Idoate[1,2] and Jose Carlos Pastor[1,2]

*Address all correspondence to: sadilauro@live.it

1 Departamento de Oftalmología, Hospital Clínico Universitario de Valladolid, Valladolid, Spain

2 Instituto de Oftalmobiología Aplicada (IOBA), Retina Group, Universidad de Valladolid, Valladolid, Spain

References

[1] Phadikar P, Saxena S, Ruia S, Lai TY, Meyer CH, Eliott D. The potential of spectral domain optical coherence tomography imaging based retinal biomarkers. International Journal of Retina and Vitreous. 2017;**3**:1. PubMed PMID: 28078103. Pubmed Central PMCID: PMC5220620. Epub: 2017/01/13. eng

[2] Lavinsky F, Lavinsky D. Novel perspectives on swept-source optical coherence tomography. International Journal of Retina and Vitreous. 2016;**2**:25. 11/0106/04/received 10/04/accepted. PubMed PMID: PMC5088466

[3] Fujimoto J, Swanson E. The development, commercialization, and impact of optical coherence tomography. Investigative Ophthalmology & Visual Science. 1 July 2016;**57**(9): OCT1-OCT13. 07/13 05/20/received 06/16/accepted. PubMed PMID: PMC4968928

[4] Pastor JC, Rojas J, Pastor-Idoate S, Di Lauro S, Gonzalez-Buendia L, Delgado-Tirado S. Proliferative vitreoretinopathy: A new concept of disease pathogenesis and practical consequences. Progress in Retinal and Eye Research. 2016 Mar;**51**:125-155. PubMed PMID: 26209346. Epub 2015/07/26. eng

[5] Ehlers JP, Dupps WJ, Kaiser PK, Goshe J, Singh RP, Petkovsek D, et al. The Prospective Intraoperative and Perioperative Ophthalmic ImagiNg with Optical CoherEncE Tomog-Raphy (PIONEER) Study: 2-year results. American Journal of Ophthalmology. 2014 Nov;**158**(5):999-1007. PubMed PMID: 25077834. Pubmed Central PMCID: PMC4250395. Epub: 2014/08/01. eng

[6] Ehlers JP, Modi YS, Pecen PE, Goshe J, Dupps WJ, Rachitskaya A, et al. The DISCOVER Study 3-year results: Feasibility and usefulness of microscope-integrated intraoperative OCT during ophthalmic Surgery. Ophthalmology. 3 Feb 2018. pii: S0161-6420(17)32218-2. PubMed PMID: 29409662. Epub: 2018/02/08. eng

[7] Ehlers JP, Uchida A, Srivastava SK. The integrative surgical theater: Combining intraoperative optical coherence tomography and 3D digital visualization for vitreoretinal surgery in the DISCOVER Study. Retina (Philadelphia, PA). 2017 Dec 18. PubMed PMID: 29256988. Epub: 2017/12/20. eng. Publish Ahead of Print

[8] Borrelli E, Palmieri M, Aharrh-Gnama A, Ciciarelli V, Mastropasqua R, Carpineto P. Intraoperative optical coherence tomography in the full-thickness macular hole surgery with internal limiting membrane inverted flap placement. International Ophthalmology. 2018 Mar 3. DOI: 10.1007/s10792-018-0880-8. [Epub ahead of print] PubMed PMID: 29502211. Epub: 2018/03/05. eng

[9] Heinrich D, Bohnacker S, Nasseri MA, Feucht N, Lohmann CP, Maier M. Intraoperative optical coherence tomography in explorative vitrectomy in patients with vitreous haemorrhage—A case series. Der Ophthalmologe: Zeitschrift der Deutschen Ophthalmologischen Gesellschaft. 2018 Feb 15. DOI: 10.1007/s00347-018-0665-5. [Epub ahead of print] PubMed PMID: 29450624. Epub: 2018/02/17. Intraoperative optische Koharenztomographie bei explorativer Vitrektomie an Patienten mit Glaskorperblutung - eine Fallserie. ger

[10] Lu CD, Waheed NK, Witkin A, Baumal CR, Liu JJ, Potsaid B, et al. Microscope-integrated intraoperative ultrahigh-speed swept-source optical coherence tomography for wide-field retinal and anterior segment imaging. Ophthalmic Surgery, Lasers & Imaging Retina. 2018 Feb 1;**49**(2):94-102. PubMed PMID: 29443358. Epub: 2018/02/15. eng

[11] Toygar O, Riemann CD. Intraoperative optical coherence tomography in macula involving rhegmatogenous retinal detachment repair with pars plana vitrectomy and perfluoron. Eye (London, England). 2016 Jan;**30**(1):23-30. PubMed PMID: 26656086. Pubmed Central PMCID: PMC4709554. Epub: 2015/12/15. eng

[12] Junker B, Maier M, Agostini H, Hattenbach LO, Pielen A, Framme C. Intraoperative optical coherence tomography in retinal detachment. Der Ophthalmologe: Zeitschrift der Deutschen Ophthalmologischen Gesellschaft. 2016 Aug;**113**(8):663-667. PubMed PMID: 27378449. Epub: 2016/07/06. Intraoperative optische Koharenztomographie bei Ablatio retinae. ger

[13] Ehlers JP, Tao YK, Srivastava SK. The value of intraoperative optical coherence tomography imaging in vitreoretinal surgery. Current Opinion in Ophthalmology. 2014 May;**25**(3):221-227. PubMed PMID: 24614147. Pubmed Central PMCID: PMC4119822. Epub: 2014/03/13. eng

[14] Carrasco-Zevallos OM, Viehland C, Keller B, Draelos M, Kuo AN, Toth CA, et al. Review of intraoperative optical coherence tomography: Technology and applications [Invited]. Biomedical Optics Express. 2017 Mar 1;**8**(3):1607-1637. PubMed PMID: 28663853. Pubmed Central PMCID: PMC5480568. Epub: 2017/07/01. eng

[15] Ehlers JP, Srivastava SK, Feiler D, Noonan AI, Rollins AM, Tao YK. Integrative advances for OCT-guided ophthalmic surgery and intraoperative OCT: Microscope integration, surgical instrumentation, and heads-up display surgeon feedback. PLoS One. 2014;**9**(8):e105224. PubMed PMID: 25141340. Pubmed Central PMCID: PMC4139373. Epub: 2014/08/21. eng

[16] Pastor-Idoate S, Rodriguez-Hernandez I, Rojas J, Gonzalez-Buendia L, Delgado-Tirado S, Lopez JC, et al. Functional characterization of rs2229094 (T>C) polymorphism in the tumor necrosis factor locus and lymphotoxin alpha expression in human retina: The retina 4 project. Clinical Ophthalmology (Auckland, NZ). 2017;**11**:973-981. PubMed PMID: 28579748. Pubmed Central PMCID: PMC5449105. Epub: 2017/06/06. eng

[17] Di Lauro S, Rodriguez-Crespo D, Gayoso MJ, Garcia-Gutierrez MT, Pastor JC, Srivastava GK, et al. A novel coculture model of porcine central neuroretina explants and retinal pigment epithelium cells. Molecular Vision. 2016;**22**:243-253. PubMed PMID: 27081295. Pubmed Central PMCID: PMC4812504. Epub: 2016/04/16. eng

[18] Pastor-Idoate S, Rodriguez-Hernandez I, Rojas J, Fernandez I, Garcia-Gutierrez MT, Ruiz-Moreno JM, et al. BAX and BCL-2 polymorphisms, as predictors of proliferative vitreoretinopathy development in patients suffering retinal detachment: The Retina 4 project. Acta Ophthalmologica. 2015 Nov;**93**(7):e541-e549. PubMed PMID: 25991504. Epub: 2015/05/21. eng

[19] Rojas J, Fernandez I, Pastor JC, MacLaren RE, Ramkissoon Y, Harsum S, et al. Predicting proliferative vitreoretinopathy: Temporal and external validation of models based on genetic and clinical variables. The British Journal of Ophthalmology. 2015 Jan;**99**(1):41-48. PubMed PMID: 25075124. Epub: 2014/07/31. eng

[20] Pastor-Idoate S, Rodriguez-Hernandez I, Rojas J, Fernandez I, Garcia-Gutierrez MT, Ruiz-Moreno JM, et al. The p53 codon 72 polymorphism (rs1042522) is associated with proliferative vitreoretinopathy: The Retina 4 Project. Ophthalmology. 2013 Mar; **120**(3):623-628. PubMed PMID: 23207172. Epub: 2012/12/05. eng

[21] Pastor-Idoate S, Rodriguez-Hernandez I, Rojas J, Fernandez I, Garcia-Gutierrez MT, Ruiz-Moreno JM, et al. The T309G MDM2 gene polymorphism is a novel risk factor for proliferative vitreoretinopathy. PLoS One. 2013;**8**(12):e82283. PubMed PMID: 24349246. Pubmed Central PMCID: PMC3857251. Epub: 2013/12/19. eng

[22] Rojas J, Fernandez I, Pastor JC, Maclaren RE, Ramkissoon Y, Harsum S, et al. A genetic case-control study confirms the implication of SMAD7 and TNF locus in the development of proliferative vitreoretinopathy. Investigative Ophthalmology & Visual Science. 2013 Mar 05;**54**(3):1665-1678. PubMed PMID: 23258148. Epub: 2012/12/22. eng

[23] Fernandez-Bueno I, Garcia-Gutierrez MT, Srivastava GK, Gayoso MJ, Gonzalo-Orden JM, Pastor JC. Adalimumab (tumor necrosis factor-blocker) reduces the expression of glial fibrillary acidic protein immunoreactivity increased by exogenous tumor necrosis factor alpha in an organotypic culture of porcine neuroretina. Molecular Vision. 2013;**19**:894-903. PubMed PMID: 23687426. Pubmed Central PMCID: 3654850

[24] Rojas J, Fernandez I, Pastor JC, Garcia-Gutierrez MT, Sanabria MR, Brion M, et al. A strong genetic association between the tumor necrosis factor locus and proliferative vitreoretinopathy: The Retina 4 project. Ophthalmology. 2010 Dec;**117**(12):2417-2423. e1-2. PubMed PMID: 20663564. Epub: 2010/07/29. eng

[25] Di Lauro S, Kadhim MR, Charteris DG, Pastor JC. Classifications for proliferative vitreoretinopathy (PVR): An analysis of their use in publications over the last 15 years. Journal of Ophthalmology. 2016;**2016**:7807596. PubMed PMID: 27429798. Pubmed Central PMCID: PMC4939352. Epub: 2016/07/19. eng

[26] Pastor JC, Mendez MC, de la Fuente MA, Coco RM, Garcia-Arumi J, Rodriguez de la Rua E, et al. Intraretinal immunohistochemistry findings in proliferative vitreoretinopathy with retinal shortening. Ophthalmic Research. 2006;**38**(4):193-200. PubMed PMID: 16679807

[27] Pastor JC, Rodriguez de la Rua E, Martin F, Mayo-Iscar A, de la Fuente MA, Coco R, et al. Retinal shortening: The most severe form of proliferative vitreoretinopathy (PVR). Archivos de la Sociedad Española de Oftalmología. 2003 Dec;**78**(12):653-657. PubMed PMID: 14689321. Epub: 2003/12/23. Acortamiento retiniano: la forma mas grave de la vitreorretinopatia proliferante (VRP). spa

12

Optical Coherence Tomography: Essential Tool in Macular Hole Management

Sana I. Tinwala

Abstract

Optical coherence tomography (OCT) is a noninvasive, diagnostic technique for accurately identifying and quantitatively characterizing macular holes. OCT is crucial in assessing fellow eyes of patients with a macular hole to detect preclinical changes leading to subsequent hole formation. The tomographic information provided by OCT, akin to an in vivo biopsy, has led to a better understanding of the pathogenesis of hole formation. The cross-sectional view produced by OCT effectively distinguishes full-thickness macular holes from mimicking conditions like lamellar holes, macular pseudoholes, and cysts, which may sometimes be difficult to differentiate clinically. This information enables early diagnosis and can guide the intervention of choice when treatment is deemed necessary. OCT is useful to prognosticate cases, thereby facilitating discussions with patients and managing visual expectations preoperatively. Intraoperative OCT (iOCT) can identify intraoperative changes in the macular anatomy during surgery that can influence functional outcomes. Postoperatively, OCT is extremely useful for documenting serial changes in the foveal architecture and is helpful in correlating functional and anatomic outcomes. As the technology continues to improve, OCT has become indispensable for all aspects of patient care for macular holes.

Keywords: OCT, macular hole, diagnosis, management, prognosis

1. Introduction

Optical coherence tomography (OCT) was developed by David Huang and colleagues at the Massachusetts Institute of Technology (MIT) [1]. Prior to its development, clinical biomicroscopic examination using the slit lamp was the mainstay for retinal structural assessment.

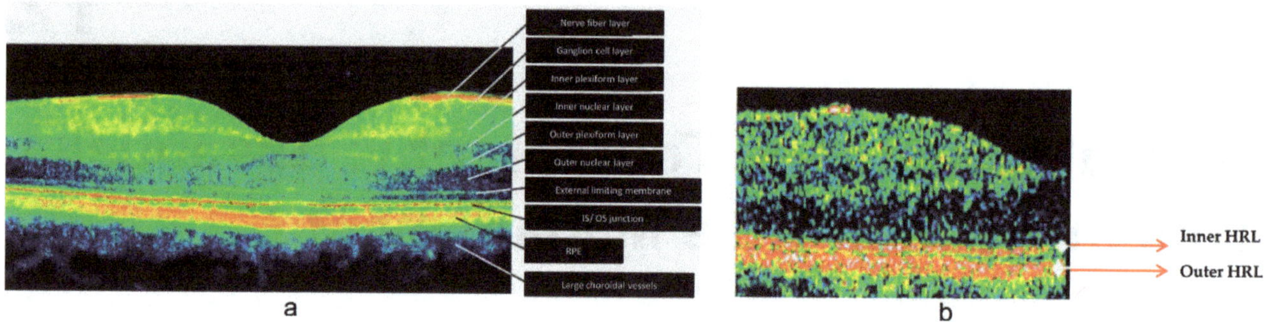

Figure 1. (a) Layers of retina. (b) The inner HRL (corresponding to the photoreceptors IS/OS junction) is thinner than the outer, which corresponds to a hyper-reflective normal complex formed by RPE and choriocapillaris.

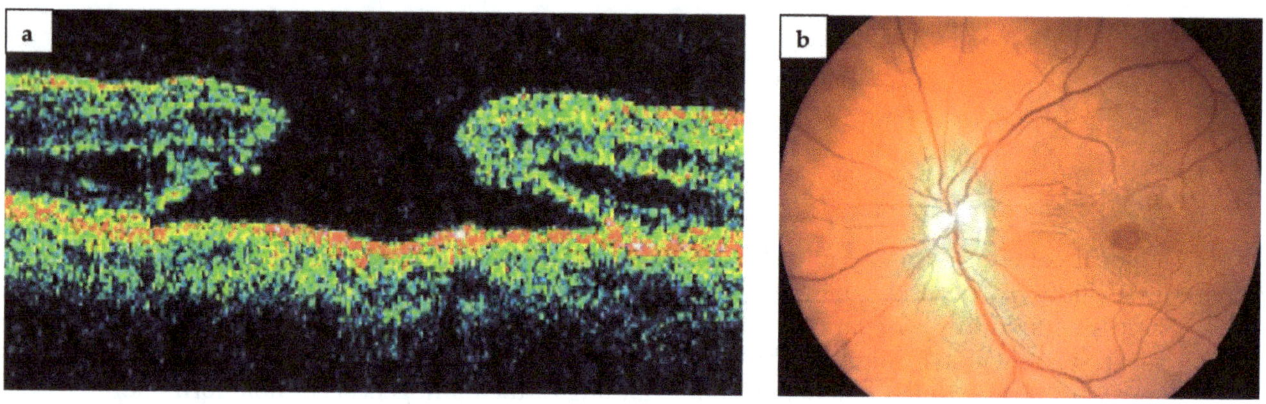

Figure 2. Full thickness macular hole (a) OCT cross sectional image; (b) color fundus photograph).

OCT is based on the imaging of reflected light. In addition to measuring transverse dimensions, it also resolves depth. OCT is akin to noninvasive tissue "biopsy"—it provides in vivo cross-sectional views (tomography) of internal tissue structures similar to tissue sections under a microscope [2, 3]. The depth resolution of OCT is typically of the order of 0.4 thousandth of an inch.

A macular hole is defined as a full-thickness defect of retinal tissue involving the anatomic fovea and primarily the foveola of the eye (**Figures 1a**, **b** and **2**). Since its development, OCT is the gold standard in the diagnosis and management of this condition. The high-resolution imaging on OCT allows cross-sectional and three-dimensional evaluation of the macula, thereby providing far greater details than what can be discerned clinically. It is helpful in detecting subtle early MHs as well as staging the more obvious and larger ones. OCT is now used to guide management of macular holes based on various parameters, as highlighted in the subsequent sections.

2. Classification of macular holes and OCT

Evolution of macular hole and *clinical appearance* of the different stages of its development has been described by Gass [4, 5]. The earliest stage is an impending hole, characterized by a yellow spot (stage 1a) or a yellow ring (stage 1b) at the fovea [4, 5]. Stage 1 macular holes are difficult to diagnose by slit lamp biomicroscopic examination alone, leading to a lot of subjective variation in diagnosis [6].

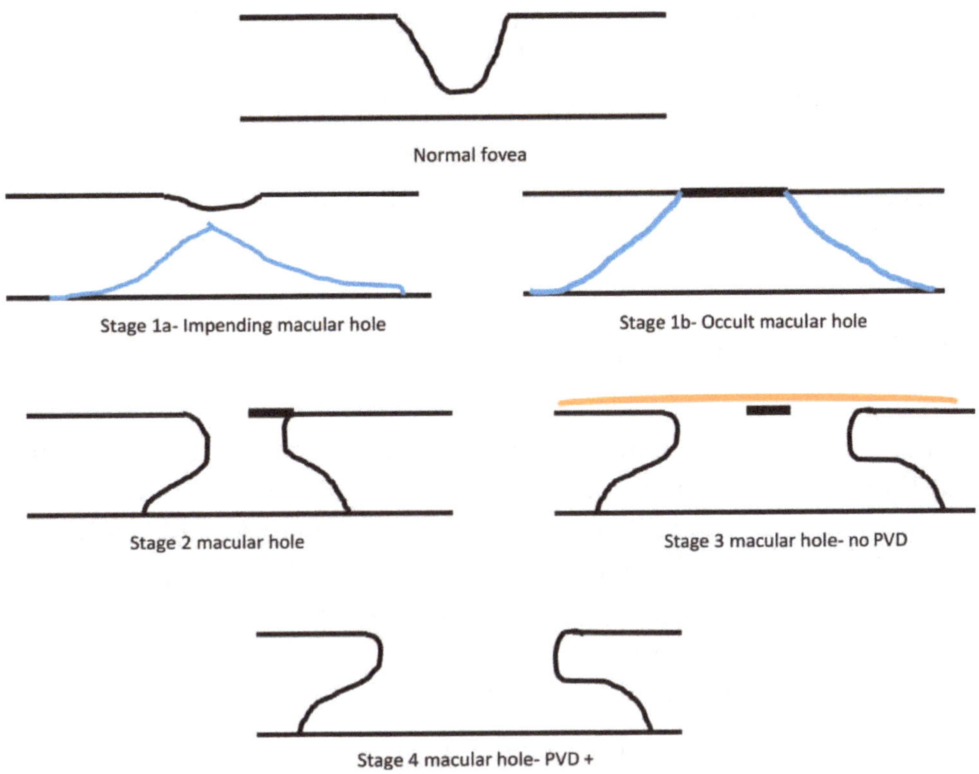

Figure 3. Grading scheme proposed and revised by Gass.

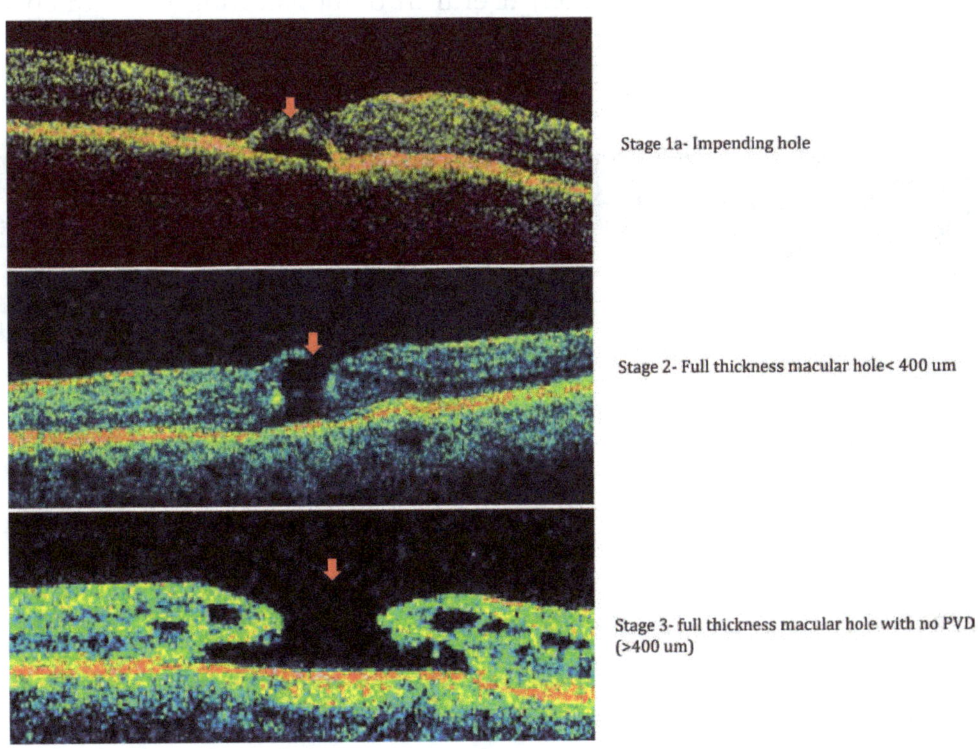

Figure 4. Stages of macular hole on OCT.

Since its introduction, OCT has been an extremely useful tool for diagnosing and staging macular holes. On OCT, a stage 1 hole appears as a cystic lesion in the inner layers of the retina (**Figure 3**) [7, 8]. *Stage 2* macular holes present as a *full-thickness defect at the fovea* (*size < 400um* in diameter). *Stage 3* macular hole is a completely evolved hole (size >400 um in diameter). In some patients, a small operculum can be seen suspended in front of the lesion. *Stage 4* macular holes appear similar to stage 3 holes except that in stage 4 holes there is *complete posterior vitreous detachment*, as frequently evidenced by a visible Weiss ring.

Hee et al. first described the use of OCT in diagnosing and monitoring macular holes [9]. Gaudric et al. later described the sequence of events in the evolution of macular holes using OCT—from anteroposterior vitreofoveal traction to full-thickness macular hole formation (**Figure 4**) [7].

3. Aiding early differential diagnosis

Diagnosing early macular hole lesions and differentiating them from other mimicking conditions are the clinical challenges in the management of macular holes. Fluorescein angiography (FA) was the earlier imaging modality of choice to identify macular holes. Although useful in characterizing full-thickness holes, this test does not help in identifying stage 1 macular holes, which are the source of clinical dilemma. The purpose of FA was largely to demonstrate other biomicroscopically similar lesions that have classic angiographic features (e.g., choroidal neovascular membranes), thereby excluding the diagnosis of macular hole.

Optical coherence tomography, as compared to FA, provides noninvasive diagnostic imaging helping early and accurate diagnosis. At the same time, it rules out other mimicking conditions, allowing the clinician to distinguish these from pseudohole and prehole conditions in almost all instances (**Figure 5**). It has been useful in demonstrating the sequence of events leading to macular hole formation over time and has thus increased our understanding of the anatomic relations in macular holes [9–11].

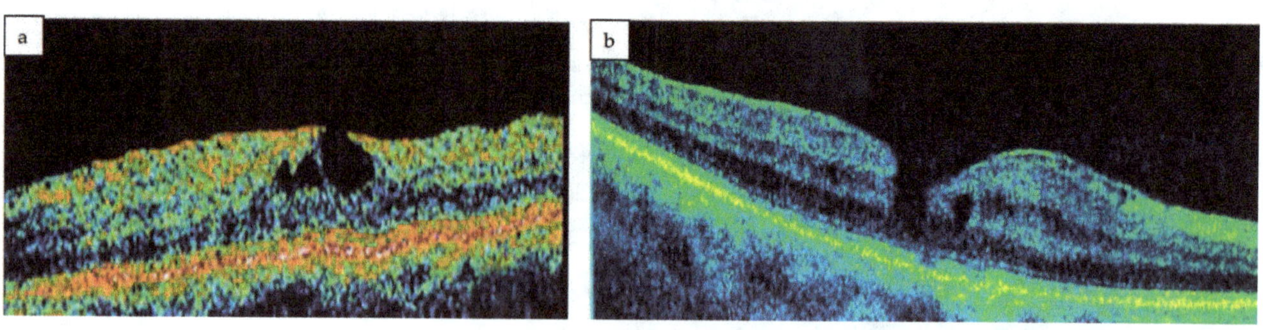

Figure 5. (a) Lamellar macular hole; (b) pseudohole.

4. Preoperative role-OCT factors

Apart from a major role in diagnosis, *preoperative OCT is an important tool for counseling patients* regarding postoperative prognosis on the basis of various OCT-based measurements (**Figure 6a–d**).

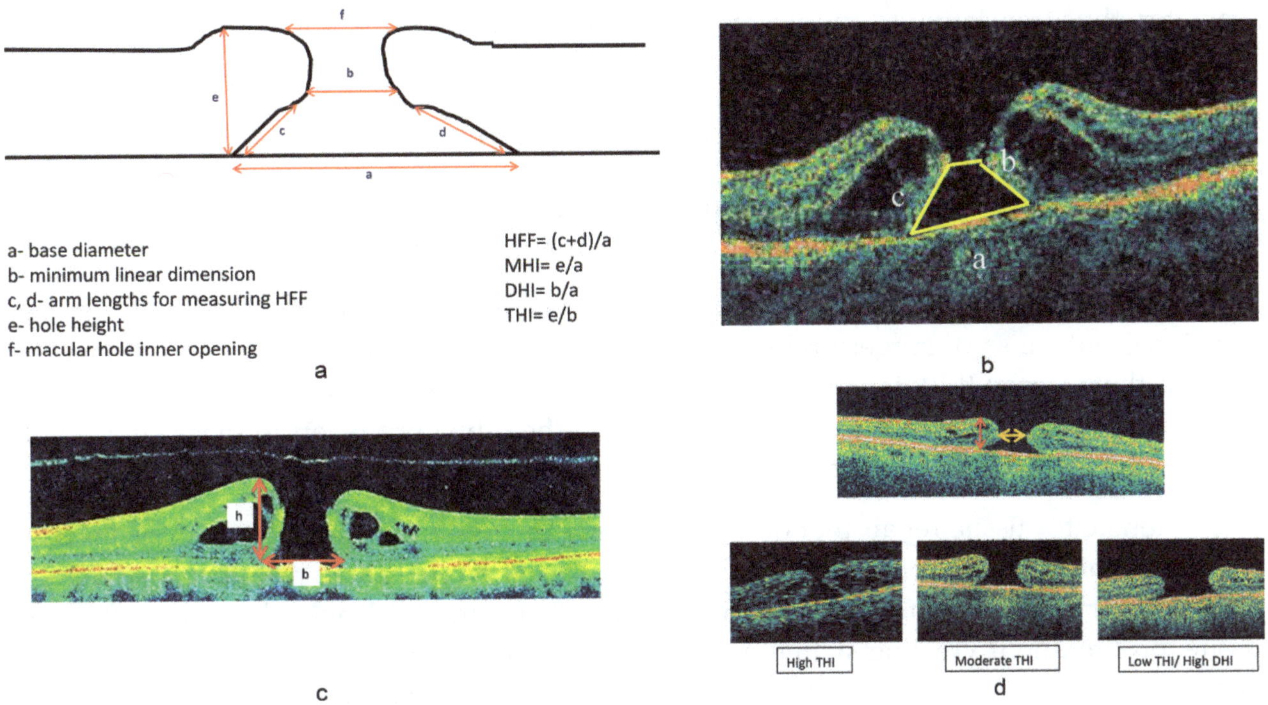

Figure 6. (a) Schematic representation of OCT factors; (b) HFF = (b + c)/a; (c) MHI = height/base (h/b); (d) Tractional hole index.

a. Hole form factor (HFF)

- It is the ratio of left arm length and right arm length to the base diameter of macular hole [10].
- In a study by Ullrich et al., it was observed that if **HFF was greater than 0.9,** the macular hole closed following a single surgical procedure, whereas if **HFF was less than 0.5,** anatomical success was achieved in 67% cases. Also, **higher HFF** preoperatively was associated with **better postoperative functional outcomes**. The base or minimum diameters were independent of the duration of the symptoms [12].

b. Macular hole index (MHI)

- It is the ratio of hole height to base diameter (ratio of perpendicular and horizontal dimensions of the hole). It can be calculated from OCT transverse images of the macular area.
- The MHI represents the **preoperative configuration** of a macular hole and is a prognostic factor for visual outcome. It was suggested that **MHI value of ≥0.5** could be used to predict better postoperative outcomes [13].

4.1. Clinical significance

In a study of large macular holes (low MHI macular holes) by Kumar et al. [14], preoperative screening for low MHI macular holes was done using spectral domain OCT. In view of large base diameters and low MHI, an additional maneuver was incorporated during surgery—intraoperative tapping of macular hole edges in all quadrants from the inner side. This leads to an in situ increase in perpendicular height of the macular hole compared with the base diameter, thus translating to an intraoperative increase in MHI and facilitating hole closure. This was done along with other surgical modifications including a large arcade to arcade ILM peel and removing any ERM associated with it. An improvement in the postoperative visual outcome was observed with large macular holes with MHI as low as 0.25.

Thus, OCT not only facilitates an accurate diagnosis, but preoperative surgical planning based on OCT factors also helps in improving anatomic and functional prognosis.

Another surgical technique proposed for large macular holes, to improve anatomic and functional outcomes of surgery by *preventing postoperative flat-open configuration* of macular holes, is the inverted ILM flap technique [15]. In this technique, after core vitrectomy and dye staining, the ILM is not completely removed from the retina but is left in place, attached to the edges of the MH. This ILM remnant is then inverted to cover and fill the MH (**Figure 7**).

The rationale for tissue repair that occurs following the use of this technique is: the inverted ILM, containing Muller cell fragments, induces glial cell proliferation, resulting in the macular hole filling with proliferating cells that enhance closure. It also works as a scaffold for tissue proliferation, creating a microenvironment that encourages correct photoreceptor alignment. This allows a near-perfect anatomic restoration, *with OCT demonstrating restoration of normal foveal architecture*. Hence, this technique results in better postoperative anatomic and functional outcome.

Also, because ILM is a basement membrane, it allows glial cell proliferation, allowing large MHs to fill with tissue over time further expanding its use to repeat MH surgery [16].

c. Diameter hole index (DHI)

   - It is the ratio of minimum diameter of MH to base diameter and is an indicator of extent of tangential traction.

d. Tractional hole index (THI)

   - It is the ratio of maximal height of MH to minimum diameter and is an indicator of AP traction and retinal hydration.

   Patients with higher THI values (>1.41) and low DHI values (<0.50) had the best post-op VA recovery [17].

As an increasing number of surgeons opt for ILM peeling to facilitate hole closure, vital dyes have become useful tools for the membrane and ensuring its complete removal [18]. Also, mixtures of dyes with high-density dextrose or polyethylene glycol (PEG) solution have improved the staining of the macula [19]. These high-density solutions when combined with the dye promote immediate settling of the dye onto the macula and minimize its dispersion throughout the vitreous cavity.

With the availability of several dyes and formulations, concerns regarding chemical or phototoxicity are always expressed. Hence, the need to develop new methods to enhance the visualization of the ILM. One example is the use of intraoperative optical coherence tomography (iOCT), which has the potential to visualize the ILM during vitrectomy with immediate surgical feedback.

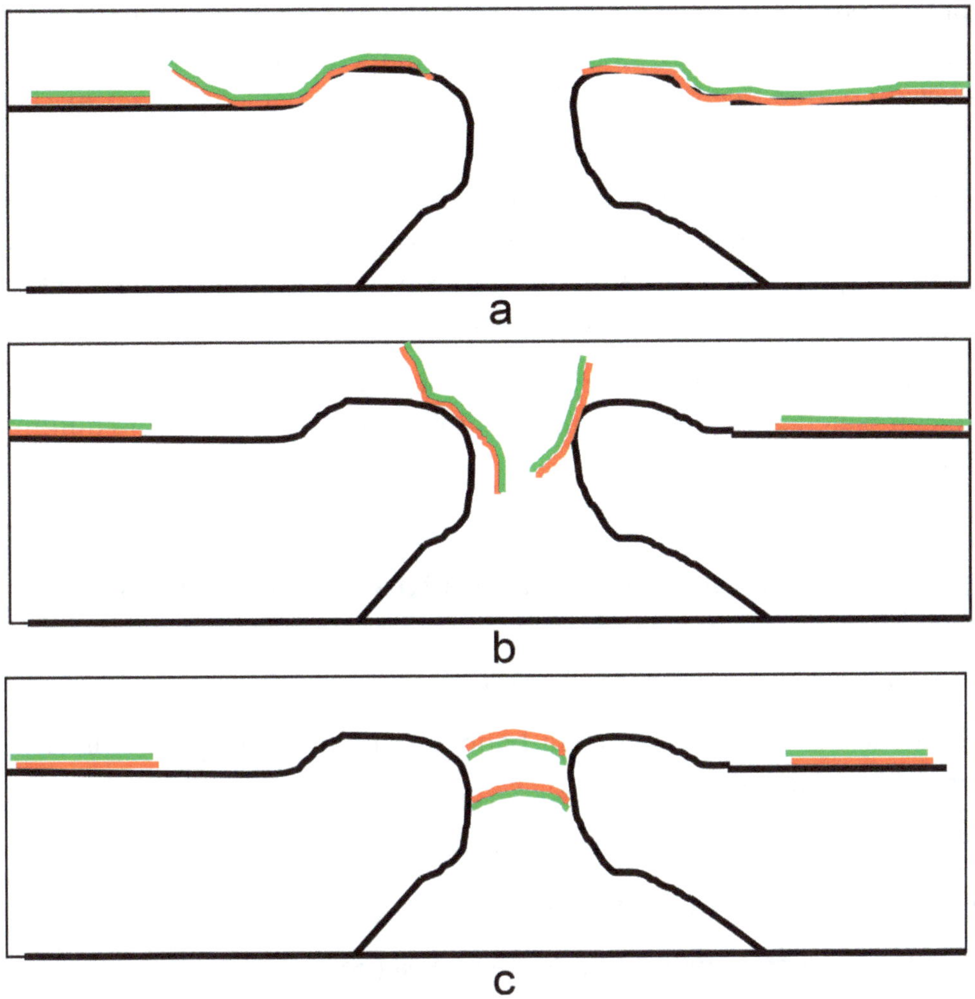

Figure 7. Line diagram demonstrating inverted ILM flap technique. (a) The surface of the ILM facing the hyaloid is depicted in green and the surface facing the retinal surface is depicted in red. (b) Trimming of the peripheral part of the ILM. (c) Inverting the central ILM flap over the macular hole. Now the surface of the ILM depicted in red faces the hyaloid and the green surface is toward the RPE-thus "inverted".

5. Intraoperative OCT (iOCT)

OCT is fundamental to our clinical decision-making for management of macular holes. It has now been incorporated as intraoperative OCT (iOCT)—supplementing surgical assessments in the operating room and guiding surgical decisions.

Intraoperative OCT consists of spectral domain optical coherence tomography (SD-OCT) on an OCT-mounted surgical microscope. It identifies intraoperative changes in the macular anatomy and provides additional information to predict visual outcomes of macular surgery. The SD-OCT scan taken immediately after ERM removal identifies a cleavage plane for the subsequent ILM peeling, allowing an accurate ILM peel causing minimum disruption of retinal architecture [20].

Intraoperative OCT has been described in several types of retinal surgeries, including vitrectomy for the macular hole. During membrane peeling, the surgeon's impression of membrane peel completeness conflicted with iOCT data in 19% of cases (e.g., iOCT displayed a persistent occult residual membrane or showed lack of residual membrane). For posterior segment surgery, it has been reported that the use of iOCT provided valuable feedback in 71% (97 of 136) of cases.

The use of iOCT, being in its early stages, has certain limitations—real-time membrane peeling using metallic instruments creates absolute shadowing. Despite this drawback, it is still useful in visualizing tissue-instrument interactions, revealing residual membranes, and confirming completion of surgical objectives in macular surgery [21, 22].

This new modality will help improve anatomic and visual outcomes by helping the surgeon ensure completeness of surgical intervention and at the same time minimizing tissue manipulation.

6. Post-op role of OCT: anatomic versus functional success

a. Photoreceptor inner/outer segment junction

- IS/OS junction is seen as the bright band proximal to the RPE. It is an indicator of photoreceptor alignment.
- Grade 0: IS/OS junction absent under the fovea.

  Grade 1: IS/OS junction present under the fovea (abnormal).

  Grade 2: IS/OS junction present under the fovea (normal).

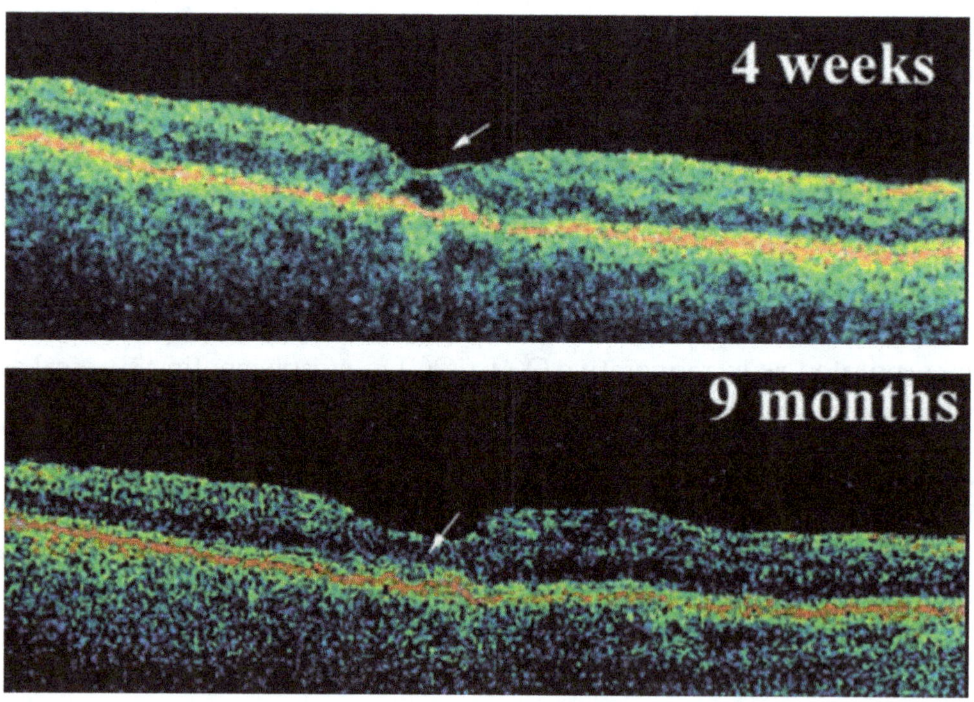

Figure 8. Spontaneous resolution of foveal lucency.

It has been noted in various studies that photoreceptor integrity is the best prognostic factor for VA.

Analysis of the inner HRL (hyperreflective layer) allows a better understanding of the outcomes of macular hole surgeries. It has been seen that anatomic success with restoration of foveal contour does not always translate to improved postoperative visual acuity. Irregularities at the level of the inner HRL after macular hole surgery may prevent visual acuity improvement. On the other hand, improvement in BCVA has been noted with IS/OS junction normalization in the postoperative period [23].

b. Foveolar gaps (lucencies) are a common occurrence post MH surgery. Conservative treatment with patient reassurance is the treatment of choice as has been demonstrated by serial OCT follow-up (**Figure 8**) [24].

c. Macular hole closure can be observed ophthalmoscopically 9–10 days after gas injection.

- Flat/open and flat/closed anatomic closure
- Elevated/open

  The closed macular holes have been variously classified based on OCT

- type 1 closure (closed without foveal neurosensory retinal defect) and type 2 closure (closed with foveal neurosensory retinal defect) (**Figure 9a**) [25]. The extent of postoperative visual improvement of type 1 closure group was larger than that of type 2 closure group. Also, only type 2 closure was associated with recurrence of the pathology. Thus, the postoperative visual prognosis directly correlated to the type of hole closure, which in turn was seen to correspond to the preoperative hole diameter [25].

  In another study by Imai et al. [26], OCT images of repaired macular holes were categorized into three patterns (**Figure 9b**).

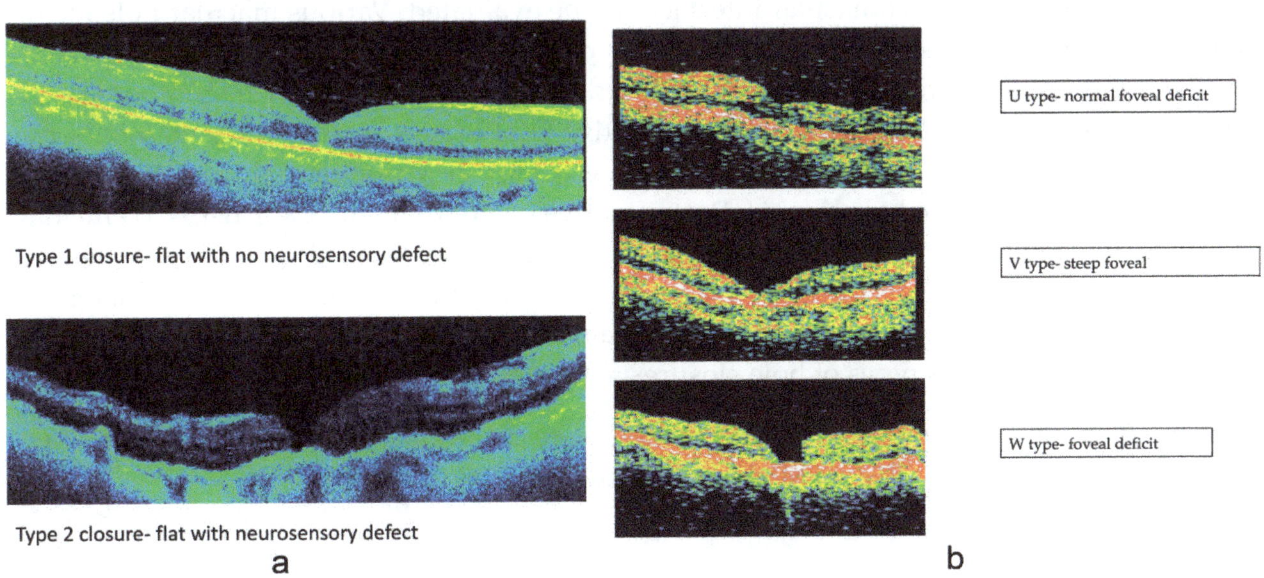

Figure 9. Types of macular hole closure on (a) OCT-Kang et al. [25] and (b) OCT-Imai et al. [26].

- U-type (normal foveal contour)—the retinal pigment epithelium and choriocapillaris layers covered by a smooth surface
- V-type (steep foveal contour)—retinal pigment epithelium and choriocapillaris layers covered with moderately backscattering layers with a notch
- W-type (foveal defect of neurosensory retina)—terminating of sensory retinal layers leading to exposure of retinal pigment epithelium and choriocapillaris layers to the surface

Postoperative acuity was well correlated with these patterns of OCT images.

7. OCT in the fellow eye

OCT can be used for serial follow-up of the fellow eye to pick up early changes. Patients with a full-thickness macular hole in one eye and foveal abnormalities in the fellow eye, consistent with a stage 1 macular hole, have a high risk of progression in the fellow eye. A close follow-up of these patients can help early intervention resulting in better visual outcomes.

8. Summary

OCT is vital for ophthalmologic clinical and surgical decision-making, in particular for macular pathologies. It complements clinical examination in diagnosing vitreoretinal interface pathologies, including macular hole [27]. OCT allows the clinician to detect initial stages of macular hole, follow its progression, and intervene early in case of progression to full-thickness holes. It can unequivocally detect the presence of a macular hole as well as changes in the surrounding retina, distinguishing it from lamellar holes and cystic lesions of the macula. Also, the status of the vitreomacular interface can be evaluated. Various macular hole factors enable the surgeon to discuss the prognosis with patients to give a more realistic expectation. Novel surgical modifications have been attempted for large macular holes diagnosed on OCT, with improved postoperative results. Intraoperative OCT is a new tool in the armamentarium helping the surgeon evaluate the completeness of ILM peel with minimal tissue disruption, thus aiding postoperative hole closure. Postoperative evaluation with OCT helps to elucidate the structural and functional changes associated with different surgical techniques. It helps us understand the mechanisms of postoperative improvement observed along with changes in the retinal architecture. OCT also helps us correlate anatomic success with functional success/failure, based on various types of hole closures and integrity of IS/OS junction.

With advances in OCT entering clinical practice, we can see an exponential expansion of our ophthalmic knowledge with a parallel improvement in patient care.

Author details

Sana I. Tinwala

Address all correspondence to: sanailyas22@gmail.com

Anuditi Eye Care, Mumbai, India

References

[1] Huang D, Swanson EA, Lin CP, et al. Optical coherence tomography. Science. 1991;**254**: 1178-1181

[2] Drexler W, Sattmann H, Hermann B, et al. Enhanced visualization of macular pathology with the use of ultrahigh resolution optical coherence tomography. Archives of Ophthalmology. 2003;**121**:695-706

[3] Potsaid B, Gorczynska I, Srinivasan VJ, et al. Ultrahigh speed spectral/Fourier domain OCT ophthalmic imaging at 70,000 to 312,500 axial scans per second. Optics Express. 2008;**16**:15149-15169

[4] Gass JD. Idiopathic senile macular hole. Its early stages and pathogenesis. Archives of Ophthalmology. 1988;**106**:629-639

[5] Gass JD. Reappraisal of biomicroscopic classification of stages of development of a macular hole. American Journal of Ophthalmology. 1995;**119**:752-759

[6] Gass JD, Joondeph BC. Observations concerning patients with suspected impending macular holes. American Journal of Ophthalmology. 1990;**109**:638-646

[7] Gaudric A, Haouchine B, Massin P, Paques M, Blain P, Erginay A. Macular hole formation: New data provided by optical coherence tomography. Archives of Ophthalmology. 1999;**117**:1744-1751

[8] Haouchine B, Massin P, Gaudric A. Foveal pseudocyst as the first step in macular hole formation: A prospective study by optical coherence tomography. Ophthalmology. 2001;**108**:15-22

[9] Hee MR, Puliafito CA, Wong C, et al. Optical coherence tomography of macular holes. Ophthalmology. 1995;**102**:748-756

[10] Puliafito CA, Hee MR, Lin CP, et al. Imaging of macular disease with optical coherence tomography. Ophthalmology. 1995;**102**:217-229

[11] Azzolini C, Patelli F, Brancato R. Correlation between optical coherence tomography data and biomicroscopic interpretation of idiopathic macular hole. American Journal of Ophthalmology. 2001;**132**:348-355

[12] Ullrich S, Haritoglou C, Gass C, Schaumberger M, Ulbig MW, Kampik A. Macular hole size as a prognostic factor in macular hole surgery. The British Journal of Ophthalmology. 2002;**86**(4):390-393

[13] Kusuhara S, Teraoka Escaño MF, Fujii S, Nakanishi Y, Tamura Y, Nagai A, Yamamoto H, Tsukahara Y, Negi A. Prediction of postoperative visual outcome based on hole configuration by optical coherence tomography in eyes with idiopathic macular holes. American Journal of Ophthalmology. 2004;**138**(5):709-716

[14] Kumar A, Tinwala SI, Gogia V, Sehra SV. Tapping of macular hole edges: The outcomes of a novel technique for large macular holes. The Asia-Pacific Journal of Ophthalmology. 2013;**2**:305-309

[15] Michalewska Z, Michalewski J, Adelman RA, Nawrocki J. Inverted internal limiting membrane flap technique for large macular holes. Ophthalmology. 2010;**117**(10):2018-2025

[16] Hayashi H, Kuriyama S. Foveal microstructure in macular holes surgically closed by inverted internal limiting membrane flap technique. Retina. 2014;**34**(12):2444-2450

[17] Ruiz-Moreno JM, Staicu C, Piñero DP, Montero J, Lugo F, Amat P. Optical coherence tomography predictive factors for macular hole surgery outcome. The British Journal of Ophthalmology. 2008;**92**(5):640-644

[18] Rodrigues EB, Maia M, Meyer CH, Penha FM, Dib E, Farah ME. Vital dyes for chromovitrectomy. Current Opinion in Ophthalmology. 2007;**18**(3):179-187

[19] Veckeneer M, Mohr A, Alharthi E, et al. Novel 'heavy' dyes for retinal membrane staining during macular surgery: Multicenter clinical assessment. Acta Ophthalmologica. 2014;**92**:339-344

[20] Pichi F, Alkabes M, Nucci P, Ciardella AP. Intraoperative SD-OCT in macular surgery. Ophthalmic Surgery, Lasers and Imaging Retina. 2012;**43**(6):S54-S60

[21] Ehlers JP, Modi YS, Pecen PE, Goshe J, Dupps WJ, Rachitskaya A, Sharma S, Yuan A, Singh R, Kaiser PK, Reese JL, Calabrise C, Watts A, Srivastava SK. The DISCOVER Study 3-year results: Feasibility and usefulness of microscope-integrated intraoperative OCT during ophthalmic surgery. Ophthalmology. 2018;**17**:32218-32212. pii: S0161-6420

[22] Ehlers JP, Tao YK, Farsiu S, et al. Integration of a spectral domain optical coherence tomography system into a surgical microscope for intraoperative imaging. Investigative Ophthalmology & Visual Science. 2011;**52**:3153-3159

[23] Baba T, Yamamoto S, Arai M, Arai E, Sugawara T, Mitamura Y, Mizunoya S. Correlation of visual recovery and presence of photoreceptor inner/outer segment junction in optical coherence images after successful macular hole repair. Retina. 2008;**28**(3):453-458

[24] Mahmoud TH, BW MC 2nd. Natural history of foveolar lucencies observed by optical coherence tomography after macular hole surgery. Retina. 2007;**27**(1):95-100

[25] Kang SW, Ahn K, Ham DI. Types of macular hole closure and their clinical implications. The British Journal of Ophthalmology. 2003;**87**(8):1015-1019

[26] Imai M, Iijima H, Gotoh T, Tsukahara S. Optical coherence tomography of successfully repaired idiopathic macular holes. American Journal of Ophthalmology. 1999;**128**(5): 621-627

[27] Mirza RG, Johnson MW, Jampol LM. Optical coherence tomography use in evaluation of the vitreoretinal interface: A review. Survey of Ophthalmology. 2007;**52**:397-421

13

Spectral Domain Optical Coherence Tomography in the Diagnosis and Monitoring of Diabetic Macular Edema

Simona Delia Nicoară

Abstract

Currently, spectral domain optical coherence tomography (SD-OCT) is a basic tool in diagnosing and monitoring diabetic macular edema (DME), which is the most frequent cause of visual impairment in the diabetic patients. OCT technology has changed the classification of DME from the traditional criteria. Macular thickness measured on OCT is considered an outcome measure to evaluate the structural and functional outcome of various therapeutic means used in DME. SD-OCT evaluates ultrastructural retinal parameters, such as the ellipsoid zone, photoreceptor outer segment length and quantifies the individual layers according to various algorithms. The aim is to present the way in which SD-OCT technology has changed our clinical practice during the last years, in diagnosing, classifying and treating DME and to illustrate its impact with practical cases.

Keywords: spectral domain-optical coherence tomography, diabetic macular edema, macular thickness, macular traction

1. Introduction

Currently, there are 400 million diabetics in the world and according to World Health Organization, by the year 2030 the population of diabetics will double [1, 2]. Diabetic retinopathy (DR) is the main cause of visual impairment within the working age population group [1, 2]. Quality of life is affected even if visual acuity decrease is mild/moderate. In the context of DR, diabetic macular edema (DME) is the most common cause of visual impairment, especially in type 2 diabetes. It is estimated that one out of four diabetics develops DME over a lifetime [1, 2].

OCT represented a breakthrough in the management of DME, both for its diagnosis and monitoring of treatment effects. OCT technology offers valuable quantitative data (macular thickness, extension of edema, macular volume) and qualitative ones (macular morphology, vitreo-macular interface) [3].

The advantages of OCT over other imaging modalities are as follows: its noninvasiveness, rapidity and safety profile [3, 4].

2. Theoretical consideration on OCT

The principle of tomography consists in the reconstruction of cross-sectional images of an object using its projections. The concept of OCT developed in 1990 and the first commercial version of OCT belongs to Carl-Zeiss in 1996. The first clinical application of OCT technology was in the field of ophthalmology. The obtained images reveal the optical properties of the scanned tissues and not the tissues themselves, and they are very similar to the histological sections.

There are two OCT methods: time domain (TD-OCT) and spectral domain (SD-OCT). The properties of the two methods are synthesized in **Table 1** [3, 4].

The most common application of OCT is the measure of macular thickness. With TD-OCT, macular thickness map is calculated from six radial scans crossing at the fovea from which result the medium macular thickness and the total macular volume. With SD-OCT, image resolution is significantly higher. Different landmarks are used to calculate macular thickness with TD-OCT and SD-OCT. With TD-OCT, photoreceptors external segments are not differentiated from the retinal pigmented epithelium (RPE) and are therefore excluded from

Property	TD-OCT	SD-OCT
Principle	Low-coherence interferometry	Fourier equation
Acquisition	An interferometer evaluates *sequentially* the back scattering of the light by the retinal structures	A spectrometer evaluates *simultaneously* the back scattering of the light by the retinal structures
Sampling	Point by point	All points simultaneously
Acquisition time	1–2 s	60 times faster
Target area	Six radial scans 20 μm wide and 6 mm long	Φ 6 mm = 65,000 scans
Acquisition rate	400 scans/s	25,000–52,000 scans/s
Display	2D	3D
Axial resolution	10–15 μ	3–7 μ

Table 1. Properties of TD-OCT and SD-OCT.

Device (company)	Axial resolution (μ)	Scans/s
Cirrus HD-OCT (Carl Zeiss Meditec)	5	27,000
Spectralis (Heidelberg Engineering)	7	40,000
RE Vue (Optovue)	5	26,000
3D OCT-1000 3D OCT-2000 (Topcon)	6	18,000
Spectral OCT/SLO (OPKO/OTI)	5	27,000
SOCT Copernicus (Optopol)	6	25,000
SOCT Copernicus HR (Canon/Optopol Inc.)	3	50,000
SD-OCT (Bioptigen)	4	20,000
Retinascans RS 3000 (Nidek)	7	53,000

Table 2. SD-OCT devices used in ophthalmology.

the evaluation of macular thickness. SD-OCT allows photoreceptors external segments be differentiated from the retinal pigmented epithelium (RPE) and are included in the value of the macular thickness [3, 4].

Many SD-OCT devices are used in the clinical practice. Their axial resolutions and scanning speeds are presented in **Table 2**.

OCT and ultrasounds are complementary methods in assessing the vitreo-retinal interface. Ultrasound scans provide a more complete image of the vitreo-retinal interface, but with significantly lower resolution. OCT offers a high resolution image of a limited area. Since OCT uses light to acquire images, its use is limited by media opacities [5, 6].

OCT is a noninvasive, well-tolerated method, easy to understand and explain. It offers qualitative information on retinal thickness, and it is reliable and reproducible. OCT reveals the presence and extension of vitreo-macular traction (VMT) [5, 6].

OCT technology holds the promise for the unprecedented capability to describe and monitor the changes in retina geometry.

3. Normal OCT aspect of the macula

The normal retinal layers have different reflectivity on OCT scans. Thus, the nerve fibers and the retinal pigmented epithelium (RPE) display high reflectivity, the plexiform and the nuclear layers have intermediate reflectivity and the photoreceptors display low reflectivity [3, 4]. The most commonly scan algorithms used in the clinical practice are the line and the volume (cube). Retinal thickness is automatically measured by the use of device software. The distance between the vitreo-retinal interface and the anterior surface of the RPE is generally comprised between 200 and 275 μm; the foveal depression ranges from 170 to 190 μm and the thickness of the peripheral retina is between 220 and 280 μm [5].

4. Macular edema

Macular edema is the main pathologic feature of diabetic maculopathy. According to ETDRS, it is defined as any detectable retinal thickening due to fluid accumulation. It may be localized in a sector of the macular region (focal) or it may be diffused. Persistent macular edema leads to the necrosis of Muller cells with subsequent formation of cystoid cavities localized mainly in the outer retinal layers (Henle's fiber, external plexiform) and sometimes in the inner plexiform layer too. In more advanced stages, the cavities may coalesce centrally forming a large hyporeflective cavity that accounts for the significant increase of foveal thickness. By consequence, beside increase of macular thickness (which is the most important OCT sign) in DME appear: large intraretinal spaces of reduced reflectivity, loss of the normal layered retinal structure and flattening of the central foveal depression. Sometimes fluid can be seen under the neurosensory retina. Hard exudates and hemorrhages are typical landmarks for DR and they appear on OCT images as small hyperreflective deposits with posterior shadowing [6].

The cysts that develop in the retina during DME vary in size. According to their size, a classification of cystoid edema was proposed by Koleva-Georgieva into mild, moderate and severe. In mild edema, cysts are small and predominantly located in the outer retinal layers. In the intermediate and severe forms, cysts are located in the outer layers, especially in the fovea. If cysts continue to increase, they occupy the whole thickness of the retina, leading to macular atrophy and profound visual loss. In mild edema, the cysts have a horizontal diameter below 300 μm, in intermediate edema the horizontal diameter of the cysts is between 300 and 600 μm and in the severe one the horizontal diameter of the cysts is above 600 μm or large confluent cavities with retinoschisis appearance are identified [6–8].

It has been shown that the status of the outer retinal layers is important for the visual outcome in patients with DME. Yohannan et al. proved that disruption of the IS/OS junction correlates well with a significant decrease of point sensitivity in patients with DME. Also, the integrity of ELM and IS/OS junctions correlates positively with visual acuity. Therefore, OCT evaluation of the outer retinal layers in patients with DME is important in predicting visual outcome [6].

Vitreo-retinal interface is very important in diabetic patients. It is known that diabetics have higher than normal vitreo-retinal adherence and that vitreo-macular traction is one of the factors explaining DME. OCT identifies various aspects: incomplete posterior vitreous detachment (PVD), epiretinal membranes (ERM) [6, 7]. OCT identifies vitreo-macular interface disorders from the preclinical stage. If posterior hyaloid is thin and partly detached from the macula, this aspect cannot be seen on biomicroscopy, but it is easily detectable on OCT. The same is true regarding the thin ERM. Thus, OCT is a very useful tool that establishes the best therapeutic option in these cases: vitrectomy with release of vitreo-macular traction/dissection of ERM, from the early stages, when the chances for a good functional outcome are the highest. Assessment of vitreo-macular interface is an important step in evaluating diabetic patients. Not only does OCT indicate the moment for vitrectomy in these patients, but it also monitors the postoperative morphological outcomes: favorable evolution (decrease of macular thickness), development of ERM or of lamellar macular hole [6].

The detached posterior vitreous face appears on OCT scans as a thin horizontal or oblique line with low/medium reflectivity in the nonreflective vitreous, above or inserting into the retina. If PVD is incomplete, it may adhere to the foveal or peripapillary region. ERM appears on OCT as a hyperreflective line on the surface of the retina. Its presence leads to retinal modifications: increase of macular thickness, loss of foveal depression, formation of intraretinal cysts and pseudoholes. The difference between PVD and ERM is made according to their reflectivity (low in PVD, high in ERM). OCT provides other details related to ERM (degree of opacity, thickness, and distance from the macula) and to its effects on the underlying retina: distortion, edema, neurosensory detachment [6].

OCT is a very reliable and reproducible method to assess and monitor macular thickness following various treatments for DME: intravitreal injections with anti-VEGF and steroids, laser photocoagulation, vitrectomy. OCT also identifies macular atrophy which explains functional failure despite resolution of edema. Monitoring patients with DME must include two major parameters: functional (visual acuity) and anatomical (OCT) [5, 6].

Cystoid macular edema (CME) appears like large ovoid spaces of low reflectivity separated by hyperreflective septae that represent intraretinal cystoid-like cavities. Posterior hyaloid traction (PHT) appears like a highly reflective band on the surface of the retina. Serous retinal detachment (SRD) appears as a dark accumulation of subretinal fluid beneath the high reflective and dome-like elevation of detached retina. The highly reflective band which represents the outer surface of the retina helps differentiating subretinal fluid from the intraretinal fluid. Tractional retinal detachment (TRD) is identified as the area of low signal underlying the highly reflective border of detached retina. It often takes the appearance of a pick-shaped configuration [5, 6].

The most common finding in diabetics is diffuse retinal thickening (DRT) [6].

There is a correlation between macular thickness and visual acuity in patients with DME. The OCT pattern that was associated with worse visual outcome is CME [6].

In DME OCT technology has significant impact at various levels: it elucidates the pathogenic mechanisms of DME; it has a major contribution in identifying hyaloid-macular traction; it identifies the subclinical DME allowing early treatment; it makes it possible to correlate macular thickness with visual acuity; it monitors the evolution of DME following treatment [5–7].

5. OCT classification of macular edema

Along with the development of OCT imaging, various classifications of DME have been elaborated. The first OCT classification of DME belongs to Otani, and it is based on morphological

Retinal thickness	No macular edema	Normal macular thickness
	Early subclinical ME	Macular thickening nondetectable clinically Retinal thickness increased on OCT
	Established ME	Retinal thickening and morphological signs of edema
Retinal morphology	Simple noncystoid ME	Increased retinal thickness; reduced retinal reflectivity; irregularities of the layered retinal structure; flattening of the foveal depression; no cystoid spaces
	Cystoid ME	Well-defined intraretinal cystoids spaces
	Serous macular detachment	Hyporeflective area under the detached neurosensory retina and over the hyperreflective line of EPR
Vitreo-macular interface	No MT	Complete PVD/no PVD/no ERM
	Questionable MT	Incomplete PVD with no detectable distortion of retinal surface contour at the point of adhesion
	Definite MT	Incomplete PVD with distortion of retinal surface contour at the point of adhesion
Retinal outer layers	IS/OS and ELM intact	IS/OS and ELM intact
	IS/OS and ELM with disrupted integrity	IS/OS and ELM with disrupted integrity

Table 3. OCT classification of macular edema (after Koleva-Georgieva).

parameters, into three categories: sponge-like swelling, cystoid edema and serous retinal detachment [5]. A fourth category was added by Trichonas et al., posterior hyaloid traction (PHT) [6]. A more detailed classification was proposed by Koleva-Georgieva, and it is based on quantitative and qualitative OCT data: retinal thickness, retinal morphology, retinal topography, macular traction, foveal photoreceptor status (**Table 3**) [8].

6. OCT-angiography

OCT-Angiography (OCT-A) enables the noninvasive visualization of 3D retinal capillary network. It correlates very well with fluorescein angiography (FA), and it is able to show even more capillaries in the pericentral macula than FA and to separate and individualize the superficial and deep capillary plexus.

7. Personal experience with SD-OCT in DME

The personal experience in using SD-OCT for the management of DME is illustrated by several cases (**Figures 1–8**).

In this case, the OCT aspect of the macula favored intravitreal injection of anti-VEGF in AO, given the absence of PHT and the high amount of fluid within the retina OS. In OD, early

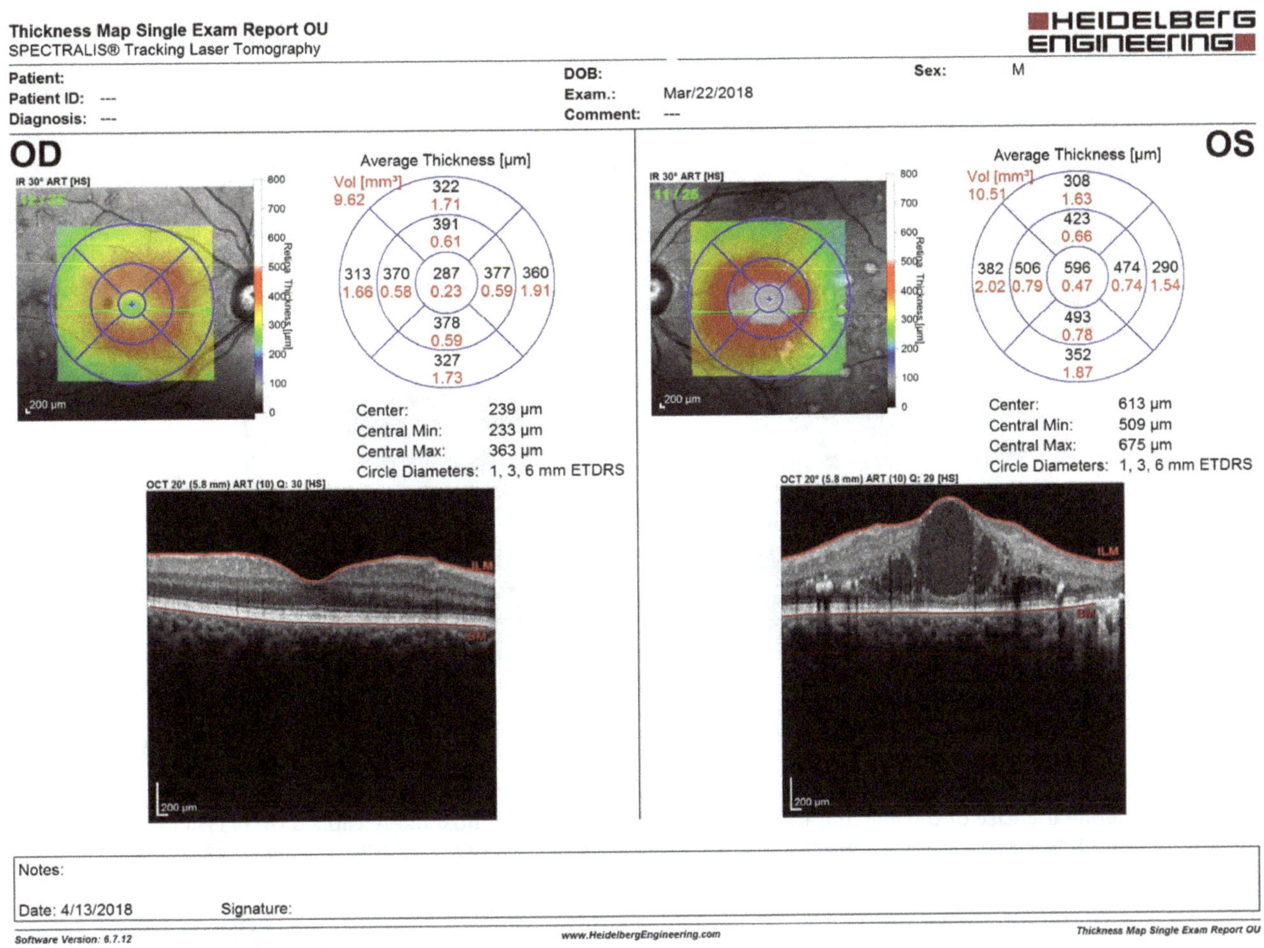

Figure 1. OD diffuse mild thickening of the macular region. OS large ovoid spaces of low reflectivity (liquid content) separated by hyperreflective septae located in the neurosensitive retina that represent intraretinal cystoid-like cavities; hyperreflective deposits with posterior shadowing (hard exudates, hemorrhages) in the neurosensory retina; no evidence of PHT; significant increase of the macular thickness, mainly centrally—on the account of the cystoids cavities.

treatment in the stage of mild edema had positive outcome. In OS, the high degree of macular disorganization prevented a significant improvement in vision (**Figure 2**).

In this case, intravitreal anti-VEGF injections alone would probably not lead to the resolution of edema, because vitreo-macular traction is also involved in its pathophysiology. Therefore, pars plana vitrectomy with dissection of the posterior hyaloid from the macular area was indicated (**Figures 3** and **4**).

In this case, anti-VEGF injections are indicated in AO, but with a much better prognosis in LE where edema is mild, as compared to RE in which the macula is disorganized (**Figures 5** and **6**).

In this case, beside anti-VEGF injections, pars plana vitrectomy appears reasonable in order to release the traction exerted by the posterior hyaloid on the macula.

Even if macular edema is mild, intravitreal anti-VEGF would prevent its progression toward more advanced stages with cystoid degeneration of the macula (**Figure 7**).

On the ground of the OCT aspect, intravitreal anti-VEGF injections are indicated in OD, but not in LE in which retinal atrophy is present (**Figure 8**).

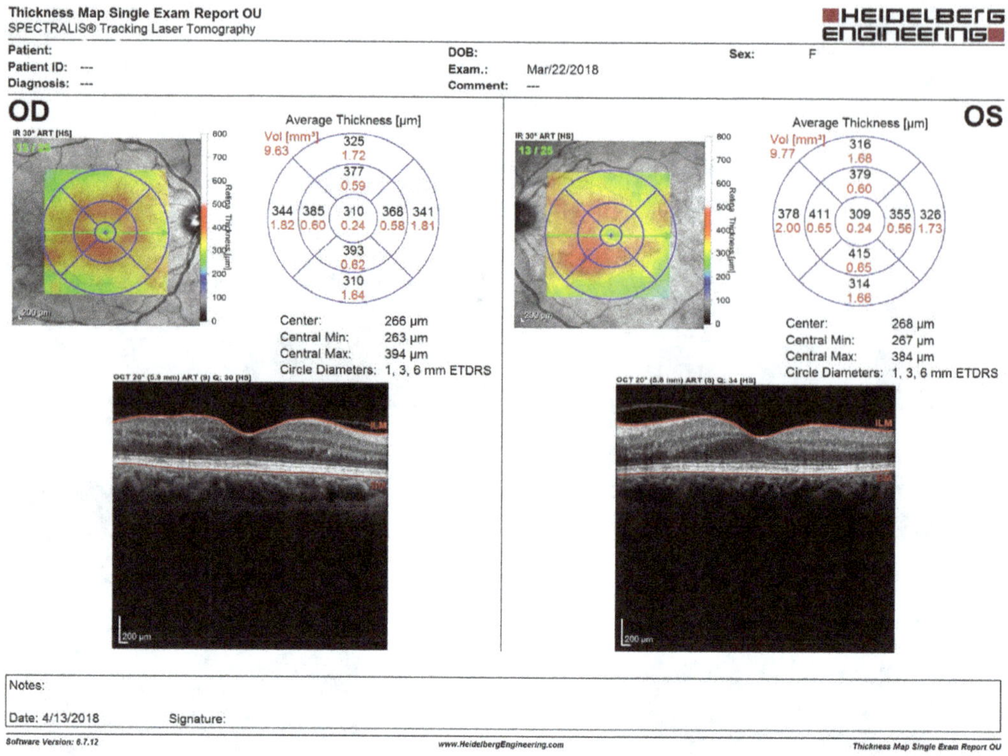

Figure 2. Moderate increase of the macular thickness in a diffuse manner, most likely caused by PHT: posterior hyaloid appears as a highly reflective band adherent to the underlying retina.

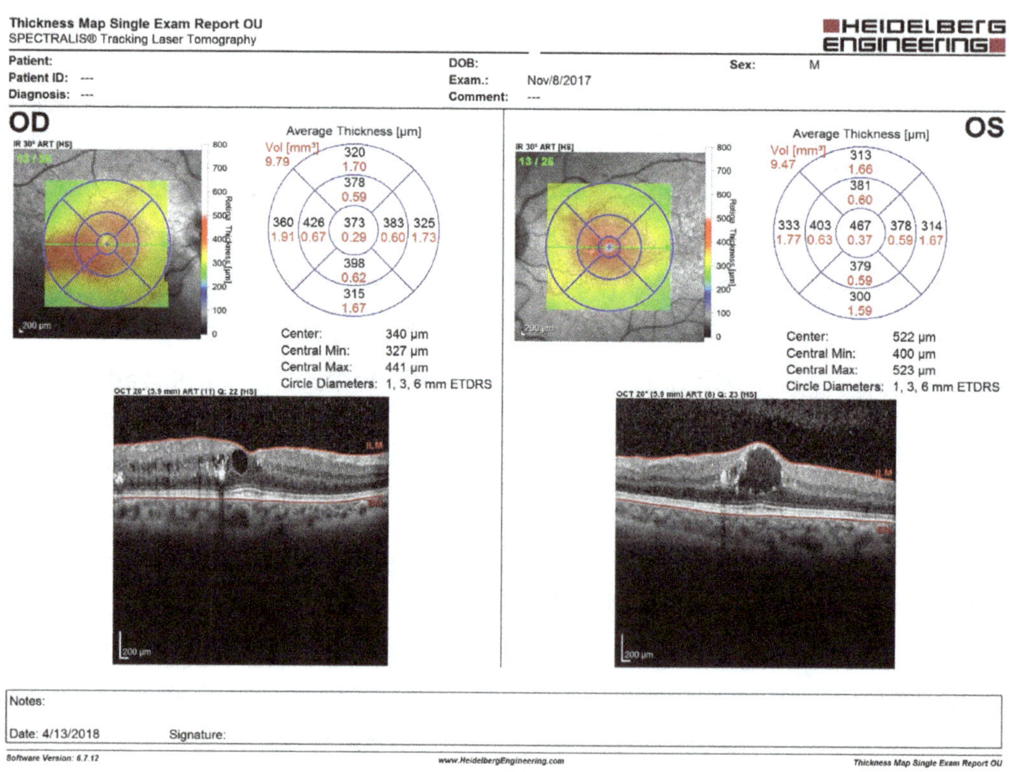

Figure 3. Diffuse DME in AO in a young patient with type 1 diabetes. Fluid is present within the neurosensitive retina in the fovea (dark spaces). PHT is not present; therefore, intravitreal anti-VEGF injections were indicated with good outcome.

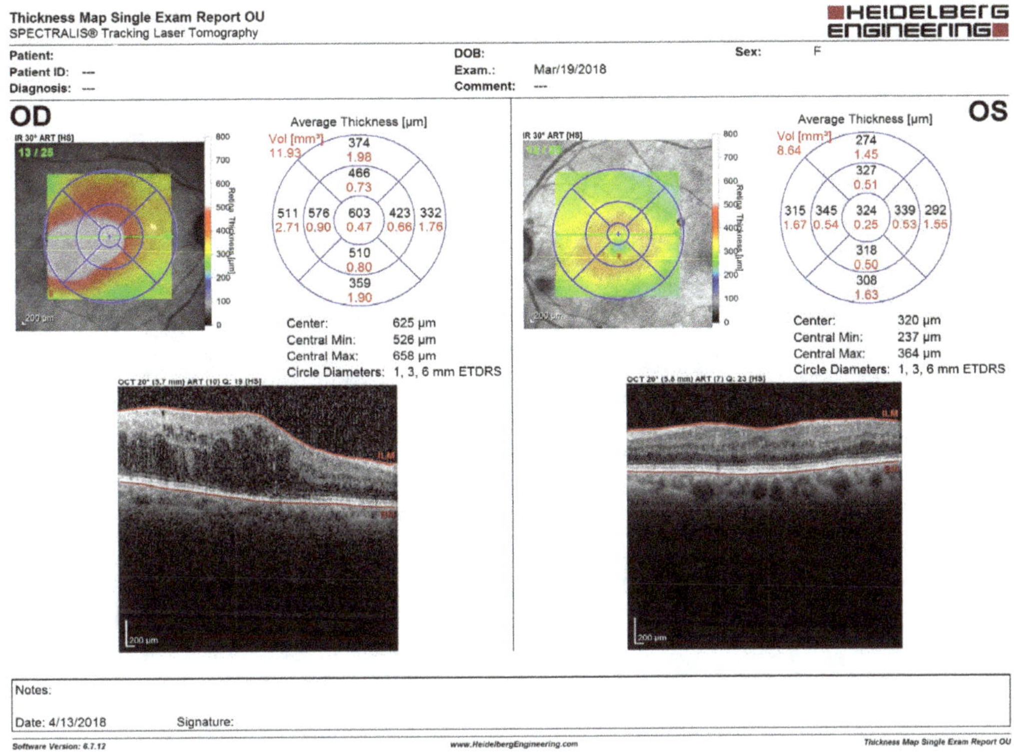

Figure 4. OD marked increase of the macular thickness, large cystoid cavities in the neurosensory retina separated by moderately reflective septae; OS slight increase of the macular thickness with diminishing of the foveal profile and tendency to flattening of the macular retina (early macular edema).

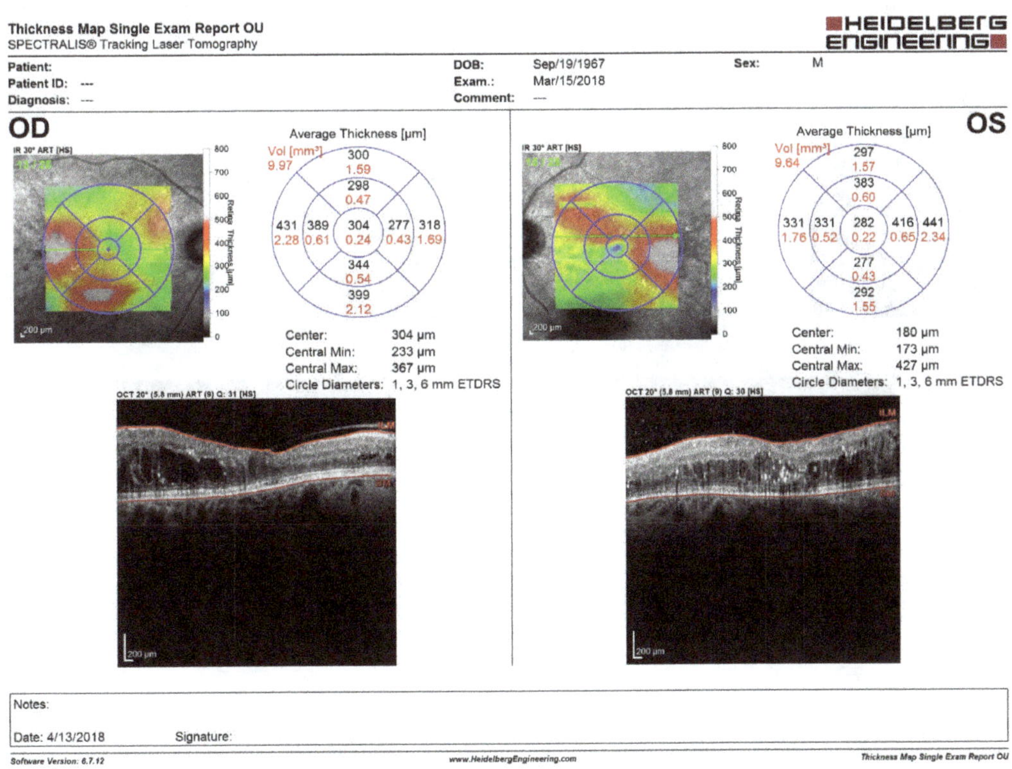

Figure 5. Focal macular edema OU: OD—beside the cystoid cavities within the neurosensitive retina, PHT is revealed; OS—smaller cystoid cavities with hyperreflective deposits and loss of normal foveal contour.

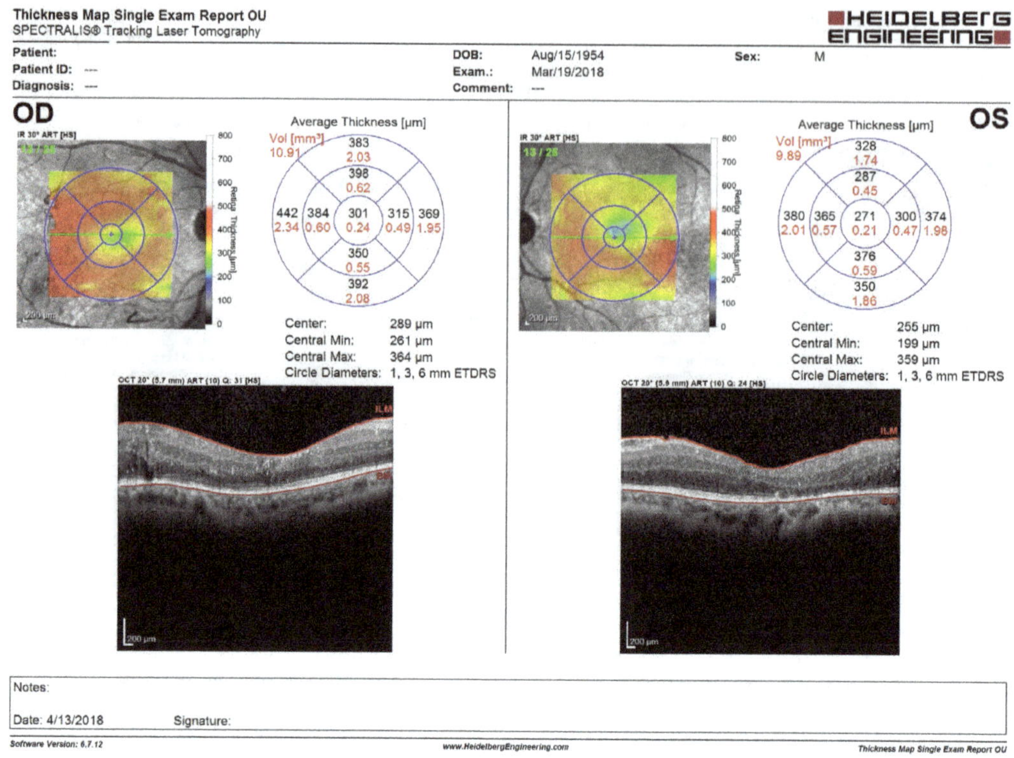

Figure 6. OD diffuse macular edema with preservation of the foveal contour and hyperreflective deposits in the neurosensory retina; OS mild focal macular edema.

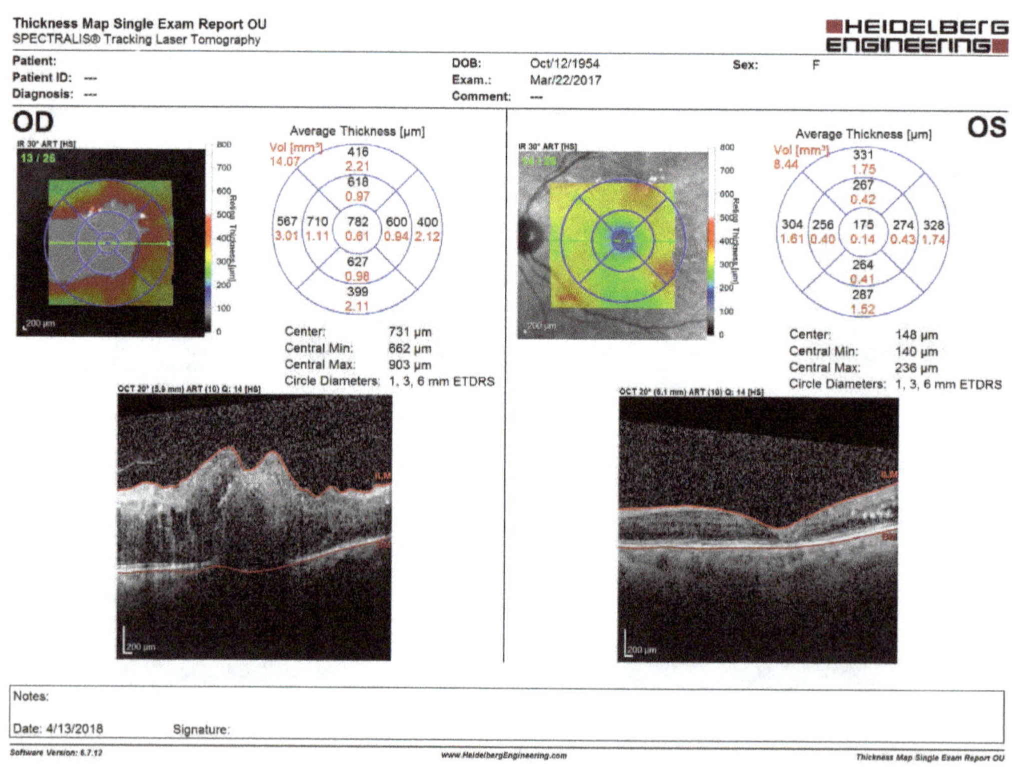

Figure 7. OD severe macular edema with considerable thickening of the macular area, cystoid cavities within the retina with involvement of the outer retinal layers and disorganization of the retinal pigmented epithelial line, PHT; OS retinal atrophy at the level of the foveal region.

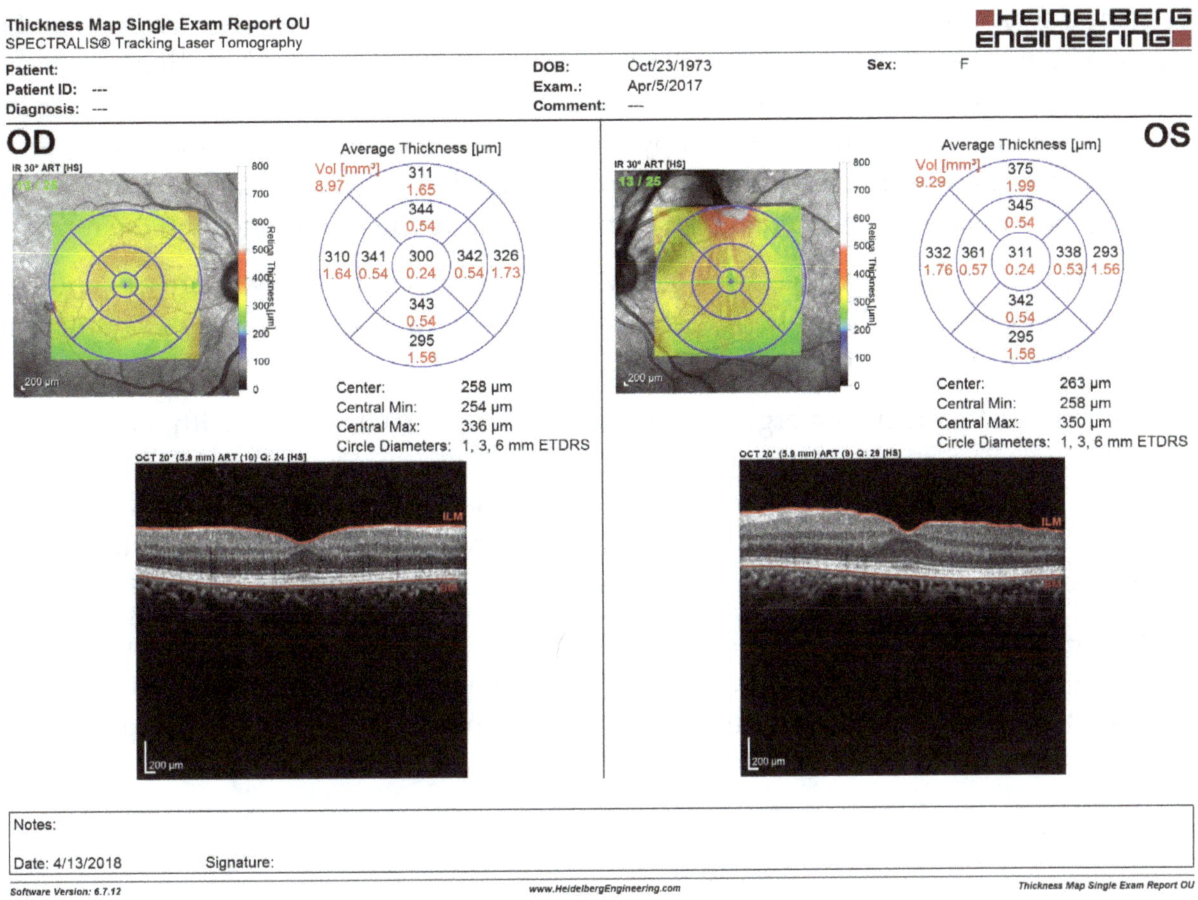

Figure 8. OD aspect following pars plana vitrectomy and dissection of the posterior hyaloid: mild diffuse macular edema, with normal foveal profile; OS mild macular edema with reflective posterior hyaloid adherent to the macula.

In LE (not vitrectomized) there is a slightly increase in macular thickness related to the traction of the posterior hyaloid on the macula. In RE, vitrectomy released the vitreo-macular traction and macular thickness is almost within the normal range.

8. Importance of OCT in selecting the appropriate therapy for DME

For many years, the only therapy of DME was laser photocoagulation which was indicated exclusively on clinical criteria, defined by Early Treatment Diabetic Retinopathy Study (ETDRS) as clinically significant macular edema [9]. Currently, therapeutic approaches of DME expanded, including anti-VEGF and steroid intravitreal injections and vitreo-retinal surgery [9]. The selection of the optimal therapy is correlated with the pathogeny of DME, which is best elucidated by OCT.

In most circumstances, DME is the consequence of internal blood-retinal barrier break-down with subsequent accumulation of fluid in the retina. Macular thickness and fluid topography are precisely evaluated by OCT. In these DME categories, the first line treatment is represented in our practice by intravitreal anti-VEGF injections. In refractory cases intravitreal steroids are considered.

OCT is the only method capable to identify and describe the aspect of the vitreoretinal interface. As such, within the DME group OCT individualizes a subgroup of patients with posterior hyaloid traction (PHT) which is often overlooked with fundus biomicroscopy. This particular form of DME is more resistant to medical therapy and vitreo-retinal surgery with membrane dissection is indicated. Intraoperative OCT is an important decision-making tool assisting the surgeon to identify the surgical planes and define the relationships of the membrane with the retina [9].

Not only does OCT identify the causes of DME, but it also allows early diagnosis and treatment of DME, before it is clinically significant [10]. This is translated in the clinical practice by better anatomical and functional outcomes.

The moment of treatment emerges from the OCT aspect correlated with visual acuity. Generally, there is a parallel correspondence between the anatomical and functional data. However, if OCT shows a slight increase in central retinal thickness (CRT) but visual acuity is 20/20, the patient is watched closely, and treatment is promptly initiated if the visual function follows a negative trend [10].

Usually, the evolution of OCT aspect of the macula is parallel to the response of visual acuity. If the increase of visual acuity does not correspond to the improvement of OCT aspect, a long time evolution of DME and/or the use of multiple treatment modalities should be considered [10].

9. Conclusions

OCT is a noninvasive, well-tolerated method, easy to understand and explain. It offers qualitative information on retinal thickness, and it is reliable and reproducible. OCT reveals the presence and extension of vitreo-macular traction.

There is a correlation between macular thickness and visual acuity in patients with DME. The OCT pattern that was associated with worse visual outcome is CME.

In DME OCT technology has significant impact at various levels: it elucidates the pathogenic mechanisms of DME; it has a major contribution in identifying hyaloid-macular traction; it identifies the subclinical DME allowing early treatment; it makes it possible to correlate macular thickness with visual acuity; it monitors the evolution of DME following treatment.

Acknowledgements

This study was funded by grant number PED 156, Executive Agency for Higher Education, Research, Development and Innovation Funding, Romania.

Conflict of interest

The author declares that there is no conflict of interest regarding the publication of this chapter.

Author details

Simona Delia Nicoară

Address all correspondence to: simonanicoara1@gmail.com

Faculty of Medicine, Department of Ophthalmology, "Iuliu Hațieganu" University of Medicine and Pharmacy, Cluj-Napoca, Romania

References

[1] Ross AH, Bailey CC. The management of diabetic macular edema. Saudi Journal of Ophthalmology. 2011;**25**(2):123-129. DOI: 10.1016/j.sjopt.2011.01.011

[2] Kiire CA, Porta M, Chong V. Medical management for the prevention and treatment of diabetic macular edema. Survey of Ophthalmology. 2013;**58**(5):459-465. DOI: 10.1016/j.survophthal.2012.10.002

[3] Țălu SD, Țălu S. Use of OCT imaging in the diagnosis and monitoring of age related macular degeneration. In: Ying G-S, editor. Age-Related Macular Degeneration – The Recent Advances in Basic Research and Clinical Care. Rijeka: In Tech; 2012. pp. 253-273. DOI: 274383296

[4] Țălu SD. New insights into the optical coherence tomography – Assessment and follow up of age related macular degeneration. In: GL Giudice, editor. Age-Related Macular Degeneration – Etiology, Diagnosis and Management – A Glance at the Future. Rijeka: In Tech; 2013. pp. 133-159. DOI: 10.5772/53357

[5] Ahmadpour-Baghdadabad M, Manaviat M, Shojaoddini-Ardekani A. Optical coherence tomography in diabetic macular edema: Patterns and related risk factors. Nepalese Journal of Ophthalmology. 2013;**5**(10):190-194. DOI: 10.3126/nepjoph.v5i2.8727

[6] Trichonas G, Kaiser PK. Optical coherence tomography imaging of the macular oedema. The British Journal of Ophthalmology. 2014;**98**(Suppl II):ii24-ii29. DOI: 10.1136/bjophthalmol-2014-305305

[7] Sikorski BL, Malukiewicz G, Stafiej J, Lesiewska-Junk H, Raczynska D. The diagnostic function of OCT in diabetic maculopathy. Mediators of Inflammation. 2013;**1**:1-12. DOI: 10.1155/2013/434560

[8] Koleva-Georgieva D. Optical coherence tomography findings in diabetic macular edema. In: Ola MS, editor. Diabetic Retinopathy. Vienna: InTech; 2012. pp. 225-249. DOI: 10.5772/30302

[9] Modi YS, Ehlers JP. Imaging modalities for the management of DME. Retina Today. 2015;**6**:66-69

[10] Kiss S. OCT useful in management of DME. Ocular Surgery News. 2016;**2**:1-3

14

Imaging the Cornea, Anterior Chamber, and Lens in Corneal and Refractive Surgery

Timo Eppig, Stephanie Mäurer, Loay Daas, Berthold Seitz and Achim Langenbucher

Abstract

Anterior segment OCT (AS-OCT) is an optical and noncontact imaging technology, which has numerous fields of application in the imaging of the cornea, anterior chamber, and the lens. In this chapter, we will present some of the application fields of AS-OCT in corneal, cataract, and refractive surgery. We will emphasize the potential of AS-OCT by several clinical examples including corneal imaging (keratoconus, keratoplasty, and refractive surgery) and intraocular lens imaging after refractive surgery. AS-OCT shows special potential for corneal imaging in case of corneal edema and for postoperative control after Descemet's membrane endothelial keratoplasty (DMEK). The postoperative follow-up of a posterior chamber Collamer lens'ses vault and measuring the anterior chamber angle could be identified as another promising field of application for AS-OCT.

Keywords: anterior segment, cataract, refractive surgery, cornea, keratoplasty, keratoconus, intracorneal ring segments, LASIK, phakic intraocular lenses

1. Introduction

Since its development in the late 1980s, optical coherence tomography (OCT) has found numerous applications not only in ophthalmology. The first ophthalmological applications were tomographical imaging of the ultrastructure of the human retina, especially the fovea. For the first time OCT allowed tomographic imaging of the retinal layers allowing detection of subretinal changes and high precision assessment of the changes in retinal nerve fiber layer thickness. The visible to near infrared wavelengths used in posterior segment OCT devices allowed high transmission in aqueous material and high reflectivity at retinal structures. At that time, the Scheimpflug imaging technology was able to provide high resolution tomographic images of the anterior segment including the lens [1]. Anterior segment biometry, such as measuring corneal thickness (pachymetry) and the depth of the anterior chamber for surgery planning in corneal refractive surgery or calculating intraocular lenses (IOL) could only be performed by ultrasound biomicroscopy or Scheimpflug imaging [2, 3]. In the 1990s, the leading research groups in OCT technology presented the first results in anterior segment imaging and biometry [4–6]. Dedicated OCT devices for tomographic imaging of the anterior segment (AS-OCT) were not available until Zeiss Meditec launched their Visante™ 1000 OCT which was based on time domain OCT technology [3]. In 2009, Tomey launched their swept-source based OCT Casia SS-1000, which was also dedicated to anterior segment imaging. Manufacturers of posterior segment OCT devices soon provided additional objective lenses allowing tomographic imaging of anterior segment structures. During the last decade, the OCT technology conquered numerous applications including corneal imaging, refractive surgery, lens imaging, glaucoma, and cataract surgery.

In this chapter, we will present and discuss applications of OCT technology in the imaging of the anterior segment of the human eye, including general imaging of anterior segment morphology as well as applications in corneal and anterior segment surgery.

2. Cornea

The cornea is the most outer structure of the human eye and contributes to about 2/3 (=48 D) of the total optical power to the eye. The cornea's structure can be subdivided into six layers with the epithelium (EP) being the outer layer which covers Bowman's layer (BL). The epithelium is covered by the tear film and consists of up to six layers of epithelial cells. Its average thickness is about 50 μm. Bowman's layer is a collagenous, acellular, nonregenerating layer and separates the epithelial cell layer from the stroma. The stroma covers 85% of the volume in the human cornea with a total thickness of about 350–450 μm [7]. The posterior limitation of the stroma is Descemet's membrane (DM), which has a thickness of about 10–15 μm [7]. The DM is the basal membrane for the endothelial cell layer, which is a single-layer of hexagonal endothelial cells with a thickness of about 4.5 μm. Dua et al. [7] identified an additional pre-Descemetal layer of 10–15 μm thickness, which they named Dua's layer (DL).

The different layers of the human cornea can be imaged in vivo by specialized ultrahigh-resolution OCT systems as shown by Werkmeister et al. [8] (**Figure 1**).

2.1. Keratoconus

Keratoconus (KC) is a corneal disease characterized by a progressive steepening and protrusion of the corneal topography accompanied by a central to paracentral thinning (**Figure 2**). Keratoconus is a bilateral disease and often manifests within the second to third decade of life. Primary diagnosis is being supported by corneal topography and corneal tomography, which both can be performed by AS-OCT. AS-OCT assists in early detection and monitoring of the progression of

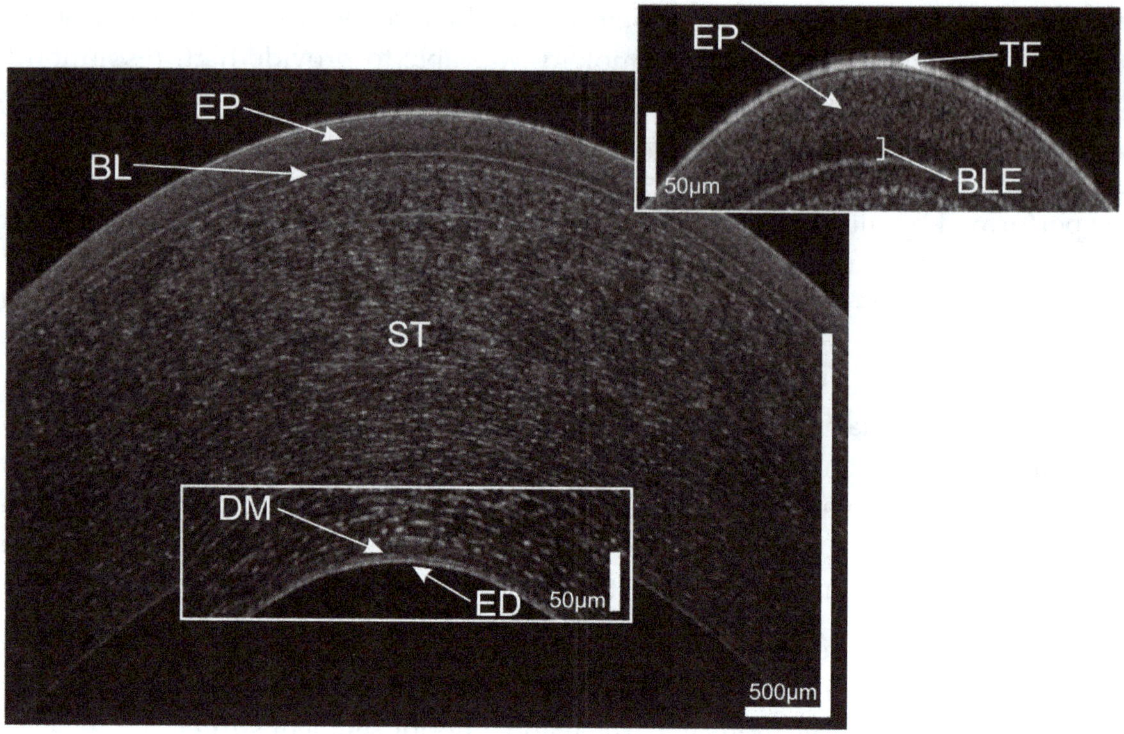

Figure 1. UHR-OCT tomogram of the central and paracentral zone of the cornea of a 38-year-old healthy male. TF, tear film; EP, epithelium; BLE, basal layer of epithelium; BL, Bowman's layer; ST, corneal stroma; DM, Descemet's membrane; ED, endothelium. Reprinted with permission from Werkmeister et al. [8], © Optical Society of America.

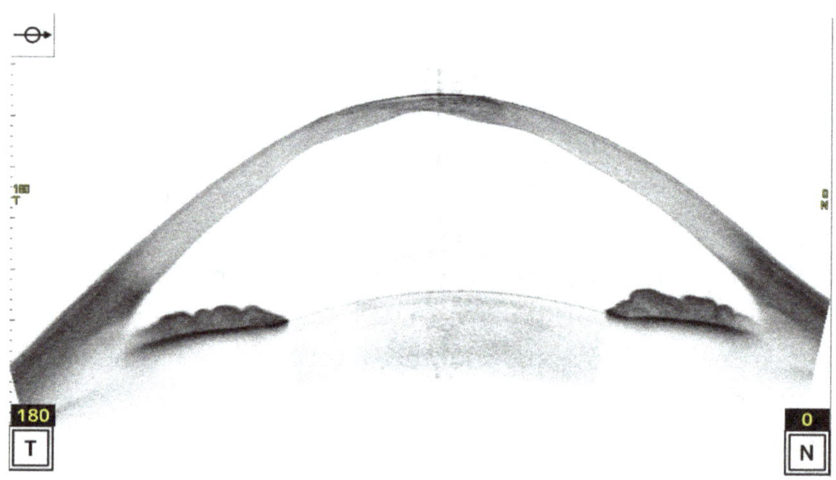

Figure 2. Horizontal image slice of an eye with keratoconus especially notable at the posterior corneal surface. Image taken with Casia 2 AS-OCT (Tomey Corp., Nagoya, Japan).

the disease in order to provide stage oriented therapeutic options. The high reliability of corneal thickness measurements make AS-OCT a useful tool for monitoring changes in corneal thickness, however measurements could not be used interchangeably with other modalities such as Scheimpflug imaging [9–11]. Schröder et al. have shown that AS-OCT technology provides a high repeatability for measuring the corneal thickness in healthy patients. They also showed that the posterior surface measurement was more reliable than with Scheimpflug technology [11].

New methods such as corneal OCT and topographic mapping of EP and BL have been proposed for early detection of keratoconus [12–15]. However, this requires high-resolution OCT technology in order to resolve EP and BL with sufficient precision.

In late, advanced stages of keratoconus, DM may tear allowing the aqueous humor to penetrate the stroma. This situation is also known as acute keratoconus, which is characterized by a corneal edema and opacification (corneal hydrops). The edema limits the visibility of structures in the anterior chamber. The development of the Descemet's tear may differ between patients, and AS-OCT is able to image through the corneal edema allowing the examiner to locate the Descemet's tear (**Figure 3**). Scheimpflug technology is limited in these cases due to increased light scattering. After the edema has diminished, the Descemet tear usually cicatrizes, affecting the patient's visual acuity. The ultimate therapeutic option is penetrating keratoplasty (PK). However, from the surgeon's point of view, the hydrops should resolve before PK should be performed [16]. AS-OCT is an ideal method for staging the disease and documenting the course of corneal hydrops (**Figure 4**) in order to define the time point when PK may be performed [17]. Pre-Descemetal sutures may be used to assist the edema in resolving and the DM in reattaching to the stroma. Therefore, the corneal hydrops is being sutured perpendicular to the DM tear [18]. Re-attachment of DM is being supported by an intracameral air bubble [18]. Despite impaired insight into the anterior chamber, AS-OCT allows taking a nearly unobstructed tomographic image of the anterior chamber including visualization of the DM tear facilitating suture planning prior to surgery [18].

In early stages of KC, when DM is unaffected and scarring has occurred in the stroma only, a deep anterior lamellar keratoplasty (DALK) may be a useful option. In this case, only the stroma (without DM) is being transplanted. AS-OCT may help to visualize pre-Descemetal scarring in order to check patients' eligibility for DALK. The utility of intraoperative AS-OCT has been proven for analyzing whether the diseased stroma has been fully removed and whether the transplant has been well integrated into the host tissue [19, 20]. In the follow-up AS-OCT again is useful to check the graft adhesion to the host's DM or to visualize DM and the anterior chamber if the view is limited due to increased light scatter caused by corneal edema (**Figure 5**). Again, OCT allows a detailed a tomographic view of the host-graft interface, which usually exhibits a high amount of scattered light.

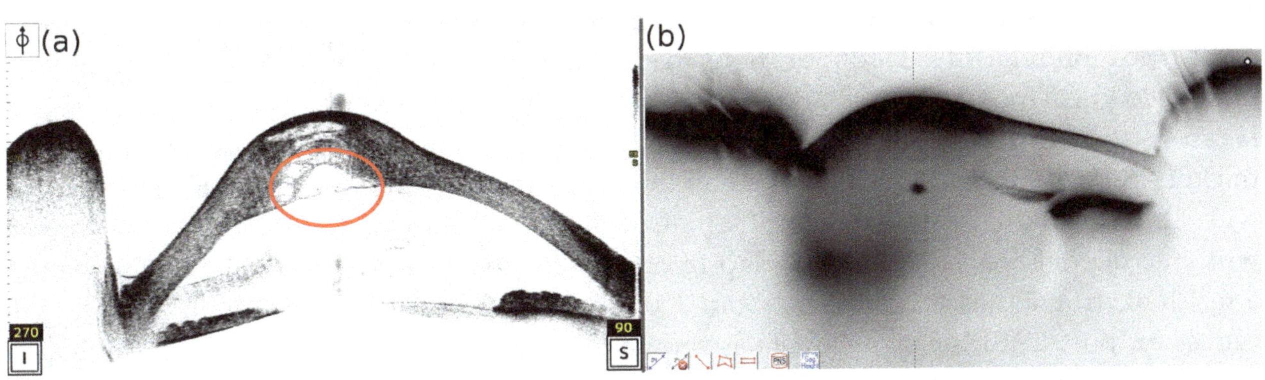

Figure 3. Eye of a 25-year-old patient with acute keratoconus (corneal hydrops). (a) The AS-OCT (Casia 2, Tomey Corp., Nagoya, Japan) image reveals the extent of the corneal edema and the location of the Descemet's rupture. The Descemet's membrane rolls are clearly visible indicating the strain of Descemet's membrane. (b) Scheimpflug imaging (Pentacam® HR, Oculus Optikgeräte GmbH, Wetzlar) is limited and cannot image the anterior chamber due to increased light scattering.

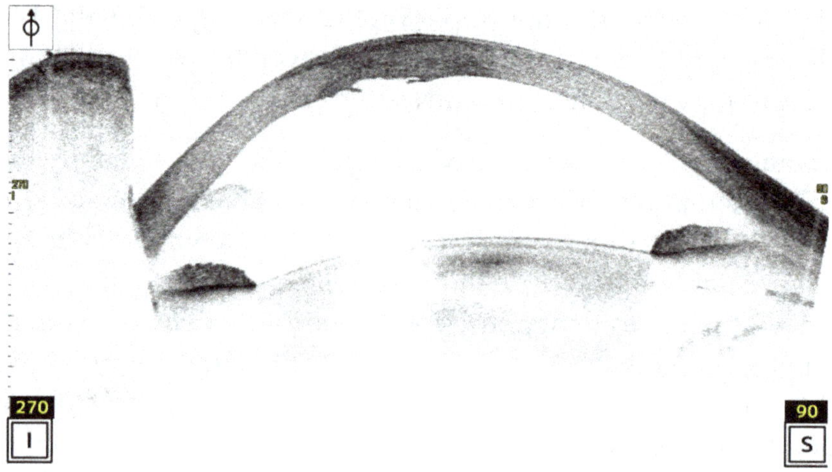

Figure 4. Eye of a 25-year-old patient 3 months after acute keratoconus (**Figure 3**) that had been treated with Muraine sutures and an air bubble in the anterior chamber. The corneal edema widely disappeared leaving a central scar including the posterior surface. The opacification is still present, visible as darker stroma in the center. Image taken with Casia 2 AS-OCT (Tomey Corp., Nagoya, Japan).

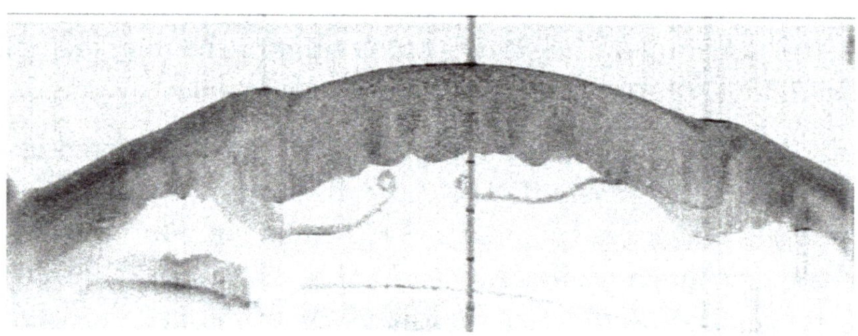

Figure 5. Descemet's rupture during DALK surgery with major edema of the full-thickness graft. Image taken with Casia SS-1000 AS-OCT (Tomey Corp., Nagoya, Japan).

2.2. Refractive surgery

The high axial resolution of AS-OCT and the capability of detecting small changes in reflectivity are ideal prerequisites for applications in corneal refractive surgery. AS-OCT is capable of imaging corneal incisions, scars, and flaps created during laser in-situ keratomileusis (LASIK). It can be used as diagnostic tool for measuring the pre- to postoperative change in corneal thickness as well as for controlling the flap thickness and flap quality. **Figure 6** shows an eye with femtosecond-laser-assisted LASIK (fs-LASIK) with a flap thickness of 120 μm. An eye with microkeratome-created LASIK-flap 18 years after surgery is shown in **Figure 7** revealing a residual stromal bed thickness of about 300 μm. AS-OCT can also assist in identifying the causes for post-LASIK corneal ectasia as shown in **Figure 8**, where we could detect a misbalanced ratio of flap to stromal bed thickness and a too thin residual stromal bed.

New methods such as small incision lenticule extraction (SMILE) could also be visualized with AS-OCT [21]. Intraoperative AS-OCT was shown to be useful in visualizing the lenticule during the management of complications in SMILE surgery [22, 23].

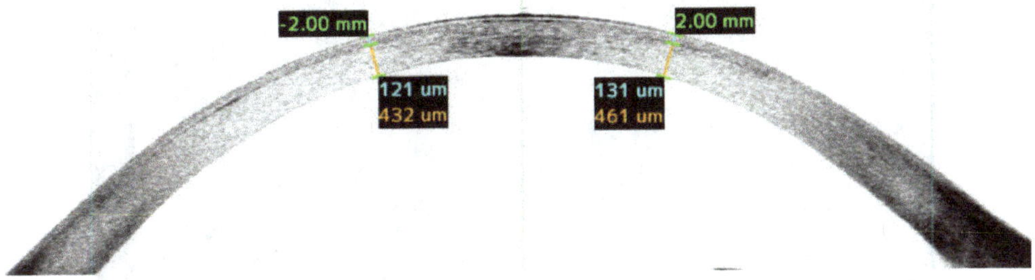

Figure 6. Right eye of a patient having received femtosecond-laser-assisted LASIK. The flap thickness of about 120 μm could be measured with the AS-OCT (Casia 2, Tomey Corp., Nagoya, Japan).

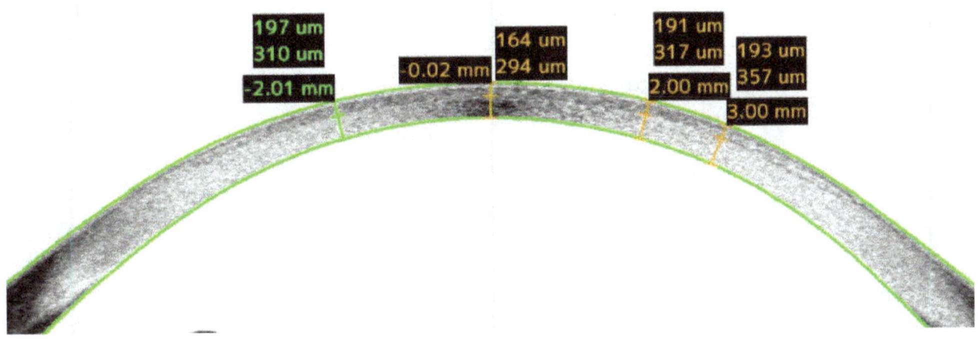

Figure 7. Left eye of a 39-year-old male with a microkeratome-created LASIK flap, which is still visible 18 years after surgery. The thickness values provided are separated into flap thickness and stromal bed thickness. The residual stromal bed is around 300 μm. Image taken with Casia 2 AS-OCT (Tomey Corp., Nagoya, Japan).

Intracorneal ring segments (ICRS) are an option for reducing the refractive power of the cornea in keratoconus if the optical center is free from scars. Therefore, a circular tunnel is being prepared within the stroma into which the plastic ring(s) are being implanted. The tunnel may be prepared mechanically or with a femtosecond-laser. However, Monteiro et al. have shown with AS-OCT that femtosecond-laser based tunnel preparation is more predictable than manual tunnel preparation [24]. Currently, there are various ICRS models on the market with different cross-sectional geometry, thickness, and arc lengths. The thickness, arc length and implantation site is usually defined by proprietary nomograms [25]. In the follow-up of ICRS, AS-OCT is useful for investigating proper placement of the ring segments, especially the distance to DM and/or BL and the epithelium [26]. In these cases, the plastic rings within the cornea will induce artifacts visible as bright stripes parallel to the line of sight. Structures lying behind these rings are subject to distortion due to the change of refractive index, which currently cannot be interpreted by clinical AS-OCT software. **Figure 9** shows an eye with intracorneal ring segments for keratoconus. Due to this image distortion, a reliable measurement of the thickness behind these structures is not feasible. However, AS-OCT is useful to follow relative changes or displacement of ICRS over time.

In patient's having received a corneal pinhole implant (KAMRA®, AcuFocus Inc., Irvine, USA), the centration and implantation of the implant beneath the femtosecond-laser-created flap is crucial and should be controlled in the OCT image. Due to the very prominent Purkinje reflex visible in the central OCT image, the assessment of proper KAMRA® implant centration could be performed at ease. However, the absorption of the pinhole implant hides any structures lying behind the implant (**Figure 10**).

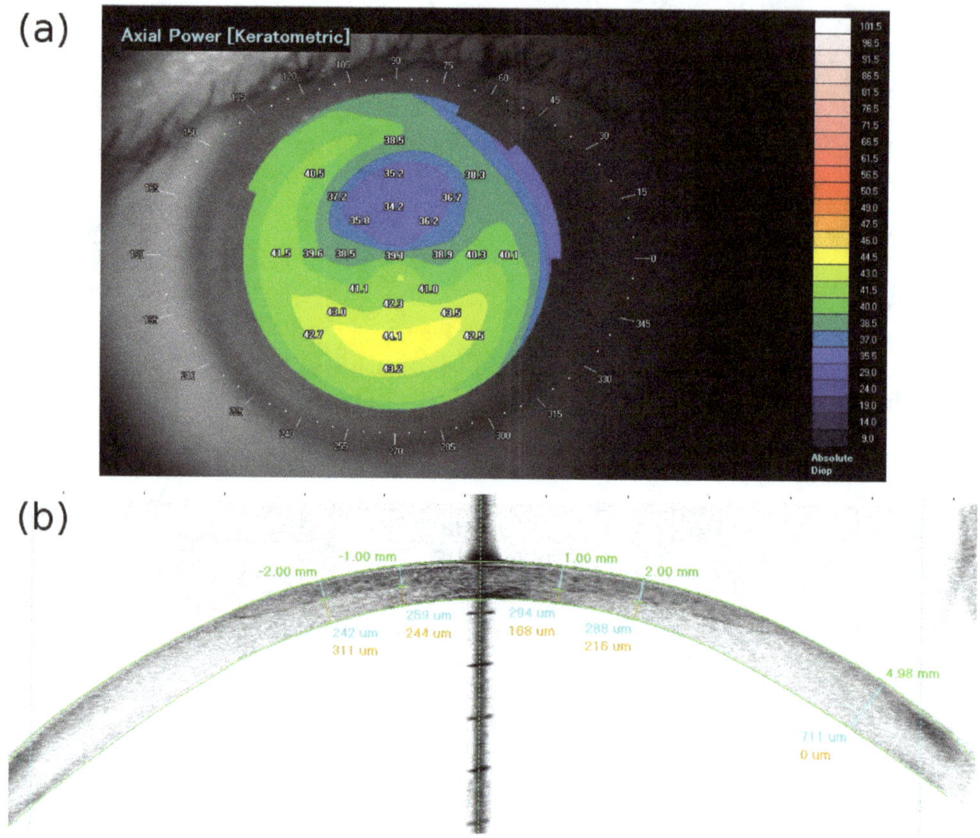

Figure 8. (a) AS-OCT-derived corneal topography in a 44-year-old patient some years after LASIK surgery. The topography reveals a decentered ablation and late onset of corneal ectasia. (b) The flap is clearly visible and the residual bed thickness was found to be less than 200 μm. Images taken with Casia SS-1000 AS-OCT (Tomey Corp., Nagoya, Japan).

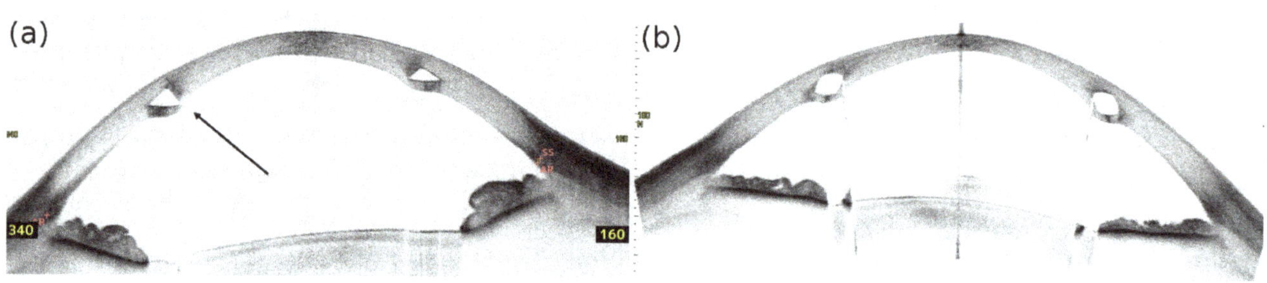

Figure 9. (a) Keratoconus eye with intracorneal ring segments (ICRS) with prismatic cross section. The sharp edge of the temporal ring (arrow) is close to the DM and should be monitored. (b) Cornea with femtosecond-laser-assisted Intacs® SK ICRS (Addition Technology Inc., Lombard, USA) implantation. The OCT image reveals the elliptic cross section of the Intacs® SK implants. The ICRS edge causes artifacts within the anterior chamber. Images taken with Casia 2 AS-OCT (Tomey Corp., Nagoya, Japan).

2.3. Corneal transplantation

The first successful transplantation of corneal tissue has been performed by Eduard Zirm in 1905 [27]. Since then, corneal transplantation has been the oldest and most successful technique of human tissue or organ transplantation. Starting from the original PK and the transfer of all corneal layers, new techniques such as lamellar transplantation have been emerging. PK has been proven to provide good optical results and excellent transplant survival depending on the initial indication for PK [28]. However, complications such as posterior step formation,

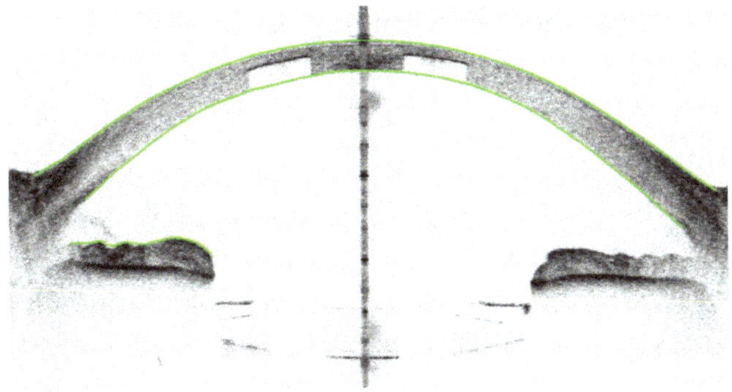

Figure 10. Pseudophakic eye with a KAMRA® intracorneal inlay for presbyopia treatment under a 200-μm femtosecond-laser flap. The central Purkinje reflex reveals that both intraocular lens and corneal inlay are well centered. Image taken with Casia 2 AS-OCT (Tomey Corp., Nagoya, Japan).

graft opacification or graft rejection may occur. In addition, a partially irregular postoperative corneal astigmatism is one of the side effects of PK. Szentmáry et al. [29] showed that nonmechanical trephination during PK yields better morphological and functional results than mechanical trephination. The immunological drawbacks could be minimized by novel lamellar techniques such as DALK, Descemet's stripping automated endothelial keratoplasty (DSAEK) or Descemet membrane endothelial keratoplasty (DMEK) [16]. AS-OCT may help in assessing the graft adhesion, the host-graft interface [30], graft thickness or step formation [31]. Yenerel et al. argued that AS-OCT may be a useful tool in monitoring the morphological results of PK and in the management of the postoperative complications after PK [32]. **Figure 11** shows two eyes after excimer-laser and top-hat profile femtosecond-laser-assisted keratoplasty illustrating the different trephination techniques.

2.3.1. *Descemet stripping automated endothelial keratoplasty (DSAEK)*

Posterior lamellar keratoplasty was originally introduced by Melles in 1998 and had continuously been improved until 2004 when Melles presented a new method for stripping the DM which led to the Descemet stripping automated endothelial keratoplasty (DSAEK) procedure

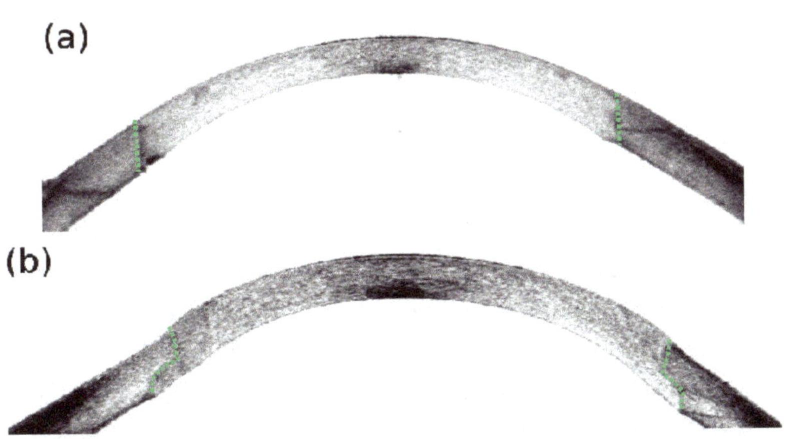

Figure 11. (a) Integrated graft in an eye after excimer-laser-assisted keratoplasty showing the straight interface and no step formation. (b) An eye after femtosecond-laser-assisted keratoplasty using a top-hat trephination profile. The dashed lines highlight the graft-host interface. Images taken with Casia 2 AS-OCT (Tomey Corp., Nagoya, Japan).

[33, 34]. The objective was to implement a technique for lamellar keratoplasty for the transplantation of endothelial cells leaving the hosts stroma in place. A thin graft of DM and stroma is being prepared from donor tissue. After stripping the host's DM the graft is placed onto the posterior side of the host cornea. Intraoperative OCT may assist in the positioning of the graft [35, 36]. Due to the thickness and geometric profile of the graft, the posterior surface of the host cornea is changed causing a change in total corneal power (**Figure 12**). This leads to invalid keratometer readings and systematic errors in intraocular lens power calculations in DSAEK eyes, leading to a hyperopic shift of up to 1.5 D [37–39]. This has to be considered in intraocular lens calculation and requires adjustment in case of combined DSAEK and cataract surgery. Therefore, corneal tomography (either AS-OCT or Scheimpflug imaging) is mandatory in these cases. In case of sequential cataract surgery in DSAEK eyes AS-OCT and Scheimpflug imaging are useful tools to calculate the total corneal refractive power instead of keratometer readings [39].

2.3.2. Descemet's membrane endothelial keratoplasty (DMEK)

Descemet's membrane endothelial keratoplasty (DMEK) was originally proposed by Melles et al. in 2006 [40] and has been increasingly performed during the last decade [41]. The indications include endothelial diseases such as in Fuchs' dystrophy when the corneal edema affects corneal transparency and visual acuity. During surgery, the DM of the host is being stripped and replaced by a donor DM with healthy endothelium. Graft attachment to the host stroma is crucial and is usually supported by a gas bubble, which is intraoperatively injected into the anterior chamber. The adhesion of the graft requires monitoring during the first days and weeks after surgery. The high resolution of AS-OCT is essential for imaging small adhesion defects and to locate the dehiscence of the graft. Especially in the short term after surgery, patients should frequently be monitored by AS-OCT in order to document graft adhesion and to determine, whether a re-bubbling is required (**Figures 13** and **14**). AS-OCT examination outperforms slit-lamp examination in the short term DMEK monitoring and the examination is quick and more comfortable for the patients than slit-lamp examination. Therefore, a three-dimensional view of the anterior segment is beneficial (video 1). Eyes after DMEK are also subject to a hyperopic shift after IOL implantation. However, the change of total corneal refractive power is markedly smaller (about 0.5 D) in DMEK than in DSAEK [42, 43].

2.3.3. Screening of corneal donor tissue

Eye banks are in charge of checking eligibility of corneal donor tissue for PK. The analysis procedure includes visual inspection, morphological and microbiological examination. One crucial parameter is the endothelial cell density, which should exceed 2000 cells/mm^2. The stroma should be free from scars for good visual rehabilitation. Corneas from donors with keratoconus or that had undergone any laser refractive surgery should not be used for PK due to the unpredictable refractive result. However, the DM might be eligible for posterior lamellar keratoplasty such as DMEK. Keratoconic and postrefractive surgery corneas could be detected by analyzing the anterior and posterior radii of curvature and the corneal thickness profile or by detecting structural changes in the corneal tissue [44]. However, in-vivo data from donors are rarely available and therefore screening of donor tissue tomography could only be performed during tissue cultivation. OCT technology allows sterile, direct noncontact tomographic imaging of corneal donor

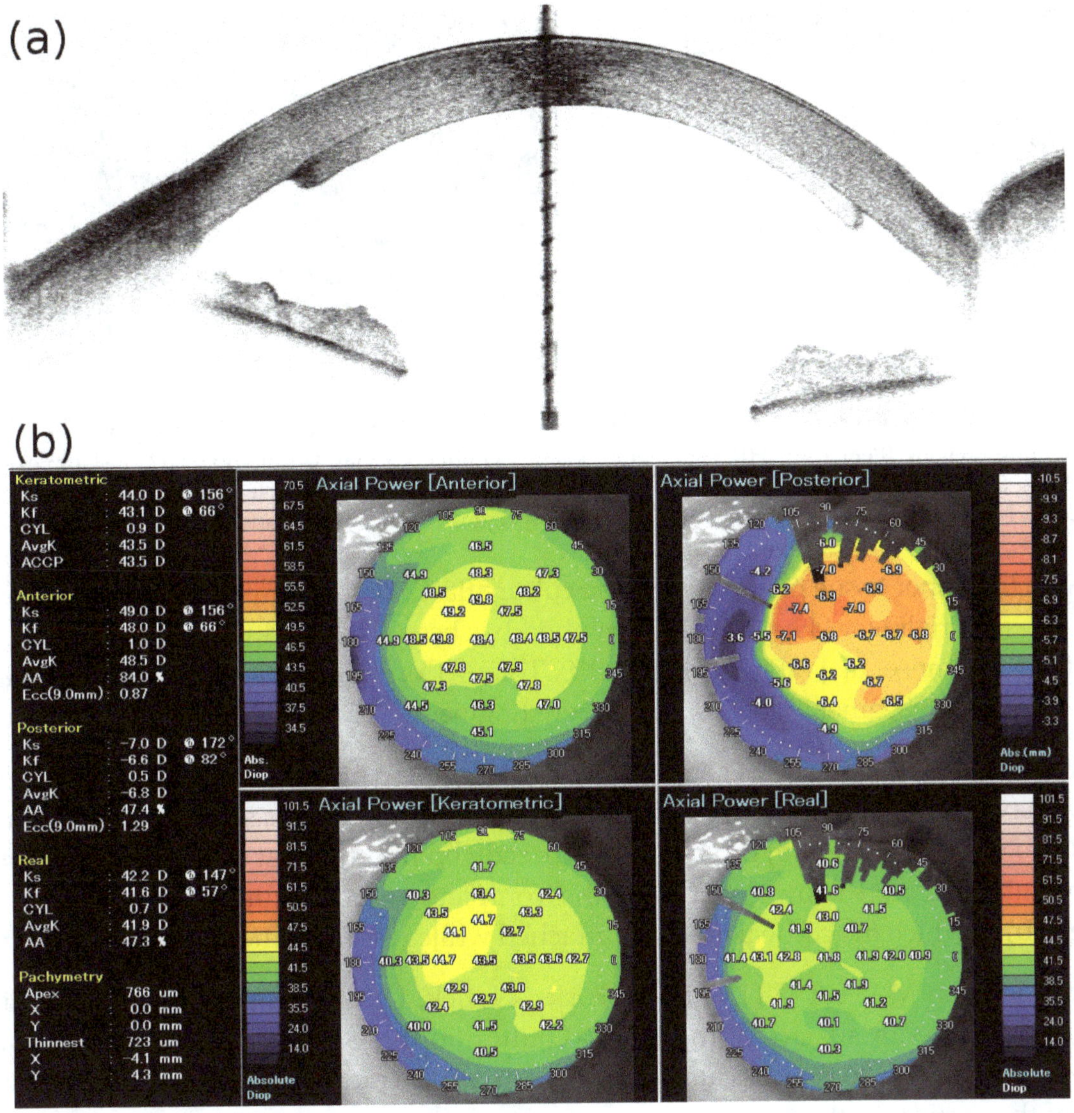

Figure 12. (a) Eye after DSAEK showing the graft well attached to the host stroma (Casia SS-1000 AS-OCT, Tomey Corp., Nagoya, Japan). The graft thickness was between 190 and 290 μm. (b) Graphical representation of the anterior and posterior refractive power as well as the keratometric power and total refractive (real) power. The values indicate that using the keratometric power, the corneal power will be over-estimated by 1.6 D (average keratometric power 43.5 D vs. real corneal power 41.9 D), which would lead to hyperopic shift after cataract surgery.

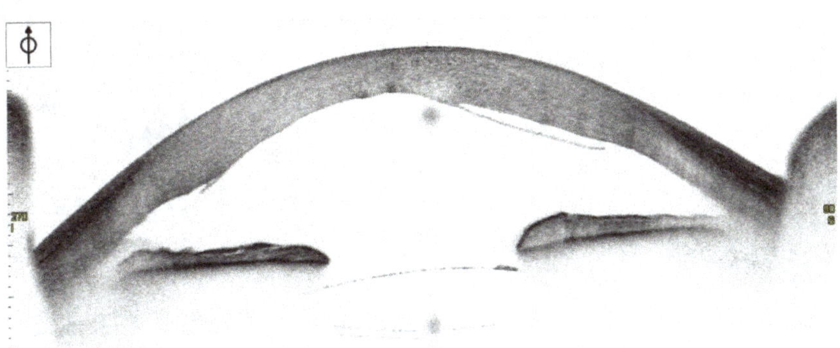

Figure 13. Vertical cross-section of a pseudophakic eye after combined DMEK and cataract surgery showing a large superior dehiscence of the graft and a partially decompensated cornea, which requires rebubbling. Image taken with Casia 2 AS-OCT (Tomey Corp., Nagoya, Japan).

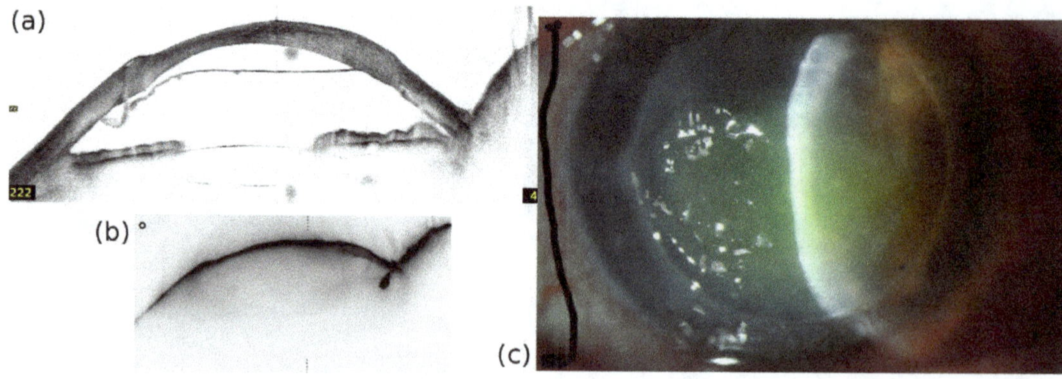

Figure 14. (a) Large area detachment of the graft after DMEK and cataract surgery. The cornea was fully opaque and (b) Scheimpflug imaging (Pentacam® HR, Oculus Optikgeräte GmbH, Wetzlar, Germany) or (c) slit-lamp examination (BX 900, Haag-Streit AG, Koeniz, Switzerland) of the anterior segment were impossible. The AS-OCT (Casia 2 AS-OCT, Tomey Corp., Nagoya, Japan) image, however, allowed analyzing the detached DM and anterior chamber.

tissue with the donor tissue placed within the culture flask. First attempts have been presented by Neubauer and Priglinger [45, 46] and the method has been enhanced with different devices and methods by Janunts et al. [47] (CASIA SS-1000, Tomey Corp., Nagoya, Japan) and Damian et al. (Spectralis Anterior Segment Module, Heidelberg Engineering GmbH, Heidelberg, Germany) [48].

Since the new AS-OCT Casia 2 (Tomey Corp., Nagoya, Japan) was launched to the market in 2016, we have developed an improved method for the tomographic screening of donor tissue. The culture flasks (**Figure 15a**) can be placed directly on the chin rest of the device (**Figure 15c**) and a volumetric scan allows capturing the complete corneal button including the holder (**Figure 15b**) to which the corneal button is attached while resting in the culture flask (**Figure 16**).

A custom written MATLAB® (The Mathworks, Natick, USA) script is then used to find the anterior and posterior surface of the corneal button in the volume dataset and a parametric surface model is fitted to the data allowing to calculate the radii of curvature and the thickness profile of the corneal button.

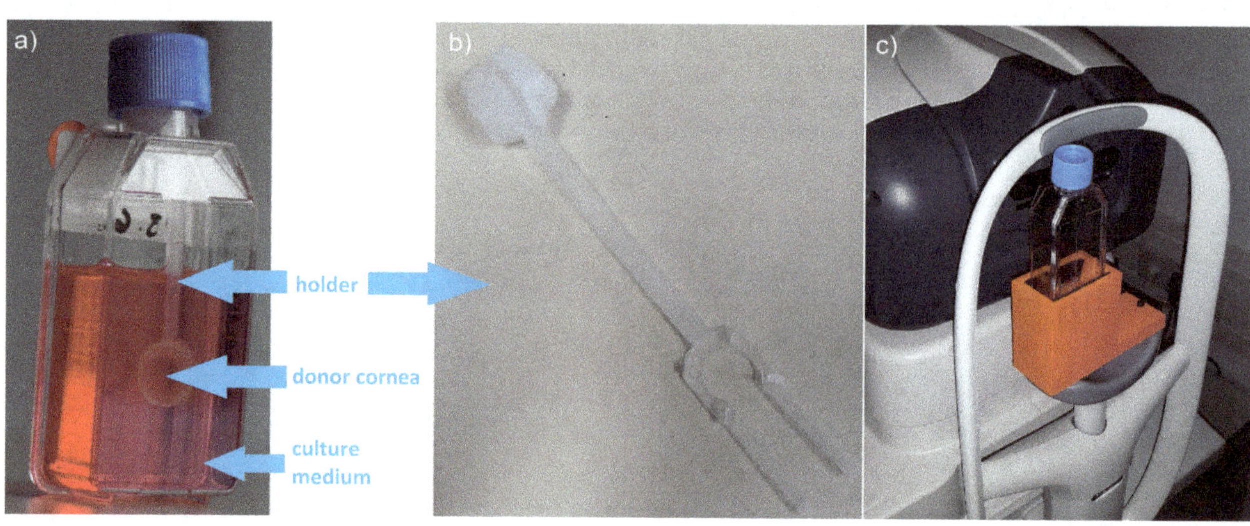

Figure 15. (a) Corneal tissue is cultivated within plastic culture flasks (adapted from Damian et al. [48]. The corneal tissue is fixed in a holder (b) to avoid free floating of the tissue in the flask. (c) The culture flask is placed on the chin rest of the Casia 2 AS-OCT with a custom made 3D-printed adaptor.

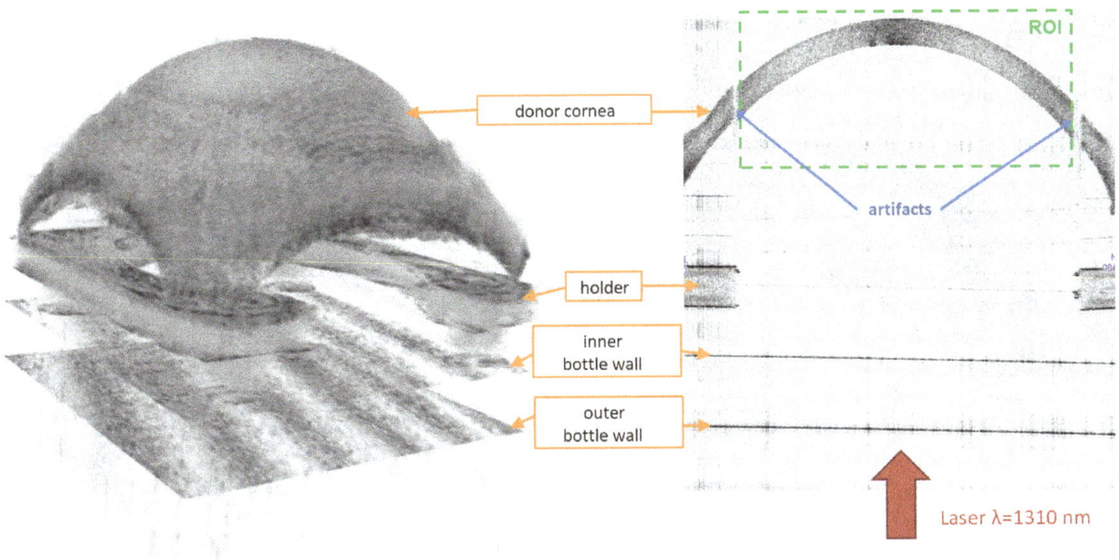

Figure 16. Volumetric dataset and central image slice from a donor cornea measured within the culture flask. The flask walls and the cornea holder are clearly visible in the image. The corneal radii of curvature can be calculated within a region of interest (ROI).

3. Phakic intraocular lenses

Precise assessment of the anterior chamber is important in glaucoma as well as in refractive surgery. Especially new concepts for refractive surgery require additional attention, such as phakic intraocular lenses. Posterior chamber implantable Collamer lenses (ICL) are a viable option for refractive surgery when corneal laser surgery is contraindicated. The most frequently used product of this type is the Visian® ICL. Such lenses are being implanted into the ciliary sulcus between the crystalline lens and the iris. The diameter of the lens has to be adapted to ciliary sulcus dimensions. The space could be estimated by using the diameter of the cornea (white-to-white diameter). Another option incorporates the use of ultrasound biomicroscopy to measure the diameter of the ciliary sulcus. The most frequent complications of early models of the ICL were a postoperative rise of intraocular pressure, angle closure, and cataract formation [49–51]. Therefore, the later models incorporated two holes within the plate haptic providing a bypass for the aqueous humor into the anterior chamber. The most recent type of ICL, the Visian® ICL V4c incorporates an additional hole in the center of the optic.

The size of the ICL is crucial to avoid contact of the ICL to the crystalline lens, which would typically happen with an undersized ICL. Oversized ICLs instead get vaulted toward the anterior chamber and may cause angle closure glaucoma [52]. Therefore, the distance of the posterior surface of the ICL to the anterior surface of the crystalline lens, the so called vault, is a key parameter to be monitored after ICL implantation. The feasibility of measuring the lens vault with AS-OCT was first shown by Bechmann et al. [53]. Several researchers reported the ICL vault to be within 90 μm and 1 mm, whereas an ideal vault is considered to be 0.5 mm [54–57]. Nakamura et al. [56] reported a method for ICL size calculation based on AS-OCT. Zhang et al. [58] compared anterior segment parameters measured with AS-OCT and ultrasound biomicroscopy. They found that AS-OCT slightly overestimated the vault and that both

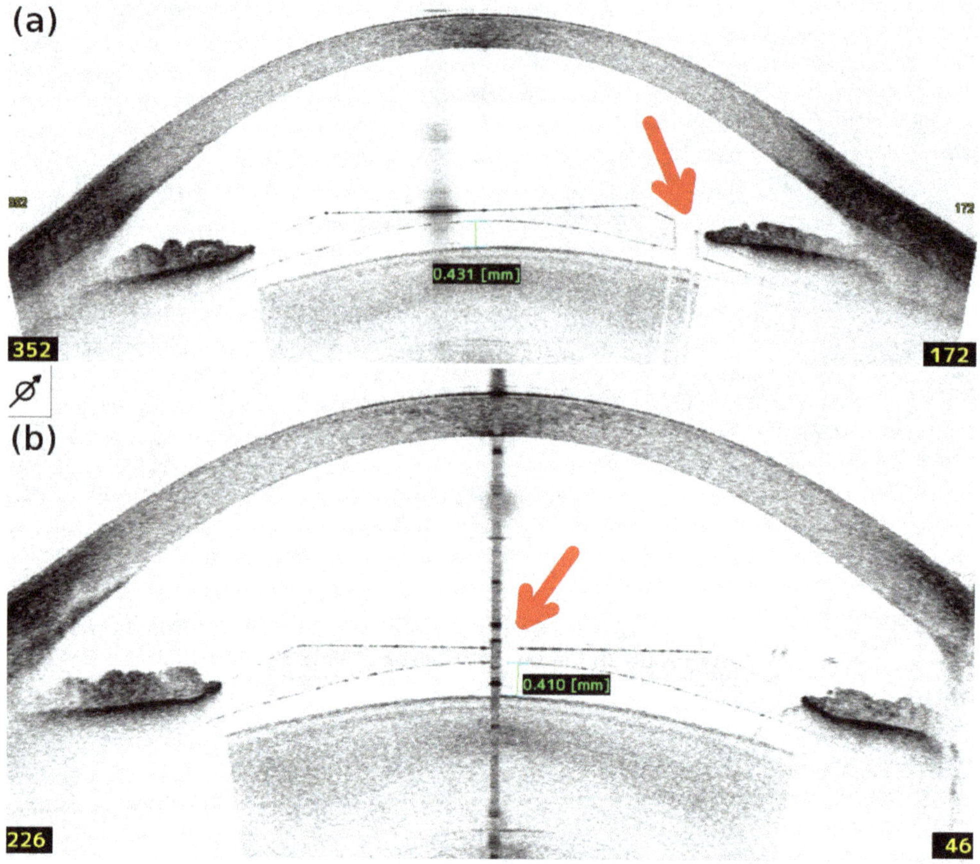

Figure 17. A myopic eye with a well-centered Visian® ICL V4c. The vault of the lens was larger than 400 μm in the center. The peripheral (top) and central (bottom) Aquaports are visible in separate image slices.

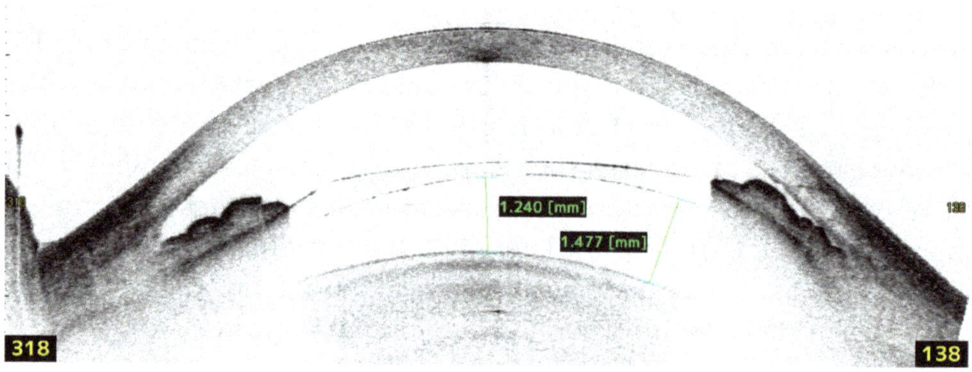

Figure 18. Angle closure at 138° after implantation of an oversized Visian® ICL V4c. The central Aquaport is visible in the image. The central vault is 1.2 mm and the peripheral vault up to 1.4 mm. Explantation of the ICL is recommended in order to prevent acute angle closure.

methods should not be used interchangeably. However, vault measurement requires manual interaction by an experienced operator as automatic analysis software is not available.

In addition, the anterior chamber angle (ACA) requires monitoring in order to detect early threat of angle closure. **Figure 17** shows a myopic eye with an ICL of the type Visian® V4c is shown in **Figure 17**, showing a well placed implant with two Aquaports and a wide ACA.

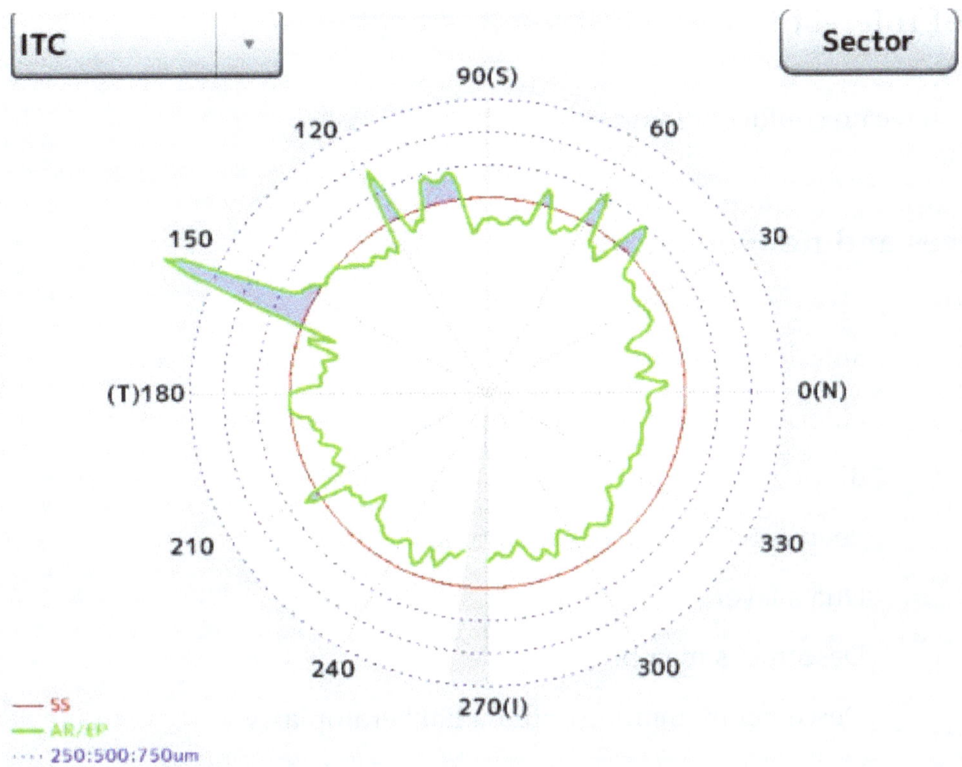

Figure 19. Star 360° analysis performed with the Casia 2 AS-OCT (Tomey Corp., Nagoya, Japan) on an eye with an oversized ICL (**Figure 18**). The green line touching the red circle and blue areas shows regions of angle closure within the circumference of the anterior chamber angle.

The application of AS-OCT in the follow-up after ICL implantation is emphasized by a case of a 26-year-old patient having undergone ICL implantation (Visian® ICL V4c) for myopia. We found a large and slightly asymmetric vault of the implant (**Figure 18**). An ACA analysis with the OCT's own software showed a threat of partial angle closure due to an oversized implant (**Figure 19**). Explantation of the ICL is recommended in order to prevent acute angle closure. The three-dimensional observation of the anterior chamber is essential.

4. Conclusions

Anterior segment OCT offers a variety of applications in corneal and refractive surgery, which need to be explored and enhanced in the future. Current analysis methods such as flap thickness or ICL vault require manual interaction by experiences operators in order to yield reproducible and representative results. The screening of corneal donor tissue allows retrieval of additional information on the tissue and may help to screen for anamnestically undetected refractive surgery such as LASIK or PRK.

Acknowledgements

The authors would like to acknowledge research funding by the Dr. Rolf M. Schwiete foundation for the development of the corneal donor screening methodology.

Conflict of interest

The authors have no conflict of interest to declare.

Appendices and nomenclature

ACA	anterior chamber angle
AS-OCT	anterior segment optical coherence tomography
D	diopter
DALK	deep anterior lamellar keratoplasty
DL	Dua's layer
DM	Descemet's membrane
DMEK	Descemet membrane endothelial keratoplasty
DSAEK	Descemet stripping automated endothelial keratoplasty
fs-LASIK	femtosecond-laser-assisted laser in-situ keratomileusis
ICL	implantable Collamer lens
ICRS	intracorneal ring segment
IOL	intraocular lens
KC	keratoconus
LASIK	laser in-situ keratomileusis
PK	penetrating keratoplasty
PRK	photorefractive keratectomy
ROI	region of interest
SMILE	small incision lenticule extraction

Author details

Timo Eppig[1*], Stephanie Mäurer[1], Loay Daas[2], Berthold Seitz[2] and Achim Langenbucher[1]

*Address all correspondence to: timo.eppig@uks.eu

1 Institute of Experimental Ophthalmology, Saarland University, Homburg, Germany

2 Department of Ophthalmology, Saarland University Medical Center UKS, Homburg, Germany

References

[1] Wegener A, Laser H. Optische Schnittbild-Vermessung des vorderen Augenabschnittes nach Scheimpflug: Möglichkeiten und Grenzen - eine Übersicht. Klinische Monatsblätter für Augenheilkunde. 2001;**218**:67-77. DOI: 10.1055/s-2001-12248

[2] Wolffsohn JS, Davies LN. Advances in anterior segment imaging. Current Opinion in Ophthalmology. 2007;**18**:32-38. DOI: 10.1097/ICU.0b013e328011550d

[3] Konstantopoulos A, Hossain P, Anderson DF. Recent advances in ophthalmic anterior segment imaging: A new era for ophthalmic diagnosis? The British Journal of Ophthalmology. 2007;**91**:551-557. DOI: 10.1136/bjo.2006.103408

[4] Drexler W, Baumgartner A, Findl O, Hitzenberger CK, Sattmann H, Fercher AF. Submicrometer precision biometry of the anterior segment of the human eye. Investigative Ophthalmology and Visual Science. 1997;**38**:1304-1313

[5] Hoerauf H, Wirbelauer C, Scholz C, Engelhardt R, Koch P, Laqua H, Birngruber R. Slit-lamp-adapted optical coherence tomography of the anterior segment. Graefe's Archive for Clinical and Experimental Ophthalmology. 2000;**238**:8-18

[6] Izatt JA, Hee MR, Swanson EA, Lin CP, Huang D, Schuman JS, Puliafito CA, Fujimoto JG. Micrometer-scale resolution imaging of the anterior eye in vivo with optical coherence tomography. Archives of Ophthalmology. 1994;**112**:1584-1589

[7] Dua HS, Faraj LA, Said DG, Gray T, Lowe J. Human corneal anatomy redefined: A novel pre-Descemet's layer (Dua's layer). Ophthalmology. 2013;**120**:1778-1785. DOI: 10.1016/j.ophtha.2013.01.018

[8] Werkmeister RM, Sapeta S, Schmidl D, Garhöfer G, Schmidinger G, Aranha Dos Santos V, Aschinger GC, Baumgartner I, Pircher N, Schwarzhans F, Pantalon A, Dua H, Schmetterer L. Ultrahigh-resolution OCT imaging of the human cornea. Biomedical Optics Express. 2017;**8**:1221-1239. DOI: 10.1364/BOE.8.001221

[9] Doors M, Cruysberg LPJ, Berendschot TTJM, de BJ, Verbakel F, Webers CAB, Nuijts RMMA. Comparison of central corneal thickness and anterior chamber depth measurements using three imaging technologies in normal eyes and after phakic intraocular lens implantation. Graefe's Archive for Clinical and Experimental Ophthalmology. 2009;**247**:1139-1146. DOI: 10.1007/s00417-009-1086-6

[10] Szalai E, Berta A, Hassan Z, Módis L. Reliability and repeatability of swept-source Fourier-domain optical coherence tomography and Scheimpflug imaging in keratoconus. Journal of Cataract and Refractive Surgery. 2012;**38**:485-494. DOI: 10.1016/j.jcrs.2011.10.027

[11] Schröder S, Mäurer S, Eppig T, Seitz B, Rubly K, Langenbucher A. Comparison of corneal tomography: Repeatability, precision, misalignment, mean elevation, and mean Pachymetry. Current Eye Research. 2018:1-8. DOI: 10.1080/02713683.2018.1441873

[12] Grieve K, Georgeon C, Andreiuolo F, Borderie M, Ghoubay D, Rault J, Borderie VM. Imaging microscopic features of Keratoconic corneal morphology. Cornea. 2016;**35**:1621-1630. DOI: 10.1097/ICO.0000000000000979

[13] Abou Shousha M, Perez VL, Fraga Santini Canto AP, Vaddavalli PK, Sayyad FE, Cabot F, Feuer WJ, Wang J, Yoo SH. The use of Bowman's layer vertical topographic thickness map in the diagnosis of keratoconus. Ophthalmology. 2014;**121**:988-993. DOI: 10.1016/j.ophtha.2013.11.034

[14] Pahuja N, Shroff R, Pahanpate P, Francis M, Veeboy L, Shetty R, Nuijts RMMA, Sinha Roy A. Application of high resolution OCT to evaluate irregularity of Bowman's layer in asymmetric keratoconus. Journal of Biophotonics. 2017;**10**:701-707. DOI: 10.1002/jbio.201600106

[15] Pircher N, Schwarzhans F, Holzer S, Lammer J, Schmidl D, Bata AM, Werkmeister RM, Seidel G, Garhöfer G, Gschließer A, Schmetterer L, Schmidinger G. Distinguishing keratoconic eyes and healthy eyes using ultrahigh-resolution (UHR)-OCT based corneal epithelium thickness mapping. American Journal of Ophthalmology. DOI: 10.1016/j.ajo.2018.02.006

[16] Seitz B, Cursiefen C, El-Husseiny M, Viestenz A, Langenbucher A, Szentmáry N. DALK und perforierende Laserkeratoplastik bei fortgeschrittenem Keratokonus. Der Ophthalmologe. 2013;**110**:839-848. DOI: 10.1007/s00347-013-2822-1

[17] Kucumen BR, Yenerel NM, Gorgun E, Dinc UA. Anterior segment optical coherence tomography findings of acute hydrops in a patient with keratoconus. Ophthalmic Surgery, Lasers and Imaging. 2010;**41**(Suppl):S114-S116. DOI: 10.3928/15428877-20101031-12

[18] Yahia Chérif H, Gueudry J, Afriat M, Delcampe A, Attal P, Gross H, Muraine M. Efficacy and safety of pre-Descemet's membrane sutures for the management of acute corneal hydrops in keratoconus. The British Journal of Ophthalmology. 2015;**99**:773-777. DOI: 10.1136/bjophthalmol-2014-306287

[19] Siebelmann S, Steven P, Cursiefen C. Intraoperative optische Kohärenztomografie bei der tiefen anterioren lamellären Keratoplastik. Klinische Monatsblätter für Augenheilkunde. 2016;**233**:717-721. DOI: 10.1055/s-0042-108588

[20] De Benito-Llopis L, Mehta JS, Angunawela RI, Ang M, Tan DTH. Intraoperative anterior segment optical coherence tomography: A novel assessment tool during deep anterior lamellar keratoplasty. American Journal of Ophthalmology. 2014;**157**:334-341.e3. DOI: 10.1016/j.ajo.2013.10.001

[21] Fu D, Wang L, Zhou X-T, Yu Z-Q. Cap morphology after small-incision lenticule extraction and its effects on intraocular scattering. International Journal of Ophthalmology. 2018;**11**:456-461. DOI: 10.18240/ijo.2018.03.16

[22] Urkude J, Titiyal JS, Sharma N. Intraoperative optical coherence tomography-guided Management of cap-Lenticule Adhesion during SMILE. Journal of Refractive Surgery. 2017;**33**:783-786. DOI: 10.3928/1081597X-20170920-01

[23] Titiyal JS, Rathi A, Kaur M, Falera R. AS-OCT as a rescue tool during difficult lenticule extraction in SMILE. Journal of Refractive Surgery. 2017;**33**:352-354. DOI: 10.3928/1081597X-20170216-01

[24] Monteiro T, Alfonso JF, Franqueira N, Faria-Correia F, Ambrósio R, Madrid-Costa D. Predictability of tunnel depth for intrastromal corneal ring segments implantation between manual and femtosecond laser techniques. Journal of Refractive Surgery. 2018;**34**:188-194. DOI: 10.3928/1081597X-20180108-01

[25] Vega-Estrada A, Alio JL. The use of intracorneal ring segments in keratoconus. Eye and vision (London, England). 2016;**3**:8. DOI: 10.1186/s40662-016-0040-z

[26] El-Husseiny M, Tsintarakis T, Eppig T, Langenbucher A, Seitz B. Intrakorneale Ringsegmente beim Keratokonus. Der Ophthalmologe. 2013;**110**:823-6, 828-9. DOI: 10.1007/s00347-013-2821-2

[27] Zirm E. Eine erfolgreiche totale Keratoplastik. Graefe's Archive for Clinical and Experimental Ophthalmology. 1906;**64**:580-593

[28] Ono T, Ishiyama S, Hayashidera T, Mori Y, Nejima R, Miyata K, Amano S. Twelve-year follow-up of penetrating keratoplasty. Japanese Journal of Ophthalmology. 2017;**61**:131-136. DOI: 10.1007/s10384-016-0489-2

[29] Szentmáry N, Langenbucher A, Naumann GOH, Seitz B. Intra-individual variability of penetrating keratoplasty outcome after excimer laser versus motorized corneal trephination. Journal of Refractive Surgery. 2006;**22**:804-810

[30] Sung MS, Yoon KC. Evaluation of graft-host interface after penetrating keratoplasty using anterior segment optical coherence tomography. Japanese Journal of Ophthalmology. 2014;**58**:282-289. DOI: 10.1007/s10384-014-0309-5

[31] Seitz B, Langenbucher A, Hager T, Janunts E, El-Husseiny M, Szentmáry N. Penetrating keratoplasty for keratoconus - Excimer versus femtosecond laser trephination. The Open Ophthalmology Journal. 2017;**11**:225-240. DOI: 10.2174/1874364101711010225

[32] Yenerel NM, Kucumen RB, Gorgun E. The complementary benefit of anterior segment optical coherence tomography in penetrating keratoplasty. Clinical Ophthalmology. 2013;**7**:1515-1523. DOI: 10.2147/OPTH.S45904

[33] Melles GRJ, Eggink FAGJ, Lander F, Pels E, Rietveld FJR, Beekhuis WH, Binder PS. A surgical technique for posterior lamellar keratoplasty. Cornea. 1998;**17**:618. DOI: 10.1097/00003226-199811000-00010

[34] Melles GRJ, Wijdh RHJ, Nieuwendaal CP. A technique to excise the Descemet membrane from a recipient cornea (descemetorhexis). Cornea. 2004;**23**:286-288. DOI: 10.1097/00003226-200404000-00011

[35] Steverink JG, Wisse RPL. Intraoperative optical coherence tomography in descemet stripping automated endothelial keratoplasty: pilot experiences. International Ophthalmology. 2017;**37**:939-944. DOI: 10.1007/s10792-016-0338-9

[36] Kobayashi A, Yokogawa H, Mori N, Sugiyama K. Visualization of precut DSAEK and pre-stripped DMEK donor corneas by intraoperative optical coherence tomography using the RESCAN 700. BMC Ophthalmology. 2016;**16**:135. DOI: 10.1186/s12886-016-0308-z

[37] Koenig SB, Covert DJ, Dupps WJ, Meisler DM. Visual acuity, refractive error, and endothelial cell density six months after Descemet stripping and automated endothelial keratoplasty (DSAEK). Cornea. 2007;**26**:670-674. DOI: 10.1097/ICO.0b013e3180544902

[38] Bahar I, Kaiserman I, Livny E, Slomovic A, Slomovic A. Changes in corneal curvatures and anterior segment parameters after descemet stripping automated endothelial keratoplasty. Current Eye Research. 2010;**35**:961-966. DOI: 10.3109/02713683.2010.506967

[39] Langenbucher A, Szentmáry N, Spira C, Seitz B, Eppig T. Hornhautbrechwert nach 'Descemet Stripping Automated Endothelial Keratoplasty' (DSAEK) - Modellierung und Konzept für die Berechnung von Intraokularlinsen. Zeitschrift für Medizinische Physik. 2016;**26**:120-126. DOI: 10.1016/j.zemedi.2015.02.003

[40] Melles GRJ, Ong TS, Ververs B, van der Wees J. Descemet membrane endothelial keratoplasty (DMEK). Cornea 2006;**25**:987-990. DOI: 10.1097/01.ico.0000248385.16896.34

[41] Flockerzi E, Maier P, Böhringer D, Reinshagen H, Kruse F, Cursiefen C, Reinhard T, Geerling G, Torun N, Seitz B. Trends in corneal transplantation from 2001 to 2016 in Germany: a report of the DOG-section cornea and its keratoplasty registry. American Journal of Ophthalmology. 2018;**188**:91-98. DOI: 10.1016/j.ajo.2018.01.018

[42] Röck T, Bartz-Schmidt KU, Röck D, Yoeruek E. Refraktionsänderung nach der Descemet-Membran-Endothelkeratoplastik. Der Ophthalmologe. 2014;**111**:649-653. DOI: 10.1007/s00347-013-2939-2

[43] Girbardt C, Oertel N, Adamek-Dyk J, Wiedemann P, Nestler A. Refraktive Veränderungen bei Triple-Descemet-Membran-Endothel-Keratoplastik. Der Ophthalmologe. 2016;**113**:217-222. DOI: 10.1007/s00347-015-0201-9

[44] Wolf AH, Neubauer AS, Priglinger SG, Kampik A, Welge-Luessen UC. Detection of laser in situ keratomileusis in a postmortem eye using optical coherence tomography. Journal of Cataract and Refractive Surgery. 2004;**30**:491-495. DOI: 10.1016/j.jcrs.2003.06.007

[45] Neubauer AS, Priglinger SG, Thiel MJ, May C-A, Welge-Lüssen UC. Sterile structural imaging of donor cornea by optical coherence tomography. Cornea. 2002;**21**:490-494

[46] Priglinger SG, Neubauer AS, May C-A, Alge CS, Wolf AH, Mueller A, Ludwig K, Kampik A, Welge-Luessen U. Optical coherence tomography for the detection of laser in situ keratomileusis in donor corneas. Cornea. 2003;**22**:46-50

[47] Janunts E, Langenbucher A, Seitz B. In vitro corneal tomography of donor cornea using anterior segment OCT. Cornea. 2016;**35**:647-653. DOI: 10.1097/ICO.0000000000000761

[48] Damian A, Seitz B, Langenbucher A, Eppig T. Optical coherence tomography-based topography determination of corneal grafts in eye bank cultivation. Journal of Biomedical Optics. 2017;**22**:16001. DOI: 10.1117/1.JBO.22.1.016001

[49] Fernandes P, González-Méijome JM, Madrid-Costa D, Ferrer-Blasco T, Jorge J, Montés-Micó R. Implantable collamer posterior chamber intraocular lenses: A review of potential complications. Journal of Refractive Surgery. 2011;**27**:765-776. DOI: 10.3928/1081597X-20110617-01

[50] Fink AM, Gore C, Rosen E. Cataract development after implantation of the Staar Collamer posterior chamber phakic lens. Journal of Cataract and Refractive Surgery. 1999;**25**:278-282

[51] Trindade F, Pereira F. Cataract formation after posterior chamber phakic intraocular lens implantation. Journal of Cataract and Refractive Surgery. 1998;**24**:1661-1663

[52] Khalifa YM, Goldsmith J, Moshirfar M. Bilateral explantation of Visian implantable Collamer lenses secondary to bilateral acute angle closure resulting from a non-pupillary block mechanism. Journal of Refractive Surgery. 2010;**26**:991-994. DOI: 10.3928/1081597X-20100521-01

[53] Bechmann M, Ullrich S, Thiel MJ, Kenyon KR, Ludwig K. Imaging of posterior chamber phakic intraocular lens by optical coherence tomography. Journal of Cataract and Refractive Surgery. 2002;**28**:360-363

[54] Alfonso JF, Fernández-Vega L, Lisa C, Fernandes P, González-Meijome J, Montés-Micó R. Long-term evaluation of the central vault after phakic Collamer® lens (ICL) implantation using OCT. Graefe's Archive for Clinical and Experimental Ophthalmology. 2012;**250**:1807-1812. DOI: 10.1007/s00417-012-1957-0

[55] Kojima T, Yokoyama S, Ito M, Horai R, Hara S, Nakamura T, Ichikawa K. Optimization of an implantable collamer lens sizing method using high-frequency ultrasound biomicroscopy. American Journal of Ophthalmology. 2012;**153**:632-7, 637.e1. DOI: 10.1016/j.ajo.2011.06.031

[56] Nakamura T, Isogai N, Kojima T, Yoshida Y, Sugiyama Y. Implantable Collamer lens sizing method based on swept-source anterior segment optical coherence tomography. American Journal of Ophthalmology. 2018;**187**:99-107. DOI: 10.1016/j.ajo.2017.12.015

[57] Tsintarakis T, Eppig T, Langenbucher A, Seitz B, El-Husseiny M. Kann die implantierbare Collamer-Linse mit Aquaport eine Winkelblockproblematik sicher verhindern? Erste Erfahrungen aus dem Homburger Zentrum für refraktive Chirurgie. Der Ophthalmologe. 2015;**112**:418-423. DOI: 10.1007/s00347-015-3237-y

[58] Zhang J, Luo H-H, Zhuang J, Yu K-M. Comparison of anterior section parameters using anterior segment optical coherence tomography and ultrasound biomicroscopy in myopic patients after ICL implantation. International Journal of Ophthalmology. 2016;**9**:58-62. DOI: 10.18240/ijo.2016.01.10

Permissions

All chapters in this book were first published in OCTAO, by InTech Open; hereby published with permission under the Creative Commons Attribution License or equivalent. Every chapter published in this book has been scrutinized by our experts. Their significance has been extensively debated. The topics covered herein carry significant findings which will fuel the growth of the discipline. They may even be implemented as practical applications or may be referred to as a beginning point for another development.

The contributors of this book come from diverse backgrounds, making this book a truly international effort. This book will bring forth new frontiers with its revolutionizing research information and detailed analysis of the nascent developments around the world.

We would like to thank all the contributing authors for lending their expertise to make the book truly unique. They have played a crucial role in the development of this book. Without their invaluable contributions this book wouldn't have been possible. They have made vital efforts to compile up to date information on the varied aspects of this subject to make this book a valuable addition to the collection of many professionals and students.

This book was conceptualized with the vision of imparting up-to-date information and advanced data in this field. To ensure the same, a matchless editorial board was set up. Every individual on the board went through rigorous rounds of assessment to prove their worth. After which they invested a large part of their time researching and compiling the most relevant data for our readers.

The editorial board has been involved in producing this book since its inception. They have spent rigorous hours researching and exploring the diverse topics which have resulted in the successful publishing of this book. They have passed on their knowledge of decades through this book. To expedite this challenging task, the publisher supported the team at every step. A small team of assistant editors was also appointed to further simplify the editing procedure and attain best results for the readers.

Apart from the editorial board, the designing team has also invested a significant amount of their time in understanding the subject and creating the most relevant covers. They scrutinized every image to scout for the most suitable representation of the subject and create an appropriate cover for the book.

The publishing team has been an ardent support to the editorial, designing and production team. Their endless efforts to recruit the best for this project, has resulted in the accomplishment of this book. They are a veteran in the field of academics and their pool of knowledge is as vast as their experience in printing. Their expertise and guidance has proved useful at every step. Their uncompromising quality standards have made this book an exceptional effort. Their encouragement from time to time has been an inspiration for everyone.

The publisher and the editorial board hope that this book will prove to be a valuable piece of knowledge for researchers, students, practitioners and scholars across the globe.

List of Contributors

Mehmet Cüneyt Özmen
Department of Ophthalmology, Faculty of Medicine, Gazi University, Ankara, Turkey

Hüseyin Baran Özdemir
Ulucanlar Eye Training and Research Hospital, University of Health Sciences, Ankara, Turkey

Elena Kiseleva, Gladkova Natalia, Streltzova Olga, Maslennikova Anna, Dudenkova Varvara and Yunusova Katerina
Nizhny Novgorod State Medical Academy, Institute of Biomedical Technologies, Nizhny Novgorod, Russia

Kirillin Mikhail and Sergeeva Ekaterina
Institute of Applied Physics of the Russian Academy of Sciences, Nizhny Novgorod, Russia

Nur Acar
School of Medicine, Acıbadem Mehmet Ali Aydınlar University, Maslak Hospital,Sarıyer, Istanbul, Turkey

Xiaogang Wang, Suhua Zhang and Bin Sun
Department of Cataract, Shanxi Eye Hospital, Taiyuan, China

Jing Dong
Department of Ophthalmology, The First Hospital of Shanxi Medical University, Shanxi, PR China

Rethabile Khutlang
Biometrics Research Group, Identity Authentication, CSIR Modelling and Digital Science, Pretoria, South Africa

Pheeha Machaka
Network Security, Network and Data Security, CSIR Modelling and Digital Science, Pretoria, South Africa

Ann Singh
Laser Sources Group, CSIR National Laser Centre, Pretoria, South Africa

Fulufhelo Nelwamondo
CSIR Modelling and Digital Science, Pretoria, South Africa

Aydin Yildiz
Department of Ophthalmology, Canakkale Onsekiz Mart University, School of Medicine, Canakkale, Turkey

Sana I. Tinwala
Anuditi Eye Care, Mumbai, India

Jorge L. Domene-Hickman
Tecnologico de Monterrey, Escuela de Medicina y Ciencias de la Salud, Monterrey,Nuevo León, Mexico

Andi Arus Victor
Department of Ophthalmology, Faculty of Medicine, Universitas Indonesia, Cipto Mangunkusumo National General Hospital, Jakarta, Indonesia

Magdy Moussa
Ophthalmology Department, Faculty of Medicine, Tanta University, Tanta, Egypt
MEDIC Eye Center, Tanta, Egypt

Mahmoud Leila
Retina Department, Research Institute of Ophthalmology, Giza, Egypt

Jorge Luis Domene Hinojosa and Nuria Judith Alemán Hurtado
Centro Medico Nacional Noreste, Monterrey, Nuevo León, Mexico

Joaquim de Moura, Jorge Novo, José Rouco, Noelia Barreira, Manuel Penedo and Marcos Ortega
Department of Computing, University of A Coruña, A Coruña, Spain
Research Center of Information and Communication Technologies (CITIC), University of A Coruña, A Coruña, Spain

Salvatore Di Lauro, Salvador Pastor Idoate and Jose Carlos Pastor
Departamento de Oftalmología, Hospital Clínico Universitario de Valladolid,Valladolid, Spain
Instituto de Oftalmobiología Aplicada (IOBA), Retina Group, Universidad de Valladolid,Valladolid, Spain

Simona Delia Nicoară
Faculty of Medicine, Department of Ophthalmology, "Iuliu Hatieganu" University of Medicine and Pharmacy, Cluj-Napoca, Romania

Timo Eppig, Stephanie Mäurer and Achim Langenbucher
Institute of Experimental Ophthalmology, Saarland University, Homburg, Germany

Loay Daas and Berthold Seitz
Department of Ophthalmology, Saarland University Medical Center UKS, Homburg, Germany

Index

www.ingramcontent.com/pod-product-compliance
Lightning Source LLC
LaVergne TN
LVHW060526210926
848485LV00005B/1154